# Depression in New Mothers

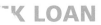
Depression is the most common complication of childbirth and results in adverse health outcomes for both mother and child. This text provides a comprehensive approach to treating postpartum depression (PPD) in an easy-to-use format. It reviews the research and brings together the evidence base for identifying and understanding the causes, as well as assessing the different treatment options, including those that are safe for use with breastfeeding mothers. Incorporating a new psychoneuroimmunology framework for understanding PPD, *Depression in New Mothers, Second edition* includes chapters on:

- negative birth experiences
- infant characteristics
- psychosocial factors, including a history of childhood abuse
- antidepressant medication for pregnant and breastfeeding women
- psychotherapy and community support
- herbal medicine, Omega-3 fatty acids, exercise, and alternative therapies
- suicide and infanticide.

Invaluable in treating the mothers who come to you for help, this helpful guide dispels the myths that hinder effective treatment and presents up-to-date information on the impact of maternal depression on the health of the mother, as well as the health and well-being of the infant.

**Kathleen A. Kendall-Tackett** is a health psychologist and an International Board Certified Lactation Consultant. She is a Clinical Associate Professor of Pediatrics at Texas Tech University School of Medicine in Amarillo, Texas. Dr. Kendall-Tackett is a Fellow of the American Psychological Association in the Divisions of Health and Trauma Psychology, and is Associate Editor of the journal *Psychological Trauma*. She is also the author of more than 220 journal articles, book chapters and other publications, and author or editor of 19 books in the fields of trauma, women's health, depression, and breastfeeding.

# Depression in New Mothers

Causes, consequences, and treatment alternatives

Second edition

**Kathleen A. Kendall-Tackett**

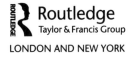
Routledge
Taylor & Francis Group

LONDON AND NEW YORK

First edition published 2005
by The Haworth Press

This edition (second) published 2010
by Routledge
2 Park Square, Milton Park, Abingdon, Oxon, OX14 4RN

Simultaneously published in the USA and Canada
by Routledge
270 Madison Avenue, New York, NY 10016

*Routledge is an imprint of the Taylor & Francis Group, an informa business*

© 2010 Kathleen A. Kendall-Tackett

Typeset in Times New Roman by
Pindar NZ, Auckland, New Zealand
Printed and bound in Great Britain by
TJ International Ltd, Padstow, Cornwall

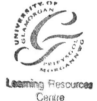

*British Library Cataloguing in Publication Data*
A catalogue record for this book is available from the British Library

*Library of Congress Cataloging-in-Publication Data*
Kendall-Tackett, Kathleen A.
Depression in new mothers : causes, consequences, and treatment alternatives /
Kathleen A. Kendall-Tackett. — 2nd ed.
    p. cm.
  Includes bibliographical references and index.
  1. Postpartum depression. I. Title.
  [DNLM: 1. Depression, Postpartum—diagnosis. 2. Depression, Postpartum—etiology.
3. Depression, Postpartum—therapy. 4. Maternal Welfare—psychology. 5. Risk
Factors. 6. Socioeconomic Factors. WQ 500 K33d 2010]
  RG852.K448 2010
  618.7'6—dc22                              2009026731

ISBN10: 0-415-77838-7 (hbk)
ISBN10: 0-415-77839-5 (pbk)
ISBN10: 0-203-86194-9 (ebk)

ISBN13: 978-0-415-77838-1 (hbk)
ISBN13: 978-0-415-77839-8 (pbk)
ISBN13: 978-0-203-86194-3 (ebk)

# Contents

# Figures and tables

## Figures

## Tables

# Foreword

To be conscious that you are ignorant is a great step to knowledge.

Benjamin Disraeli

Denial and ignorance are two of the barriers in recognizing and treating women suffering from perinatal mood disorders. After more than a quarter century in the field, I am pleased that we're making progress in both areas. There is much less public denial surrounding this topic. The amount of scientific research about maternal mental illness has increased. I believe that knowledge is power. Without accurate information consumers become passive victims and professionals may give their patients poor care. To become more knowledgeable, we need books with up-to-date, research-based studies. *Depression in New Mothers: Causes Consequences and Treatment Options* provides us with more than statistics and information. This is a book with a heart. It is written by a mother who understands motherhood. Each chapter in *Depression in New Mothers* has summaries of thought-provoking international research studies. The depth of the science is staggering and fascinating. We still don't understand all that neuroscience tells us about the brain but we have many clues. When I was first exposed to postpartum psychiatric illness in 1984 it was described as a "picture puzzle". The pieces are beginning to fit together and at the same time, we continue to ask more questions. Your knowledge quotient is going to increase dramatically from reading this second edition of a landmark contribution to the literature.

Dr. Kathleen Kendall-Tackett has been a pioneer educator in the field of maternal mental health since her first book, *Postpartum Depression*, was published in 1993. In this new volume she expands upon her knowledge of the complexities and interrelationships that exist in the field of maternal depression. Her goal is to equip her readers with the information needed to make a real difference in the lives of mothers and babies. She has achieved this goal through a systematic framework that will help you understand the topic and how to communicate effectively with postpartum mothers.

Myths about motherhood are also barriers to seeking appropriate care during pregnancy and the postpartum period. Dr. Kendall-Tackett has identified six distinct myths about postpartum depression that are pervasive. Misperceptions about depression are dangerous! We cannot effectively provide adequate assistance if healthcare providers and the public continue to perpetuate them. In Chapter 2, she demonstrates how expensive misperception is because of the harm untreated depression causes to mother and baby. We cannot afford NOT to get involved. Infanticide and maternal suicide are the most shocking reactions to postpartum illness. I agree with her message that we must get serious, seek the truth, and act on this knowledge.

Chapter 3 is about depression and breastfeeding. Dr. Kendall-Tackett has devoted an entire chapter to this important topic because *"When providers urge mothers to quit who want to continue, breastfeeding can become a barrier to treatment."* Sadly, there are many well-meaning care providers who are not listening to the mothers. I hope that Dr. Kendall-Tackett's summary of recent research will change this behavior. We know that you cannot tell if someone is depressed by "just looking". In Chapter 4, the topic of screening and the challenges of assessment are covered.

Dr. Kendall-Tackett tackles neuroscience and psychoneuroimmunology in Chapter 5. The amount of research that has taken place in the past five years is encouraging. There are now excellent studies on the physiological phenomenon effect on the mental well-being of mothers.

In Chapter 6 the research literature on negative birth experiences and untreated previous trauma are given the attention they deserve. The concluding message is one of hope: people can and do recover from traumatic events. More specifics on trauma-related treatment are found in Chapter 12.

The topic of infant characteristics and depression in their mothers as described in Chapter 7 is not discussed often enough. Infant crying, sleep habits, prematurity, chronic illness or disability can also affect mothers' moods. This seems rather obvious but for years developmental psychologists dismissed their importance. Another reason for this "disconnect" was that the researchers and clinicians in reproductive and infant psychology were not sharing their findings with the scientists actively researching postpartum psychiatric illness, and visa versa. Fortunately, this has changed. If your professional interest is the baby, my hope is that you'll begin to turn your attention to the mother's emotional needs as well. The baby needs her to be healthy. Make certain that she is not still grieving for the baby she perceived would be born without special challenges. Look into her eyes with an open heart, ask a caring question about how she is feeling.

Chapters 8 and 9 delve into the psychological and social components of postpartum depression. Dr. Kendall-Tackett summarizes the large body of literature on the psychological factors – including self-esteem, self-efficacy, and expectations – that are involved. In addition, she describes research on previous psychiatric history, depression during pregnancy, violence against women, the connection between childhood and domestic abuse, parenting difficulties, abuse and breastfeeding, and loss. Since my personal bias is towards social risk factors, I couldn't agree more with her sentence "women do not become mothers in a vacuum."

A major challenge facing us is a mother's own denial. I've spoken on the telephone with and have emailed depressed mothers and their families for over 25 years. These women are not in denial and, frankly, I don't worry about them. I am deeply troubled, however, by our inability to engage in a dialogue with those who never reach out for help. Plainly put, we can't treat her if she doesn't perceive any need – I speak from personal experience as well. My own denial lasted far too long. It is very tricky, but again, I believe that education is the key. If we can routinely start talking about negative emotions related to childbearing as naturally as we do about pain in labor and sore nipples, then there will be progress in improving maternal mental health.

Chapters 10, 11, 12 and 13 offer comprehensive descriptions of alternative and complementary treatments including Omega-3s, SAM-e, exercise, bright light, herbs and combined modalities, psychotherapy, community interventions and antidepressants. Dr. Kendall-Tackett covers each of these thoroughly, citing the most recent research. Mothers ask, "what can I do? Will I ever be myself again?", "Do I have to take medicine?" and some state emphatically, "I won't take anything." I don't have a medical background and yet by having a better understanding of therapies, I can direct mothers and their families towards learning about treatment options. The goal is the same. Healthy mothers mean healthy families.

After reading so much science, it is both touching and refreshing to conclude with the words of one mother, Jenny, who has "been there". There is no substitute for truth and honesty. When it comes to feeling equipped to help others, it truly begins with being satisfied that you know your own comfort level with mental illness. It is my hope that after reading this important book you will, indeed, be ready to make a difference in the lives of mothers and babies. Dr. Kathleen Kendall-Tackett, as author and educator, surely is an inspiration to all of us.

Jane Honikman, M.S.
Founder
Postpartum Support International
Santa Barbara, California

# Preface

The world has changed much since I began work on my first book on postpartum depression in 1991. I was a new mother with a recently acquired Ph.D. in developmental psychology. In trying to make sense of my own postpartum experience, I started to read the research literature on postpartum depression. I was stunned at how different it was from what I was reading about postpartum depression in the popular press. I realized that depression in new mothers was far more complex, and far more interesting, than I had realized. Armed with this knowledge, I put together a book proposal. And the rest, as they say, is history. *Postpartum Depression: A Comprehensive Approach for Nurses* was published in 1993. The revised version, *Depression in New Mothers*, was published in 2005.

Working on these volumes has given me a front-row seat, as it were, to what is happening in the field. The sheer number and quality of studies has continued to amaze me. We now know substantially more about depression than we did even a decade ago, allowing us to be more effective in identifying and treating it than ever before.

One of the more exciting shifts in postpartum depression research comes from the field of psychoneuroimmunology (PNI). PNI research examines the role of stress, depression and other negative mental states on the immune system. Both physical and psychological stress increase systemic inflammation, which, in turn, increases the risk of depression. At first glance, this may not seem particularly relevant. But as I describe in Chapter 5, having this knowledge marks a critical shift in how we understand depression. Inflammation is not simply *a* risk factor for depression. It is *the* risk factor for depression, the one that underlies all the others (Kendall-Tackett, 2007). The discussion of individual risk factors is still relevant, but the integration of PNI research provides a unifying framework for understanding why we see what we see. PNI research also informs treatment decisions and help us understand why the broad array of modalities used to treat depression are all effective.

Another striking feature of recent research is its international scope. There are studies from literally around the world. The large increase in studies on the assessment and treatment are recent – and welcome – additions to this literature. I've expanded the discussion to include the new research on the use of antidepressants in pregnant and postpartum women. The literature on the role of breastfeeding in depression has increased to the point where it warranted a separate chapter. In addition, new studies on mothers' sleep and fatigue offer some surprising findings.

The book you are about to read is essentially a new volume. I have preserved some of the studies cited in the earlier two volumes for continuity, and because they are good studies. I have also included the mothers' stories from the original edition because they are timeless, and continue to illustrate points in a way that no mere review of the literature can. With the emphasis today on evidence-based care, the goal of this book is to provide you with the evidence in an easy-to-use format. Some of the newer findings have changed the way we think about depression and the field is continuing to evolve.

When I speak at conferences, participants often tell me that the topic of depression in new mothers is more interesting than they imagined. I hope that this will be true for you as well. I also want to encourage you to get involved with this population. No matter what your role, there is a way you can help. The late Ray Helfer, a pediatrician and co-author of the first article on child maltreatment, once described the perinatal period as a "window of opportunity" in our work with families. At no other time are they as interested and willing to learn. You have before you an opportunity to make a real difference in the lives of mothers and babies. My goal is to equip you to do just that.

Kathleen A. Kendall-Tackett
Amarillo, Texas

# Part I

# Overview

# 1 Depression in new mothers

## Myths vs. reality

I never thought I would have postpartum depression. After two years of trying to conceive and several attempts at in vitro fertilization, I thought I would be overjoyed when my daughter, Rowan Francis, was born in the spring of 2003. But instead I felt completely overwhelmed. This baby was a stranger to me. I didn't know what to do with her. I didn't feel joyful. I attributed feelings of doom to simple fatigue and figured that they would eventually go away. But they didn't; in fact, they got worse.

I couldn't bear the sound of Rowan crying, and I dreaded the moments my husband would bring her to me. I wanted her to disappear. I wanted to disappear. At my lowest points, I thought of swallowing a bottle of pills or jumping out the window of my apartment.

Brooke Shields, *New York Times*, July 1, 2005

Depression in new mothers is one of the most common complications of childbirth. Yet it is still subject to many myths and misperceptions among professionals and lay people alike. This misinformation can be a particular problem because it means that practitioners – and mothers themselves – do not recognize it when they see it.

The truth is that postpartum depression isolates mothers when they most need the help of others. Mothers may be ashamed to admit that life with a new baby is not always bliss. They may assume that everyone has made a smoother transition to motherhood than they have. And they may be truly embarrassed that they are not able to "cope" better, as Beck (2006: 40) describes:

Postpartum depression is a serious mood disorder that can cripple a woman's first months as a new mother. I have described it as "a thief that steals motherhood." Without appropriate clinical intervention, postpartum depression can have long-ranging implications for both mother and child.

## Myths about postpartum depression

Misperceptions abound regarding depression in new mothers. In a summary of websites related to postpartum depression, Summers and Logsdon (2005) found that 11 of the 34 websites they reviewed contained little or no useful information about depression. Some even contained information that was potentially harmful. Unfortunately, myths and misperceptions can keep mothers from receiving the attention they need. Here are some of the most common ones.

### *Myth #1: Depression in new mothers is not serious*

One of the most prevalent myths is that postpartum depression is not serious. Fewer people voice this myth today in the wake of the Andrea Yates case. Andrea Yates was the mother in Texas who drowned her five young children in the bathtub while suffering from postpartum depression and psychosis. She was convicted of murder, and her conviction was eventually overturned.

What many fail to realize is that depression that does not end in infanticide can still be quite harmful to both mothers and babies. We will visit this topic again in Chapter 2.

### *Myth #2: Postpartum depression is caused by shifts in estrogen and progesterone*

Medical students and women who had experienced postpartum depression were asked what causes it. The differences in their responses were rather striking (Small, *et al.*, 1997). The medical students were more likely to attribute depression to hormonal factors (notably, estrogen and progesterone) and to women's "tendency to depression." In contrast, the women themselves were more likely to attribute depression to social, physical health, and life-event factors that included lack of time/space for themselves, feeling unsupported, being isolated, financial stress, and poor physical health.

The women had it right. As you will see, the hormonal hypothesis for postpartum depression has not aged well. Reproductive hormones have, at best, a tangential role in depression in new mothers. However, we now know that a variety of psychological, social, and immunologic factors have an important role to play in the development of depression. In fact, the knowledge base on this topic has rapidly expanded, presenting a more wholistic and fascinating picture of what happens in both the antenatal and postpartum periods.

### *Myth #3: Postpartum depression is more common in white middle-class women*

There is a prevailing belief that postpartum depression is something that only afflicts affluent white women (Martinez, *et al.*, 2000). Revelations of postpartum depression by such well-known women as Brooke Shields, Marie Osmond, and the late Princess Diana, have been undeniably helpful in that they have increased awareness. The one downside, however, is that they have inadvertently reinforced the notion that postpartum depression is a condition of privilege. As you shall see, postpartum depression affects women in many different cultures, and across all income levels. And poor women are actually at higher risk.

### *Myth #4: We don't really know what causes postpartum depression*

I have to admit, this one mystifies me. Whenever I hear it, my prompt response is "yes, we do." The causes of depression vary from woman to woman. But we have identified the major risk factors for depression. And because we do know what causes it, we are more effective in treating it than ever before.

*Myth #5: Postpartum depression will go away on its own*

Unfortunately, untreated postpartum depression can last for months – or longer. Zelkowitz and Milet (2001) identified 48 couples where one or both partners was suffering from postpartum mental illness. Four months later, 54% of the mothers, and 60% of their partners, still had psychiatric diagnoses. In a second study, mothers were assessed at two, three, six, and twelve months postpartum. Mothers who depressed at two months continued to be depressed at each subsequent assessment point throughout the first year (Beeghly, *et al.*, 2002).

*Myth #6: Women with postpartum depression cannot breastfeed*

Sadly, many women, when they seek help for depression, are told that they must wean their babies so they can take medications. For some mothers, weaning is no problem. But for others, weaning is experienced as a significant loss. The good news is that almost all treatments for depression are compatible with breastfeeding, and there are sound medical reasons to support mothers who want to continue. Treatments for depression are described in Chapters 10 to 13.

## Assumptions about postpartum depression

So how do we begin to think about postpartum depression? Below is a framework I've found helpful in my work with new mothers. It provides a way of talking with mothers about what is going on in their lives, and a framework for understanding their responses.

*Becoming a mother is a stressful life event*

This first assumption seems obvious in one way, but we often do not keep this in mind. We need to acknowledge that becoming a mother turns a woman's world upside down. It changes almost every aspect of her life: her work, her home, and even her ability to do something as simple as taking a shower.

*Depression is within the normal range of responses following a*
*stressful event*

That being said, we also need to acknowledge that when exposed to a stressful life event, a certain percentage of people are going to become depressed. This assumption is helpful because it normalizes depression. (But that is different from saying it is of no consequence.) When we accept that depression can be part of life, it makes it more comfortable for us to discuss it with mothers. On the other hand, if we treat depression as a freak occurrence, we are going to be uncomfortable, and the mother is likely to feel shame.

*The causes of postpartum depression vary from woman to woman*

It is also important to keep in mind that postpartum depression has many possible causes. There is not a one-size-fits-all explanation for depression in new mothers. The factors underlying postpartum depression vary from woman to woman, and understanding the multiple causes allows us to be more targeted with our interventions.

**Postpartum depression is not limited to the first six weeks postpartum but can occur any time in the first year**

Some people think that "postpartum" only includes the first four to six weeks. But this is not the way it is described in the research literature. "Postpartum depression" includes the entire first year. We should not be surprised that a woman with a four-month-old, or a nine- or ten-month-old baby is depressed.

## Symptoms of depression

Postpartum depression can manifest in a wide variety of symptoms. These include moods of sadness, anhedonia (the inability to experience pleasure), low self-esteem, apathy and social withdrawal, excessive emotional sensitivity, pessimistic thinking, irritability, sleep disturbance, appetite disturbance, impaired concentration, and agitation. These symptoms are common to other forms of depression as well (Preston and Johnson, 2009; Rapkin, *et al.*, 2002). They may feel mentally foggy, anxious, angry, guilty, or that their lives will never be normal again (Beck, 2002). Depression might present with somatic complaints as the predominant symptom, including pain, fatigue, sleep and appetite disturbances (Alexander, 2007).

When discussing symptoms of depression, there are some that are especially concerning. These symptoms could indicate a more serious manifestation of depression, and are listed in Table 1.1.

## Diagnostic criteria for major depressive disorder

While many mothers may exhibit symptoms of depression, major depression is a more serious manifestation of depressive symptoms that has specific diagnostic criteria. For a diagnosis of major depression, patients must have at least five of the following symptoms during the same two-week period:

1   depressed mood most of the day;
2   anhedonia most of the day;
3   significant weight loss when not dieting, or weight gain, or change in appetite;
4   insomnia or hypersomnia;
5   activity disturbance, psychomotor agitation or retardation;

*Table 1.1* Symptoms that raise concern

- She reports that she has not slept in two to three days.
- She is losing weight rapidly.
- She cannot get out of bed.
- She is ignoring basic grooming.
- She seems hopeless.
- She says that her children would be better off without her.
- She is actively abusing substances.
- She makes strange or bizarre statements (e.g. plans to give her children to strangers).

6   abnormal fatigue or loss of energy;
7   feelings of worthlessness or excessive guilt;
8   diminished ability to think or concentrate or make decisions;
9   recurrent thoughts of death, or recurrent suicidal ideation, with or without a specific plan.

The symptoms listed above should not be due to psychosis and the woman should never have had a manic or hypomanic episode. Further, the woman's symptoms should not be due to physical illness, alcohol, medication or illegal drugs, or normal bereavement. In addition, these symptoms must represent a change in previous functioning, and must include at least depressed mood and anhedonia. These symptoms can be by subjective report or observation of others, and must occur nearly every day (American Psychiatric Association, 2000).

## Dysthymic disorder

Depression can also manifest as dysthymic disorder, which is a chronic low grade of depression or depressed mood. It lasts for at least two years, for most of the day, and for more days than not (Alexander, 2007). For a diagnosis of dysthymia, at least two of the following symptoms should be present:

- poor appetite or overeating
- sleep disturbances
- fatigue
- low self-esteem
- poor concentration and difficulties making choices
- feelings of hopelessness.

Dysthymic disorder tends to be more chronic than major depression, but most people with dysthymia have also suffered from major depression (Alexander, 2007).

Even depression that does not meet full diagnostic criteria for major depression, however, should not be ignored. Weinberg and colleagues (2001) compared women with subclinical depression to three groups: depressed pregnant women, women with postpartum major depression, and non-depressed women. Women with subclinical depression had poorer psychosocial functioning than non-depressed women, and were comparable to those with major depression. Moreover, they had more negative and less positive affect, had poorer self-esteem, and less confidence as mothers. Donna describes how her symptoms came on suddenly after the birth of her daughter.

> I never really went into labor. They did three inductions … I knew I was going to have a c-section. When they said it was a girl, I just went numb. I just didn't feel like I had given birth. I felt disconnected from my body. I was up for 24 hours. I was crying hysterically. She wanted to eat a lot. I never was able to breastfeed. I was in the hospital crying. I didn't feel like her mother. I was very disconnected. I was freaking out. My friends kept telling me that it was the baby blues.

## Is postpartum depression a distinct condition?

When discussing postpartum depression, professionals frequently raise the question of whether it is distinct from non-puerperal mental illness. Some have argued that puerperal and non-puerperal mental illnesses are similar in terms of their symptomatology and factors predicting onset, and that the *only* distinguishing characteristic of puerperal mental illness is an onset and triggers that are specific to new motherhood (e.g. infant characteristics, sleep deprivation, and birth experience). At the present time, there is no specific diagnostic category for postpartum illness in the *Diagnostic and Statistical Manual* (DSM IV). However, the specifier "with postpartum onset" can be added to the following conditions: major depressive disorder; manic or mixed episode in major depressive disorder; bipolar I or II disorder, or brief psychotic disorder if these conditions occur in the first four weeks after birth (Rapkin, *et al.*, 2002).

## Incidence

Incidence of postpartum depression ranges quite a bit between various studies, but the typical range is 12% to 25% of new mothers (Beck and Gable, 2001a; Centers for Disease Control, 2008; Moses-Kolko and Roth, 2004; Rapkin, *et al.*, 2002), with rates in some high-risk groups being as high as 35% or more. Some estimates in the U.S. indicate that 500,000 American women experience postpartum major depression annually (Moses-Kolko and Roth, 2004). Studies with higher percentages may have included both major depression and depressive symptoms in their totals. If the "depressed" group in a study included those with depressive symptoms, then the percentage of mothers is going to be higher than if only women with a formal diagnosis of major depression are included. Similarly, the percentage will be higher if those with major and minor depression are included in the "depressed" group.

In a large U.S. population study of pregnant and postpartum women, 14,093 women 18 to 50 years old were interviewed about past pregnancy status (Vesga-Lopez, *et al.*, 2008). The main outcomes of the study were Axis I psychiatric disorders, substance abuse, and treatment seeking. In this sample, currently pregnant women had lower risk of any mood disorder than non-pregnant women, but there were significantly higher rates of postpartum major depression compared with other time periods. Age, marital status, health status, stressful life events, and history of traumatic experiences were all associated with psychiatric disorders in pregnant and postpartum women.

The Centers for Disease Control published prevalence data on self-reported depressive symptoms in 17 U.S. states (Centers for Disease Control, 2008). The prevalence ranged from 11.7% in Maine to 20.4% in New Mexico. In this sample, younger women, women with lower levels of education, and women who received Medicaid benefits for their delivery were more likely to report depressive symptoms. Postpartum depressive symptoms were associated with smoking during the last trimester of pregnancy and three types of stress during pregnancy (partner-related, traumatic, or financial). In a smaller number of states, NICU admission was associated with depressive symptoms, as was low birth-weight delivery, and emotional stress. Depression was assessed using the two-item screen: *Since your new baby was born, how often have you had little interest or little pleasure in doing things? And since your new baby was born, how often have you felt down, depressed, or hopeless?*

In a sample drawn from a national evaluation of the Healthy Steps for Young Children program, 4,874 mothers completed interviews at two to four months (McLearn, *et al.*, 2006a). They found that 17.8% reported depressive symptoms as indicated by the Center for Epidemiologic Studies Depression Scale. Compared with non-depressed mothers, depressed mothers were less likely to continue breastfeeding, show their infants a book at least once a day, play with their infant at least once a day, talk to their infants while working, or follow two or more routines. The authors concluded that depression is common in the early postpartum period and can lead to unfavorable parenting practices.

## U.S. ethnic group differences

Several recent studies have found that incidence of depression varies by ethnicity within the U.S. A study from North Carolina compared rates of depression in new mothers (N=586) among four American ethnic groups: Hispanics, Native Americans, African Americans, and whites (Wei, *et al.*, 2007). They found that Hispanic women had by far the lowest rates of depression, with a rate of only 2.5%. In contrast, Native Americans had the highest rates of major depression (18.7%), and an average rate of minor depression (10.5%). White women had the second-highest rates of major depression (17.6%) and the highest rate of minor depression (19.6%). The rate for African Americans was 14.8% and 9.9% for major and minor depression, respectively. There was a strong association between rates of depression and breastfeeding, and Hispanic women had the highest breastfeeding rate, which the authors thought explained the ethnic-group difference. The sample overall demonstrated strong associations between symptoms of postpartum depression and history of depression, history of treatment, and breastfeeding.

A study of 218 low-income Hispanic mothers of babies or toddlers in the U.S. found a rate of depression at 23%, with only half of the women indicating that they had needed help for sadness or depression since their child's birth (Chaudron, *et al.*, 2005). They defined "high levels of depressive symptoms" as a score of 10 or higher on the Edinburgh Postnatal Depression Scale (EPDS) (see Chapter 4). Using the more stringent cut-off of 13 or higher, the rate of depression was 13%. In this sample, the only demographic characteristic related to depression was being an adolescent.

In a prospective of 1,735 women, Mora and colleagues (2009) described the trajectories of depressive symptoms in a sample of low-income, multi-ethnic, inner-city women. Seventy percent of the women were African American, 17% were Latina, and the remaining 13% were white or from other ethnicities. The women were recruited during pregnancy and interviewed once during pregnancy, and at three postpartum interviews up to two years later. Based on their analyses, the researchers grouped the women into five distinct groups: chronically depressed (7%); antenatal depression only (6%); postpartum only – resolves in the first year postpartum (9%); late, present at 25 months postpartum (7%); and never having been depressed (71%). The authors designed their study to examine the timing and overall exposure to symptoms, noting that most studies are cross-sectional and do not allow for understanding the pattern of depression across time. One of the findings the authors identified as remarkable was that 71% had no symptoms at any assessment, and that a further 15% had transient symptoms. Depression across the three classes shared some risk factors, including a high level of objective stress and fair/poor self-rated emotional health. High parity was associated with chronic depression, and ambivalence about pregnancy was associated with both antenatal and chronic depression.

## International incidence of postpartum depression

Postpartum depression is not limited to white middle-class American women. It is relatively common in other countries as well. For example, in a study of mothers from Costa Rica and Chile, one-third of the mothers were dysphoric after childbirth, and 35% to 50% had had at least one episode of major depressive disorder (MDD) in their lifetimes. All the mothers were low-income and had at least one child under the age of 3 (Wolf, *et al.*, 2002).

A Norwegian study of 259 followed mothers longitudinally through pregnancy and the first year postpartum (Eberhard-Gran, *et al.*, 2004). Using a cut-off of greater than 10 on the EPDS, women had the highest odds of depression in the last trimester of pregnancy and the first eight months postpartum. Women in the second and third trimesters had the highest rates. This association remained even after for controlling for other risk factors in depression including a high score on the life-event scale, a history of depression, and a poor relationship with their partners.

In a sample of 892 women from nine countries, the rates of depression were highest in non-whites from Asia and South America (Affonso, *et al.*, 2000). Europeans and Australians had the lowest rates. The rate for American mothers was somewhere in between. The countries included were the U.S., Guyana, Italy, Sweden, Finland, Korea, Taiwan, India, and Australia.

Postpartum depression occurred in comparable rates in mothers from Turkey. In a study by Danaci and colleagues (2002), 14% of 257 mothers were depressed at six months postpartum. Risk factors for depression included a higher number of living children, living in a shanty, being an immigrant, having a baby with a serious health problem, a previous history of psychiatric illness for herself or her husband, and poor relationships with her spouse or his family. The relationship with the husband's family may be particularly salient for women in traditional cultures who are often living with them (Danaci, *et al.*, 2002).

Mothers in India (N=252) also suffered from postpartum depression. They were interviewed during their third trimester, at six to eight weeks and six months postpartum. Twenty-three percent were depressed, and 78% of these women had "substantial" clinical morbidity. Their risk factors for depression included economic deprivation, poor marital relationships, and gender of the infant. These risk factors were similar to those found in Western samples, especially poverty and poor marital relationships (see Chapter 9). The factor unique to this culture was gender of the infant; mothers were more likely to become depressed if they had a girl (Patel, *et al.*, 2002).

Mothers in Nepal had surprisingly low rates of depression (Regmi, *et al.*, 2002): 12% at two to three months postpartum. The authors were surprised at this low rate, and pointed out that Nepal is one of the poorest countries in the world, with an infant mortality rate of 75 per 1,000.

### *Summary*

The above-cited studies indicate that postpartum depression occurs in many different countries, and in all ethnic groups in the U.S. It is not entirely clear from these studies which ethnic group is most at risk, but what we do know is that postpartum depression can affect mothers from a broad range of backgrounds, ethnicities, and nationalities.

## Postpartum psychosis

Postpartum psychosis is the most serious form of postpartum mental illness. Although postpartum psychosis is not the focus of this book, it is important to mention it because of its severity, and its co-occurrence with depression. It occurs in 0.1% to 0.2% of all new mothers, and most episodes begin abruptly between days three and fourteen postpartum (Rapkin, *et al.*, 2002).

In two studies of women hospitalized for severe postpartum illness in Edinburgh, Scotland (Davidson and Robertson, 1985), and Kaduna, Nigeria (Ifabumuyi and Akindele, 1985), the three most common diagnoses were unipolar depression, bipolar depression, and schizophrenia. Transient organic psychosis was also a diagnosis for a small percentage of subjects in both studies.

Miller (2002) noted that the most common differential diagnoses for postpartum psychosis include major depression with psychotic features; bipolar disorder; schizoaffective disorder; schizophrenia, and brief reactive psychosis. Some medical conditions can be related to post-partum psychosis, and should be ruled out before diagnosing these symptoms as due to mood disorders. Such other conditions include thyroiditis, hypothyroidism, B12 deficiency, and adult $GM_2$ gangliosidosis. Substances that can trigger a psychotic episode include bromocrip-tine, metronidazole, and addictive substances including LSD, PCP, and ecstasy.

## *Bipolar disorder*

One type of postpartum psychosis is bipolar disorder. The initial course of bipolar disorder leads to a rate high of misdiagnoses because it usually manifests in the puerperium as major depression without psychosis (Beck, 2006). With this disorder, women may experience hypo-manic episodes that include inflated self-esteem, increased talkativeness, decreased sleep, racing thoughts, and increased goal orientation. Unlike the mania that occurs in bipolar I disorder, hypomania is not socially disabling. Differentiating major depression from bipolar disorder, particularly bipolar disorder II, can be challenging. But bipolar disorder is associated with a significantly earlier age of onset, more recurrences, atypical and mixed depressions, and a family history of bipolar disorder or completed suicide compared with major depression (Beck, 2006; Yatham, *et al.*, 2009). The Canadian Network for Mood and Anxiety Disorder's (CANMAT) guidelines noted that postpartum is a time when rates of hypomania may be at their highest levels (Yatham, *et al.*, 2009).

In a study of 30 bipolar women who had children, 66% had a postpartum mood episode (Freeman, *et al.*, 2002). Most of these episodes were exclusively depressive. Of the women who became depressed after their first child, all became depressed after subsequent births. Depression during any pregnancy also increased the risk of postpartum depression.

Birth can also trigger episodes of psychosis in bipolar women with a family history of postpartum psychosis (Jones and Craddock, 2001). One study examined 313 deliveries of 152 women with bipolar disorder. Twenty-six percent of the deliveries were followed by an episode of puerperal psychosis, and 38% of the women had at least one puerperal psychotic episode. Family history also increased risk. There were 27 women with bipolar disorder who had a family history of postpartum psychosis. Seventy-four percent of these women developed postpartum psychosis. In contrast, only 30% of the women with bipolar disorder, but without a family history of postpartum psychosis, had a postpartum psychotic episode.

Antidepressants should be used cautiously in women with postpartum depression due to the risk of inducing postpartum psychosis, mania, and rapid cycling (Freeman, *et al.*, 2002; Moses-Kolko, *et al.*, 2005). In published case reports, induction of mania happened in the absence of family history of psychiatric disorder, but with a family history of bipolar disor-der (Yatham, *et al.*, 2009). For these women, the anti-convulsant medications may be more appropriate in that they have both mood-stabilizing and antidepressant effects (Leibenluft, 2000).

## Conditions comorbid with postpartum depression

In addition to bipolar disorders, which can occur with or without psychosis, there are several other conditions that can co-occur with postpartum depression including postpartum anxiety disorders, eating disorders, and substance abuse. These are described below.

## Postpartum anxiety disorders

Postpartum anxiety disorders include panic disorders, generalized anxiety disorder, social phobia, obsessive-compulsive disorder, and posttraumatic stress disorder. Several factors appear to contribute to postpartum anxiety disorders including additional responsibilities, and changing social, family, and professional roles (Rapkin, *et al.*, 2002).

A study of 207 mothers in Australia examined the relationship between depression and anxiety in pregnancy and postpartum, noting that this relationship is often bidirectional (Skouteris, *et al.*, 2009). In this study, depressive symptoms in early pregnancy predicted anxiety symptoms in later pregnancy, and anxiety in later pregnancy predicted depressive symptoms postpartum. These relationships were present even after controlling for social support, prior depression, and sleep quality. Skouteris and colleagues (2009) found that anxiety scores were more stable than depression scores across the multiple assessment points, and suggested that clinicians should screen not only for depression but for anxiety as well.

Cohen, *et al.* (1994) found that the impact of pregnancy on panic disorder was mixed. In this study, the researchers retrospectively followed the clinical course of 49 women who had panic disorder before pregnancy. Seventy-eight percent of these women had either no change, or a slight improvement, while pregnant. For 27% of the women, their panic disorder became more severe during pregnancy. It appeared that patients with milder symptoms either improved or stayed the same during pregnancy. In contrast, women with more severe illness needed to continue treatment with anti-panic medication during their pregnancies.

## Obsessive-compulsive disorder

Obsessive-compulsive disorder (OCD) is another anxiety disorder that often co-occurs with postpartum depression. It is characterized by recurrent, unwelcome thoughts, ideas, or doubts that give rise to anxiety and distress (obsessions). These obsessions lead to excessive behavioral or mental acts (Abramowitz, *et al.*, 2002). The exact incidence of postpartum OCD is not known, but birth of a child, particularly with high rates of obstetric complications, is one of the known triggers of symptoms (Maina, *et al.*, 1999).

In postpartum women, obsessional thoughts are often focused on infant harm. Some concern fears of harming the baby with knives, throwing the baby down stairs or out of a window, or other types of harm (Abramowitz, *et al.*, 2002). Other types of compulsions concerned repetitive thoughts of their babies dying in their sleep; that they would sexually misuse their babies, or physically misplace them. In a study of 15 women with postpartum-onset OCD, all suffered from disabling intrusive obsessional thoughts of harming their babies. Most of these women were also depressed (Sichel, *et al.*, 1993). Not surprisingly, obsessive thoughts can be very troubling to mothers, as DeeDee describes.

> My postpartum depression was basically weird thoughts toward the baby, and he was a wonderful baby. The perfect baby. One time I had him on the bathroom floor with me. All of the sudden, I had this thought to kick the baby. This was the first weird thought I had toward him. My pediatrician told me that this was very normal. "You had a traumatic delivery." I would have weird thoughts when I was breastfeeding. I was constantly worried that the baby would hit his head on the table. I was also scared to walk through the doorway, that he would hit his head. These thoughts would become obsessive. I was afraid if I told anyone, they'd take the baby away. I finally told my mom. She said it was normal and not to worry. This lasted around five months. If I was ironing, I'd be terrified

that the baby would be burned. Even if he was upstairs asleep in his bed. Then I would start to analyze my thoughts. "Am I thinking he'd be burned because I wanted him to be burned?" I was also scared of knives … I didn't want to do these things. I couldn't understand why I was thinking this way. These thoughts happened every day, all the time. Slowly, I had fewer thoughts. I'd think "there's no way he can hit his head when I'm holding him." The hardest thing was I couldn't find anyone who had this experience. I knew about it, but I couldn't seem to find anyone who had been through it.

Wisner, *et al.* (1999) compared women with postpartum depression and women with non-postpartum depression. In both these groups, there were high rates of OCD that co-occurred with depression. Fifty-seven percent of the postpartum women had OCD symptoms, as did 36% of the non-postpartum depressed women. The authors concluded that childbearing women are more likely to experience obsessional thoughts and compulsions when experiencing major depression.

A study of four men revealed that they too experienced postpartum OCD that coincided with their wives' deliveries. These obsessions were very similar in content to the obsessional thoughts of new mothers. And the men responded with feelings of shame and guilt (Abramowitz, *et al.*, 2001).

Beck (2002) identified anxiety, relentless obsessive thinking, anger, guilt, and contemplating self-harm as part of her "spiraling down" dimension of postpartum depression. This dimension was part of a metasynthesis of 18 qualitative studies of postpartum depression. Obsessive thoughts were so intrusive for the women in Beck's (2002) studies, that they often became intolerable. Women tended to ruminate over feelings of failure as a mother, fearing that they or their babies might be harmed, wondering if they would ever feel normal again, and constantly worrying about the baby. These mothers tended to self-silence and to isolate themselves because they were sure no one would understand what they were going through.

*Responding to concerns about infant harm*

Descriptions of thoughts about harming the baby must also be handled with great care. Women I've spoken with indicated that professionals either reacted with great alarm, or assured them that the thoughts were "normal." The women who were troubled by these thoughts indicated that one of the worst reactions people had was to become alarmed, and express great concern that they would kill their babies. This reaction did not stop the thoughts, but actually fed into them and made them more intense.

Abramowitz, *et al.* (2002) distinguished obsessive thoughts of infant harm from psychosis. In psychosis, thoughts of harm are consistent with a person's delusional thinking. A person acts out aggressive behavior because she believes she has to do it. (There is more on these types of thought in Chapter 2.) In contrast, obsessive thoughts do not increase risk of infant harm. These thoughts are unwanted and inconsistent with a person's normal behavior, and so distressing that people suffering from OCD will go to great lengths to keep these bad things from happening.

It is also unhelpful when professionals dismiss these thoughts as "normal" because the women themselves know that they are not. They may be fairly commonplace, but that doesn't mean they are normal. When speaking to a mother, you can say something like this: "It must be very distressing to you to have such thoughts. Many other women have these thoughts and they do not mean that you are a bad mother or that you will harm your baby. These thoughts usually mean that you are under some type of stress, and it may help to talk with someone about it." Then you can offer some names of people who can help. This type of approach validates the mother's experience while at the same time taking the problem seriously.

In more serious cases, you may need to take additional action. If the mother refuses help, or if you fear that the baby is in danger, you may be legally obligated to make a report to the department of social services or your local child protective agency.

### *Posttraumatic stress disorder*

Another co-occurring anxiety disorder is posttraumatic stress disorder (PTSD). Women may come into the postpartum period with pre-existing PTSD that could be due to prior trauma, such as previous abuse or sexual assault, or that could be caused by the birth itself. Even if women do not meet full criteria for PTSD, they may have troubling symptoms. In a study of Vietnamese and Hmong women living in the U.S., Foss (2001) found that posttraumatic stress disorder was highly correlated with depression in this sample. PTSD in postpartum women will be described more fully in Chapters 6 and 8.

### *Eating disorders*

Eating disorders can also co-occur with depression during pregnancy and the postpartum period. In one recent study, active bulimia nervosa also increased the risk of postpartum depression, miscarriage, and preterm birth (Morgan, *et al.*, 2006). In this study, a cohort of 122 women with active bulimia while pregnant were compared with 82 pregnant women with quiescent bulimia. The risk of depression (odds ratio (OR)=2.8, CI=1.2–2.6), miscarriage (OR=2.6, CI=1.2–5.6), and preterm birth (OR=3.3, CI=1.3–8.8) were all increased among with women with active bulimia. These effects were not explained by the confounding factors of laxative misuse, demographic differences, alcohol/substance abuse, cigarette use, or absolute weight difference.

In a sample of 49 women with eating disorders who had recently given birth, the rate of postpartum depression was 35% (Franko, *et al.*, 2001). The majority of these women had had normal pregnancies, but three of the women had babies with birth defects. Among the women in the study, those who had active symptoms of either anorexia or bulimia during pregnancy were at increased risk for postpartum depression. The authors recommended close monitoring of women with past or current eating disorders during pregnancy and in the postpartum period.

Binge eating and vomiting before pregnancy predicted postpartum depression in another study of 181 women. Mothers whose eating disorders were active during pregnancy were the most distressed in this sample, particularly those with a binge or purge type of eating disorder. However, low-intensity exercise was associated with less distress (Abraham, *et al.*, 2001).

### *Substance abuse*

Finally, substance abuse can also co-occur with postpartum depression. In a review of 17 studies, Ross and Dennis (2009) found that women who were actively abusing substances were at increased risk for postpartum depression. Regarding substances, alcohol, cocaine, and illegal drugs were the substances specifically considered.

In another study (Pajulo, *et al.*, 2001a), 8% of 391 pregnant women were depressed. Substance abuse and life stress both predicted depression in pregnancy, as did difficulties with their social networks (friends, partners, and the women's own mothers). A second study by these same authors (Pajulo, *et al.*, 2001b) compared 12 mothers who abused substances and 12 control mothers, in their emotional health and interactions with their babies at three and six months postpartum. Not surprisingly, the substance-abusing mothers were significantly more depressed, had less social support, and more life stress than the control mothers. Their interactions with their babies were also less positive.

Substance abuse is obviously a serious problem for both mothers and babies. If women abuse substances during pregnancy, the state may intervene and remove the baby from the mother's care after delivery. For substance-abusing mothers, intervention for depression alone would be incomplete. Mothers who abuse substances also need referrals to programs that can directly address their substance abuse.

## Summary

Postpartum depression is responsible for a wide range of symptoms, and can co-occur with other conditions such as anxiety disorders, eating disorders, and substance abuse. Bipolar disorder can also appear in the postpartum period, and may manifest as major depression or postpartum psychosis.

In the next chapter, I describe why depression is harmful for mothers and babies.

# 2 Why depression is harmful for mothers and babies

Depression affects babies in every aspect of their development: emotional, social, cognitive, and behavioral. Mothers, too, are negatively affected by depression and this is reflected in their higher healthcare costs. A study from Canada found that depressed mothers had healthcare costs that were twice those of non-depressed mothers. Mothers who were very depressed had costs that were five times higher (Roberts, *et al.*, 2001). These findings on mothers and babies indicate that depression is far too serious to ignore.

## Why depression is bad for mothers

In adults, depression increases the risk of a number of serious diseases including coronary heart disease, myocardial infarction, chronic pain syndromes, premature aging, impaired wound healing, and even Alzheimer's disease (Kiecolt-Glaser, *et al.*, 2005). Most of these diseases won't affect mothers in the perinatal period, but they can be the long-term effects of untreated depression.

Of particular interest is the link between depression and cardiovascular disease. This link is important because it gives us insight into the physiological processes involved in depression. Depression is a risk factor for cardiovascular disease (Frasure-Smith and Lesperance, 2005), and patients who become depressed after a myocardial infarction are two to three times more likely to have another one. They are also three to four times more likely to die (de Jonge, *et al.*, 2006; Lesperance and Frasure-Smith, 2000). The risk exists not only for those suffering from major depression, but also for those who have milder forms as well.

Kop and Gottdiener (2005) hypothesized that depression in early adulthood may promote vascular injury, and that the immune system may increase further early-stage cardiovascular disease by encouraging lipid and macrophage deposits. For people with pre-existing cardiovascular disease, depression-related chronic inflammation can reduce the stability of plaque, which can lead to acute cardiac episodes. The inflammation-depression connection will be described in more detail in Chapter 5.

Depression is also related to health behaviors. In a review of the literature, depression was correlated with poor eating habits, use of tobacco, and abuse of alcohol and drugs. People may use these harmful behaviors as a way to cope with negative emotions. Depressed people even ate more chocolate (Salovey, *et al.*, 2000).

Depression can also impair women's relationships. Depressed women report more communication problems with their partners, and have marital dysfunction that persists long after the depression has resolved (Roux, *et al.*, 2002). One study compared women who were currently depressed, those with a history of depression, and those with no history of depression. The depressed and formerly depressed women were impaired on every measure of interpersonal behavior, had less stable marriages, and reported lower levels of marital satisfaction than women with no history of depression (Hammen and Brennan, 2002).

These studies indicate that depression has serious health implications for mothers, including increased risk of cardiovascular diseases, a suppressed immune system, and decreased health behaviors. These effects may not manifest immediately, but it is important to acknowledge them, because they indicate that depression is too serious to simply hope that it will resolve on its own.

Unfortunately, depression in mothers also affects babies, and these effects appear in a relatively short time.

## Why maternal depression is bad for babies

There has been a large number of studies over the past 30 years demonstrating the harmful effects of maternal depression on children, from the neonates to young adults. Below is a summary of these findings, starting with the *in utero* effects of untreated depression.

### *The impact of untreated depression on fetal development*

The impact of maternal depression on infants begins during pregnancy. Several studies have demonstrated that depression during pregnancy is a strong risk factor for preterm birth. In a recent review, Field and colleagues (2006a) noted that depressed women are more likely to deliver prematurely and that they often have neonates who require intensive care for serious postpartum complications, such as bronchopulmonary dysplasia and intraventricular hemorrhage. Depressed mothers are also at increased risk of having babies who have a low birth weight and are small for gestational age.

In a prospective cohort study of 681 women from France, the rate of spontaneous preterm birth for depressed women was more than double that of non-depressed women (9.7% vs. 4%; OR=3.3; Dayan, *et al.*, 2006). A study in Goa, India (N=270) found that mothers who were depressed during their third trimester were significantly more likely to have low-birth-weight babies than their non-depressed counterparts. The most-depressed mothers were at highest risk (OR=2.5). This was true even after controlling for other factors that influence birth weight, such as maternal age, maternal and paternal education, and paternal income (Patel and Prince, 2006).

Anxiety can also increase the risk of preterm birth. A study of 1,820 women from Baltimore found that women with high levels of anxiety about their pregnancies were significantly more likely to have their babies prematurely (Orr, *et al.*, 2007). Indeed, women with the highest levels of pregnancy-related anxiety had three times the risk of preterm birth compared with women with low anxiety. These findings were true even after controlling for traditional risk factors for preterm birth including first- or second-trimester bleeding, drug use, unemployment, previous preterm or still birth, smoking, low body mass index, maternal education, age, and race.

Another study of 415 pregnant women from L.A. had similar results (Glynn, *et al.*, 2008). In this study, pregnant women were assessed at 18 to 20 and 30 to 32 weeks' gestation. The sample was 23% Hispanic, 48% white, 14% African American, and 15% from other ethnic groups. Elevated risk for preterm birth was associated with increased stress and anxiety. These findings persisted even after controlling for obstetric risk, pregnancy-related anxiety, ethnicity, parity, and prenatal life events. The authors concluded that prenatal stress is an important predictor of preterm birth.

In a study of 279 pregnant women, state anxiety, perceived stress, life-event stress, and pregnancy-specific stress were examined for their potential effects on preterm birth (Lobel, *et al.*, 2008). The researchers found that pregnancy-specific stress predicted birth outcomes better than other forms of stress or when they were all combined. After controlling for obstetric risk, they found that pregnancy-specific stress was related to increased smoking, caffeine consumption, and unhealthy eating, and was inversely related to healthy eating, vitamin use, and exercise. The authors concluded that pregnancy-specific stress contributed directly to preterm birth and indirectly to low birth weight through smoking.

Not every study has found a relationship between depression and low birth weight or prematurity, however. In a large cohort study of 10,967 women, investigators found that women depressed during pregnancy were significantly more likely to have low-birth-weight babies (Evans, *et al.*, 2007). However, once the investigators controlled for confounding factors, with smoking being the largest, this relationship disappeared. The authors concluded that there was no independent effect of depression on low birth weight. However, given that depressed women are more likely to smoke, and that depression may mediate smoking, the authors' statement about lack of a relationship may be premature.

### Possible underlying mechanisms for preterm birth and other effects

Some of the increased risk of preterm birth may be due to elevated levels of stress hormones. In a study of 70 depressed and 70 non-depressed women (Field, *et al.*, 2004), participants were assessed during their second trimester of pregnancy and during the neonatal period. None of the women were in treatment for depression or taking psychotropic medications. Mothers with depressive symptoms had higher prenatal cortisol and norepinephrine levels, lower dopamine and serotonin, and a higher percentage of depressed mothers (34%) had babies who had a low birth weight compared with the non-depressed mothers (14%). The infants also had higher cortisol levels, and lower levels of dopamine and serotonin. They also had less optimal habituation, orientation, motor, range of state and autonomic stability on the Brazelton Scale.

Mothers with high levels of urinary cortisol were significantly more likely to have premature babies in a study of 300 women in their last trimester of pregnancy (Field, *et al.*, 2006b). These infants also had lower habituation and high reflex scores on the Brazelton Assessment Scale. Using discriminate function analysis, the researchers found that cortisol levels more accurately predicted short gestation and low birth weight than did scores on the depression inventory.

Depression has several possible ways to influence birth weight and gestational age. Cortisol changes the placental environment and directly crosses the placenta. CRH, a precursor hormone to cortisol, induces vasodilatation, causing the uterine artery to constrict, reducing blood flow to the fetus. This may restrict oxygen and nutrient delivery, and has been associated with preterm birth. CRH also triggers parturition. Norepinephrine can affect fetal growth via its effects on the cardiovascular system. It is related to uterine artery resistance and indirectly to blood flow and fetal growth in animal studies. But it does not cross the placenta (Dayan, *et al.*, 2006; Field, *et al.*, 2004, 2006a). These hormone levels can also be influenced by other mood states that are often co-morbid with depression, such as stress and anxiety.

Another possible pathway by which depression increases the risk of preterm birth involves the immune system (see Chapter 5). Depression activates the proinflammatory cytokines, such as interleukin (IL)-6 and tumor necrocis factor (TNF)-alpha, and prostaglandin E2, which is secreted in response to cortisol and proinflammatory cytokines. Prostaglandin E2 plays a major role in uterine contractions (Dayan, *et al.*, 2006). IL-6 and TNF-$\alpha$ are elevated in

depressed mothers and also ripen the cervix before delivery. In a study of 30 p
Coussons-Read and colleagues (2005) found that TNF-α and IL-6 levels v
higher and the anti-inflammatory cytokine IL-10 was significantly low
were stressed compared with mothers who weren't. The authors hypoth
mation was the likely mechanism to explain the relationship between
preterm birth. They noted that high levels of inflammation (particularly IL-
were associated with pre-eclampsia and premature labor. Infection also increases the
preterm delivery, and TNF-α is released in response to both viral and bacterial infections.
They concluded that high levels of proinflammatory cytokines may, in fact, endanger human
pregnancies. (The role of the immune system in depression is described in more detail in
Chapter 5.)

### Effects of maternal depression on infants

After babies are born, mothers' depression can still affect them. A number of physiological
indicators are more common in infants of depressed mothers. For example, abnormalities
in electroencephalograms (EEGs) have been observed in infants of depressed mothers at
three to six months. Babies of depressed mothers had depressed affect and right frontal EEG
asymmetry as early as three months (Field, *et al.*, 1995). The mothers were all low-income,
single adolescents of African American or Hispanic ethnicity (N=32). The babies were all
full-term with no medical conditions. Right frontal asymmetry is an abnormal pattern found
in chronically depressed adults, and is a physiologic marker of depression in babies (Field,
*et al.*, 2006a).

Another study of 48 neonates (Field, *et al.*, 2002a) found that babies with greater relative
right frontal EEG activation had elevated cortisol levels, showed more variability in state
changes during sleep/wake observations, and had less than optimum performance on the
Brazelton Neonatal Behavior Assessment Scale. Their mothers also had lower prenatal and
postnatal serotonin levels and higher levels of cortisol (both consistent with depression).
The authors concluded that greater relative right frontal activation may place these infants at
increased risk for developmental problems.

In a study from Finland of 520 mothers, data were collected in the second trimester of
pregnancy and at two and twelve months postpartum (Punamaki, *et al.*, 2006). Mothers'
prenatal depression and anxiety predicted infants' developmental problems at twelve months.
Babies of depressed mothers had poor neonatal health and increased birth complications. Their
mothers were also more likely to use assisted reproductive technology and have a history of
infertility. Among the mothers who used assisted reproductive technology, prenatal depressive symptoms predicted postpartum depression at two months and depressive symptoms at
twelve months. Postpartum depression at two months was related to infant developmental
problems and difficult child characteristics at twelve months.

Chronicity and severity of depression also influences the amount of its negative impact.
Diego and colleagues (2005) recruited four groups of mothers (N=80) in their second trimester
of pregnancy: non-depressed women, women only depressed during pregnancy, women only
depressed postpartum, and women who were depressed during both pregnancy and postpartum. They found that babies born to mothers with prenatal depression spent more time fussing
and crying, and showed more stress behaviors than babies whose mothers were not depressed
or who were only depressed postpartum. The authors concluded that infants are influenced
by the timing and duration of depression, not simply by its mere presence.

A truly frightening finding had to do with postpartum depression in the neonatal period and increased risk of SIDS (Sanderson, *et al.*, 2002). In this cohort study of 32,984 births in Sheffield, UK, from 1988 to 1993, there were 42 infant deaths attributed to SIDS. Multivariate analyses identified three significant risk factors for SIDS: smoking (OR=7.24); a high score on the Edinburgh Postnatal Depression Scale (OR=3.2), and living in a poor area (OR=2.33). The authors concluded that a high EPDS score, and by implication high depressive symptoms, were possibly implicated in SIDS.

## Effects of maternal depression on toddlers and preschoolers

Toddlers were observed in a clean-up task with their adolescent mothers in order to observe parenting styles (Pelaez, *et al.*, 2008). There were 17 depressed and 19 non-depressed mothers. The parenting styles were classified as: (1) authoritative – mother provides firm control and set limits in a warm, respectful manner; (2) authoritarian – mother shows verbal or physical rejection or control, or lacks positive encouragement; (3) permissive – mother provides positive verbal communication, but sets no limits or provides no instructions, and (4) disengaged – mother is uninvolved, unresponsive or avoidant, and has flat affect. Depressed mothers were more likely to be classified as authoritarian or disengaged. Mothers' depression also appeared to impact their children's behavior. The toddlers of depressed mothers spent less time following instructions, displayed aggressive play for a greater percentage of time, and had less time on-task than toddlers of non-depressed mothers.

In a secondary analysis of data from the Healthy Steps National Evaluation, McLearn, *et al.* (2006a; 2006b) examined whether depression at 2 to 4 months, or current depression, predicted poorer parenting at 30 to 33 months. The analysis included data from 3,412 mothers. They found that mothers with depressive symptoms at 2 to 4 months were less likely than non-depressed mothers to participate in infant safety activities including using a car seat and lowering the water heater temperature. They were also less likely to play with their children at 30 to 33 months. Mothers with current depression had reduced odds of using electric outlet covers, using safety latches, talking with their children, limiting TV or video watching, following daily routines, and being nurturing. In addition, currently depressed mothers had increased risk of using harsh punishment, slapping the child's face, or spanking with an object. The study authors indicated that current depression had a stronger influence on parenting behaviors, but that early depression may set a negative pattern that carries through early childhood.

Maternal depression can also affect preschoolers. In a study of 112 mother-infant dyads, the researchers found that brief maternal depression did not negatively impact infant performance at either 12 or 15 months (Cornish, *et al.*, 2005). However, chronic maternal depression was related to lower infant cognitive and psychomotor development, with similar effects for boys and girls. One out of four infants whose mothers were chronically depressed scored in the mildly-to-significantly delayed range on psychomotor development. Infants of chronically depressed mothers were also less likely to be walking competently by 15 months. Contrary to expectation, chronic maternal depression was not related to delays in infant language development.

In a study of 4- to 5-year-olds born to adolescent mothers, Black and colleagues (2002) found that maternal depression, and the mother's perceptions of her partner, influenced children's behavior problems. This was a high-risk sample: 42.4% of the children had been maltreated; 36% had externalizing scores in the clinical range, and 10.8% had internalizing scores in the clinical range. When mothers were depressed, they perceived the quality of their relationship with their partner more negatively, and their children showed more symptoms.

Unfortunately, children who were premature may be more susceptible to the negative effects of maternal depression. In a series of two studies, researchers compared children's cortisol levels after interacting with their depressed or non-depressed mothers (Bugental, *et al.*, 2008). The children were 14 to 16 months old. Preterm infants were more reactive to their mothers' depression than infants who were full term, with higher cortisol levels when interacting with their depressed mothers and lower cortisol levels when interacting with a non-depressed mother. The authors concluded that premature infants were more sensitive to the emotional environment of their homes, and that there were possible implications for their developmental outcomes.

## Effects of maternal depression on school-age children

The negative impact of maternal depression has been documented in children of elementary-school age. In an American study of 5,000 mother-infant pairs, children of depressed mothers had more behavior problems and lower vocabulary scores at age 5 than did other children (Brennan, *et al.*, 2000). In this study, mothers were assessed for depression during pregnancy, immediately postpartum, and when their children were 6 months and 5 years old. Severity and chronicity of depression were related to more behavior problems, as were more recent episodes of maternal depression.

Murray and colleagues (2001) found that children of depressed mothers were more likely, at age 5, to express depressive cognitions, such as hopelessness, pessimism, and low self-worth, especially when exposed to a mild stressor. The authors noted, however, that much of this relationship can be accounted for by current maternal hostility toward the child. In another study, maternal depression during the child's first two years of life was the best predictor of elevated baseline cortisol in response to a mild stressor at age 7 (Ashman, *et al.*, 2002).

Children of mothers who had postpartum depression had lower social competence scores at ages eight to nine in a study from Finland (Luoma, *et al.*, 2001). Social competence included parents' reports of children's activities, hobbies, tasks, and chores; functioning in social relationships; and school achievements. Mothers were assessed for depression prenatally, postnatally, and when their children were 8 to 9 years old. Mothers' current depression was also associated with low social competence and low adaptive functioning.

Negative findings also appear at age 11 (Hay, *et al.*, 2001). In this study, women were assessed for depression at three months postpartum (N=149). At age 11, 132 of these children were tested. Children of mothers who were depressed at three months postpartum had significantly lower IQ scores and had a number of problems in school including attentional and mathematical-reasoning difficulties. They were more likely to be in special education. The effects were particularly pronounced for boys. The links between postpartum depression and IQ were not accounted for by social disadvantage or by mothers' later mental health problems.

## Effects of maternal depression on young adults

There is also increased risk of depression in offspring of depressed mothers that lasts well into adulthood. In a study of 2,427 young adults (Lieb, *et al.*, 2002), depression in either their mothers or fathers increased the risk of depression in the subjects. Interestingly, paternal depression was associated with an earlier onset of depression, and increased severity, impairment, and recurrence in their children.

A study of 150 pregnant women found that antenatal and postpartum depression predicted smoking in adolescent offspring (Hay, *et al.*, 2008). In this study, 31% of the mothers were depressed during pregnancy and 22% were depressed at three months postpartum. Mothers who were depressed at either of these time points were more likely to be depressed at subsequent assessment points. The authors concluded that mothers' lifelong symptoms of depression created a risky environment before birth and in the postpartum period. Depression in the perinatal period was a robust predictor of child behavior problems. The exact chain of causal events is unknown, but perinatal depression predicted cumulative stress for families, which promoted adolescent disorder, including teen smoking.

A 20-year follow-up of children of depressed mothers and fathers compared them with a matched group of children whose parents had no psychiatric illness. The adult children of depressed parents had three times the rate of major depression, anxiety disorders, and substance abuse compared with children of non-depressed parents. In addition, children of depressed parents had higher rates of medical problems and premature mortality (Weissman, *et al.*, 2006b).

## The interaction styles of depressed mothers

Depression in mothers can lead to long-lasting and serious effects in their babies. The next logical question to ask is why this occurs. To understand why, it's instructive to look at the interaction styles of depressed mothers. Depressed mothers tend to have one of two basic interaction styles: avoidant and angry-intrusive (Beck, 1995; Field, 1992; Tronick and Weinberg, 1997). These styles are described below.

---

### Characteristics of positive mother-infant interaction

An effective (or synchronous) mother–child interaction contains many components (Capuzzi, 1989). The mother and infant must give clear cues to each other, the mother must be responsive to the infant's cues, the infant must respond to the mother's caregiving, and the environment must be supportive of and facilitate this interaction. This is the process by which mothers become attached to their infants. When this process breaks down, it can lead to insecure attachments between mothers and babies, and maternal depression.

---

### *Avoidant and angry–intrusive interaction styles*

In the avoidant style, mothers spend approximately 80% of their time disengaged from their babies, ignoring their cues. Mothers with this style are unresponsive, have flat affect, and do not support their infants' activities; and they only respond to infant distress. Babies react to this style by trying to engage their mothers in interaction. Unfortunately, they are generally not successful. Lack of maternal responsiveness is highly stressful for babies, as demonstrated by elevated cortisol levels and abnormal EEG patterns. These infants protested about 30% of the time, and watched their mothers less than 5% of the time. They became disengaged, and engaged in self-comforting, self-regulatory behaviors such as thumb sucking, looking away, passivity, and withdrawal to help them cope with their state. When they cannot engage their mothers, they often respond by "shutting down" (Field, 1992).

In the angry-intrusive style, mothers are more engaged with their babies, but the interactions are characterized by hostility and intrusiveness. In this style, mothers expressed anger and irritation, and roughly handled their babies approximately 40% of the time. These mothers also ignore their babies' cues. Mothers with the angry-intrusive style spoke in an angry tone, poked at their babies, and interfered with their babies' activities (Tronick and Weinberg, 1997). Rather than interacting in a give-and-take fashion, these mothers dominated the relationship. Babies react to this style by trying to disengage from their mothers approximately 55% of the time (e.g. arching, looking or pushing away). They only protest about 5% of the time. These infants are often angry, and show frustration easily in anticipation of their mothers' intrusiveness (Tronick and Weinberg, 1997). Mothers may interpret this behavior as rejection (Field, 1992).

In Beck's (1996a) phenomenological study of 12 mothers with postpartum depression, the themes of anger and avoidance are woven throughout the mothers' accounts. Participants indicated that they were overwhelmed by their childcare responsibilities. Their day-to-day interactions with their children were filled with guilt, irrational thinking, loss, and anger. One mother, who was experiencing detachment from her baby, reported the following.

> The baby would be on the table looking at me, dressed, washed, cooing and laughing and smiling, and I just looked at her.
>
> (Beck, 1996a: 100)

Another mother reported how depression made her feel extremely angry.

> I felt so much anger inside of me. I had to stop and think that this little baby doesn't know any better. I looked up and saw my husband in the doorway, and I said, "Get the baby away!"
>
> (Beck, 1996a: 100)

## The still-faced mothers studies

The still-faced mother paradigm has been used in many studies to demonstrate – under laboratory conditions – the effects of maternal depression. Tronick and colleagues asked mothers to pretend that they were depressed when interacting with their three-month-old babies. These mothers spoke in a monotone, had little or no facial affect, and seldom touched their infants. It only took about three minutes before the infants became distressed at the way their mothers were acting. The infants became wary, and tried to engage their mothers in their normal affective states. The infants continued to be wary even when mothers returned to their normal affect (Weinberg and Tronick, 1998). This paradigm was designed to assess infants' reactions to a break in normal social interaction. Infants often responded by trying to elicit responses from their mothers by smiling briefly. However, when their mothers did not respond, the infants became distressed within a few interaction cycles (Moore, *et al.*, 2001).

One study also tried to predict infant response to maternal interaction style predicted problems in later development. In this study, 129 mother-infant pairs participated. Approximately half of the mothers met criteria for major depressive disorder. The infants were assessed at two, four, and six months (Moore, *et al.*, 2001). The infants' responses predicted internalizing and externalizing behaviors at 18 months. The findings of Moore and colleagues demonstrated that infants are sensitive to disruptions in social reciprocity as early as two months of age.

## Intervention for depressed mothers

Researchers have also examined the impact of intervention on the mother–infant relationship. Does mother–baby interaction improve when depression resolves? Conversely, does depression remit when the interaction improves? These questions have important clinical applications and the findings so far have been mixed. In a study of 117 postpartum women with depressive symptoms (Horowitz, *et al.*, 2001), half of the women were assigned to a treatment group where they were coached to improve in their responsiveness to their infants. At the end of the intervention, mothers in the intervention group did show significantly higher levels of maternal responsiveness, but the intervention had no effect on their depressive symptoms.

At least two studies from the U.K. have found that infant massage can help with maternal depression and the effects may be due to improved mother–infant interactions. The first was a small pilot study with 12 mothers in the massage group and 13 in the control group (Glover, *et al.*, 2002). All the mothers had scored over 13 on the EPDS. At the end of the trial, depressive symptoms improved more for the mothers in the massage group than for mothers in the control group (although both improved). In addition, mothers' interactions with their babies had improved. The authors highlighted that massage relaxed mother and baby, increased maternal confidence, increased mothers' understanding of babies' cues, and released oxytocin, which promoted bonding.

The second study assigned 34 mothers who were depressed to infant-massage or support-group conditions (Onozawa, *et al.*, 2001). There were five weekly sessions. The EPDS scores fell in both groups by the end of five weeks, with a larger effect in the infant-massage group. There was also significant improvement in mother–infant interaction in the massage group. The mothers in the massage condition were specifically taught how to read their babies' cues.

A study of 151 mother–infant pairs examined the impact of antidepressants on mother and child psychopathology (Weissman, *et al.*, 2006a). They found that remission of maternal depression was associated with a reduction of child symptoms and diagnoses. A maternal response of at least 50% was required to see an improvement in the child.

A question a recent study asked is whether treating depression is sufficient to help with maternal role functioning (Logsdon, *et al.*, 2009). In this study, mother–infant interaction was taped for 27 women and their infants. The women completed a measure of maternal-role gratification and the Infant Care Survey. The researchers found that antidepressants did improve maternal gratification and overall functioning, but did not have an effect on maternal self-efficacy or maternal–infant interaction. The percentage of positive infant affect did improve over time. Self-efficacy increased for the mother when the infant demonstrated a higher percentage of positive affect. But the correlation was not significant. McLennan and Offord's (2002) review raised similar concerns about whether targeting postpartum depression alone was sufficient to ameliorate negative child outcomes. Depression and negative interaction style may need to be addressed separately.

Another study examined the impact of breastfeeding on infants of depressed mothers (Jones, *et al.*, 2004). This study compared four groups of postpartum women: depressed women who were either breast- or bottle-feeding, and non-depressed women who were either breast- or bottle-feeding. The outcome was babies' EEG patterns. In this study, babies of depressed, breastfeeding mothers had *normal* EEG patterns. In contrast, babies of depressed, non-breastfeeding women did not. In other words, breastfeeding protected babies from the harmful effects of maternal depression. The authors observed that depressed, breastfeeding mothers touched, stroked, and made eye contact with their babies more than depressed, non-breastfeeding women because these behaviors are built into the breastfeeding relation-ship. This is one more reason to encourage and support breastfeeding in depressed mothers.

What these above-cited studies indicate is that it is possible to reverse the harmful effects of maternal depression on infants and children. However, particularly when symptoms are long-lasting, both the depression and the dysfunctional interaction need to be addressed.

In the next section, I describe two of the most serious and disturbing forms of mother and infant harm: infanticide and maternal suicide.

## Infanticide and maternal suicide

The most serious manifestations of postpartum illness are when a mother takes her own life or that of her baby. Fortunately, the incidence of these responses is rare. Unfortunately, most of what we know about infanticide and maternal suicide is based on case studies and anecdotal evidence. Nevertheless, some small studies shed some light on these frightening responses.

### *Infanticide*

As I described in Chapter 1, thoughts of infant harm can be fairly common among depressed mothers. But most obsessive thoughts do not involve the mother thinking of actually harm-ing her baby. Rather, they are obsessive concerns for infant safety, and thoughts about what may happen to the baby. More concerning are women's specific thoughts of harming their infants. Even when women have these thoughts, most never act on them. A qualitative study of 15 women with non-psychotic depression in Brisbane, Australia, explored the themes that mothers presented regarding their thoughts of infanticide (Barr and Beck, 2008). Although mothers with no psychotic symptoms have a lower risk of actual physical harm to their infants, we know little about the thought processes of mothers who have infanticidal thoughts with no intention to act. This study was implemented in order to explore the characteristics of infanticidal thoughts. All of the women had babies 0 to 12 months old. The authors found specific themes regarding their thoughts of infanticide.

- *Experience of horror*: Women experienced horror regarding their thoughts of harming their babies.
- *Distorted sense of responsibility*: Women felt despondent and that their situation was hopeless. Infanticidal thoughts occurred alongside suicidal thoughts.
- *Consuming negativity*: This was reflected by anger and hatred towards their babies that were associated with infanticidal thoughts.
- *Keeping secrets*: All of the participants indicated that they were ashamed of their thoughts and kept them from family and healthcare providers.
- *Managing the crisis*: A theme for some of the women was related to arranging circum-stances to keep their infants safe at times when they might harm them (e.g. scheduling help at high-stress times of day).

Barr and Beck (2008) summarized their findings by noting that recurring obsessional thoughts of infant harm were commonly experienced by depressed mothers, and that women with non-psychotic depression may not be at increased risk of infanticide. However, Barr and Beck urged healthcare providers to assess women for psychotic or delusional symptoms and/or behavior that puts the infants at risk, and concluded that women experiencing infanticidal thoughts need to seek help.

Chandra and colleagues (2002) studied 50 Indian women who had been admitted to a psychiatric hospital postpartum. They collected data from three sources: the mother's partner, nursing observations made during the first week in the hospital, and the psychiatric assessment within the first week of admission. In this sample, 43% reported infanticidal thoughts, 36% reported infanticidal behavior, and 34% reported both infanticidal thoughts and behavior. Infanticidal ideas and behavior tended to co-occur. In a logistic regression, depression and psychotic ideas predicted infanticidal ideation. Psychotic ideation also predicted infanticidal behavior.

A study from Korea included 45 women who either killed or attempted to kill their infants. Women were included in the sample if they had diagnoses of either major depression or bipolar disorder (Kim, *et al.*, 2008). The data were collected via chart review and the researchers were interested in whether depressive symptoms at admission could predict later diagnoses of bipolar disorder. They found that while only 24% of the patients had a diagnosis of bipolar disorder at admission, 73% had this diagnosis at discharge. Among women admitted with a diagnosis of major depression, 65% were later reclassified based on the appearance of hypomanic or manic episodes. Thirty-six percent of their sample had attempted suicide immediately after committing filicide. They suggested that healthcare providers consider the diagnosis of bipolar disorder when examining filicidal depressive mothers. They also noted that treating women who had bipolar disorder with antidepressants could be detrimental for patients. Indeed, 77% of their subjects had been treated with unopposed antidepressants with or without anti-psychotics.

A study from Finland (Haapasalo and Petaja, 1999) examined mental state examination reports from 48 mothers who killed or attempted to kill their children. In this study, the researchers differentiated between neonaticides (within the first 24 hours) and subsequent deaths for children under the age of 12. The majority of these non-neonatal killings were children under the age of 4 (N=33). The non-neonaticide killings are of most interest to our present discussion. The women who killed their babies in the first 24 hours tended to be young, unmarried women who denied that they were pregnant. In contrast, the non-neonatal killings were committed by married women, living with a spouse, who were significantly more likely to be homemakers. Two-thirds of these women had documented psychological problems including depression (81%); anxiety and fear (45%); psychosis (30%), and somatization and eating disorders (27%). Only 9% had obsessional thoughts. Sixty-three percent of these mothers had a history of some form of child maltreatment. The most common was psychological abuse (44%), followed by physical abuse (25%), neglect (10%), and sexual abuse (6%). Only 15% of these killings were due to postpartum depression. The others were joint suicide-homicide attempts, impulsive aggression, psychotic episodes, and abusive acts. Before the homicides, most of these mothers were reported to be "perfect" mothers who had taken good care of their children.

Meyer and Oberman (2001), in their book on mothers who kill their children, noted that in the case of infanticide, it is often difficult to distinguish "mad" from "bad." There are often elements of both. In some cases, there are clear indications of postpartum psychosis, such as delusional thinking. But in other cases, there are often pre-existing life stresses, such as past or current abuse, substance abuse, or some other impairing factor.

## Maternal suicide

Maternal suicide is another frightening response to postpartum depression. In a study from the Danish Psychiatric Case Register and the Danish registers of birth and causes of death

(1973–1993), a total of 1,567 women had been admitted to psychiatric hospitals during the postpartum period. Of these women, 107 (6.8%) had died. The authors concluded that suicide risk among the general population of postpartum women is low. However, among the population of hospitalized postpartum women, the risk of suicide is high, especially in the first postpartum year when suicide risk is increased 70-fold (Appleby, *et al.*, 1998).

Fortunately, completed suicide is relatively rare. However, as with thoughts of harming the baby, we do not know the incidence or prevalence of suicidal ideation. In a sample of hospitalized women in Australia (Fisher, *et al.*, 2002b), 5% reported suicidal ideations. Four mothers I've spoken with indicated that they had these types of thoughts.

> I'm still dealing with the sexual abuse [her own past history]. I hadn't dealt with it before the birth. I told my husband [for the first time] in the hospital. I was hysterical. I was afraid of being alone so my husband stayed the night. If I could've opened the window, I would have jumped out. [Val]

> I had breastfeeding problems. He was colicky. I was afraid I wouldn't be able to comfort him. I didn't have thoughts of hurting him, but I thought of suicide. That's how depressed I was. [Elizabeth]

> The severe depression would come on and go away. One time I was sorting through all our medicines, sorting the ones that were very lethal into a pile. The severe episodes only lasted about 1/2 minutes, but the moderate depression stayed. I couldn't be left alone. [Melissa]

> My husband and sister thought they would take care of me. I started having visions of my own funeral. I was having all kinds of scary thoughts. At that point, they decided I needed to go into the hospital. The week after my daughter's birthday, I was acutely suicidal. I packed some clothes and my pills. I was going to go to New York City, rent a hotel room and kill myself. My husband said I was rambling and saying please take care of her. As I was getting on the train, my husband was at the train station because they found my car. [Donna]

When postpartum depression leads to suicide, it leaves behind a heartbroken family. Depression activist Joan Mudd writes, "In 2001 my dear daughter, Jennifer Mudd Houghtaling, lost her battle with postpartum depression." A tribute to Jennifer described her as follows.

> No one would be more stunned by the turn of events that created the Jennifer Mudd Houghtaling Postpartum Depression Foundation than Jennifer. Her ebullient joy and laser beam of personal interest and insight was her gift to everyone she knew and loved. Carefree, energetic, devoted and nonjudgmental, Jennifer would want to know what she could do to help this cause, how does this terrible disease occur, and most of all, what needs to be done to solve it. It was her generosity of spirit that was so special.
>
> Be it, being an active member of the "Big Sister" program, or teaching adults to read, or keeping in touch with an aged friend who had become blind, or trying to convert her dog (unsuccessfully) to being a vegetarian, Jennifer made all those around her feel like they mattered.
>
> That light should have shone brightly on her much desired and cherished baby boy Brandon. More than anything, Jennifer wanted Brandon. When she found out that she

was carrying a baby boy she named him immediately and changed the password in her computer to Brandon so she could see his name and say it everyday.

In 2004, Joan and her husband founded the Jennifer Mudd Houghtaling Foundation to increase awareness of postpartum depression among healthcare providers, increase screening for new mothers, and save other women from Jennifer's fate.

Towards that end I describe (in Chapter 4) some general screening questions for suicide risk and need for hospitalization. Care must also be used in medication choice for mothers at risk for suicide. Safer choices for potentially suicidal mothers are described in Chapter 13. If identified in time, maternal suicide can be prevented.

## Conclusions

Depression causes more harm to mother and baby than people generally realize. These effects provide ample reason to take depression seriously, and to encourage mothers to seek treatment. In working with mothers, however, you must be careful with the information about infant harm. While it can be helpful in motivating women to seek services, we must never communicate that their depression has somehow "ruined" their babies or children. Many times mothers fear this, and this belief has been a motivating factor in some cases of infanticide. We can, however, use this information to gently encourage mothers to get help because when they get better, it will also be good for their babies.

# 3 Depression and breastfeeding

Some providers and advocates caring for women with postpartum depression consider breastfeeding a risk factor for depression. Based on this belief, mothers are often urged to quit in order to recover. While this advice is well-intended, we need to question whether it is medically sound. Do women need to wean in order to recover from depression? And what do mothers want to do? Some of these same providers argue that even if mothers want to continue, what we really need to do is give them "permission" to quit. When actress Brooke Shields experienced postpartum depression, her family strongly urged her to stop breastfeeding. She adamantly refused because she felt that breastfeeding was the one thing that was helping her to hang on to her sanity.

> If I were to eliminate that [breastfeeding], I might have no hope of coming through this nightmare. I was hanging on to breastfeeding as my lifeline.
> (Cited in McCarter-Spaulding and Horowitz, 2007: 80)

When providers urge mothers to quit who want to continue, breastfeeding can become a barrier to treatment. Mothers may delay or avoid treatment because they believe that they will be told to wean. In my experience, this fear is realistic – and unfortunate and unnecessary because almost all treatments for depression are compatible with breastfeeding. In addition, this view does not take into account recent research demonstrating breastfeeding's protective effect on maternal mental health. This research is summarized below.

## The adaptiveness of breastfeeding

A recent review found that rates of depression are lower in breastfeeding mothers than their non-breastfeeding counterparts (Dennis and McQueen, 2009). This is not to say that breastfeeding mothers never get depressed – for they certainly do. This is also not to say that we should ever coerce a mother into breastfeeding when she is simply too overwhelmed to deal with it. On the other hand, some depressed mothers report that breastfeeding is the only thing going well for them, so we should not be cavalier about chucking it aside as if it were of no consequence. Recent studies indicate is that there are very good reasons to support mothers who want to continue breastfeeding and that it can become an important part of their recovery.

In Chapter 4, I describe the results of studies from the field of psychoneuroimmunology (PNI) and the role of the stress response in depression. Researchers in PNI have discovered that breastfeeding is protective of maternal mental health because it downregulates the stress response. This down-regulation confers a survival advantage by protecting the breastfeeding mother and directing her toward milk production, conservation of energy, and nurturing behaviors (Groer, *et al.*, 2002). Hormones related to lactation, such as oxytocin and prolactin, have both antidepressant and anxiolytic effects (Mezzacappa and Endicott, 2007).

Mezzacappa and Katkin (2002) presented data from two studies that indicated that breastfeeding buffers mothers against negative mood. In the first study, they compared 28 breastfeeding and 27 bottle-feeding mothers on levels of perceived stress in the past month. As predicted, the breastfeeding mothers reported less stress, even after controlling for possible confounding variables.

The second study included 28 mothers who were both breast- and bottle-feeding (Mezzacappa and Katkin, 2002). The researchers measured mothers' stress levels immediately before and after both types of feeding. This study was a major methodological improvement over previous studies in that women served as their own controls. Since there were not pre-existing differences between breast- and bottle-feeding mothers, it was possible to attribute the observed difference in mood to feeding method alone. The researchers found that breastfeeding decreased negative mood and bottle feeding decreased positive mood in the same women.

A study of 43 breastfeeding women found that both breastfeeding and holding their babies without breastfeeding significantly decreased adrenocorticotropic hormone (ACTH), plasma cortisol, and salivary free cortisol (Heinrichs, *et al.*, 2001). Breastfeeding and holding the infant led to significantly decreased anxiety, whereas mood and calmness improved only in the breastfeeding group. In response to an induced stressor, breastfeeding exerted a short-term suppression of the hypothalmic-pituitary-adrenal (HPA) axis response to mental stress. The authors concluded that suckling provided a short-term suppression of the stress-related cortisol response and HPA-axis response to mental stress. They argued that this short-term suppression provided several evolutionary and biological advantages. It isolated the mothers from distracting stimuli; facilitated their immune system; protected the babies from high cortisol in the milk, and prevented stress-related inhibition of lactation.

In a study of lab-induced stress, breastfeeding women had a significantly attenuated stress response (Altemus, *et al.*, 1995). There were 10 breastfeeding and 10 non-breastfeeding women who were all 7 to 18 weeks postpartum. They performed a 20-minute treadmill exercise program at 90% of maximal oxygen capacity in order to measure stress. Plasma ACTH, cortisol, and glucose were significantly lower in the breastfeeding than in the non-breastfeeding mothers. The same was true of basal norepinephrine. However, overall sympathomedullary responses were similar in both groups. Prolactin levels were elevated throughout the exercise condition for breastfeeding women and there was a difference in prolactin levels over time between the groups. Oxytocin levels did not change.

Another study compared stress levels of three groups of women: women who were exclusively breastfeeding (N=84), women who were exclusively formula feeding (N=99), and non-postpartum healthy volunteers (N=33). The researcher found that breastfeeding women had lower perceived stress, depression and anger, and more positive life-events than the controls. Serum prolactin was inversely related to stress and mood in formula-feeding mothers, but this was not true for the breastfeeding mothers (Groer, 2005). More recently, the same researcher and a colleague (Groer and Morgan, 2007) found in a study of 200 women at four to six weeks postpartum, that depressed women were significantly less likely to be breastfeeding and that they had significantly lower serum prolactin levels. The researchers also reported significantly more life stress and anxiety.

Groer and Davis (2006) examined the question of whether breastfeeding protected mothers from the deleterious effects of stress on immunity. They specifically examined levels of interferon-gamma (IFN-γ) and the ratio of IFN-γ/interleukin (IL)-10. They noted that when formula-feeding mothers were exposed to stress, depression, anxiety, anger, and negative life-events, they had decreased IFN-γ and a decreased serum ratio of IFN-γ/IL-10. Breastfeeding mothers were protected from these effects. The researchers' findings suggested that formula-feeding mothers had potentially diminished cellular immunity when they experienced stress.

Breastfeeding's down-regulation of the stress response appears to have long-term effects, and it probably explains another set of recent finding regarding cardiovascular disease (Schwartz, *et al.*, 2009). This study included 139,681 postmenopausal women (Mean age=63 years). The researchers found that women with a lifetime history of breastfeeding for more than 12 months were less likely to have hypertension, diabetes, hyperlipidemia, or cardiovascular disease than women who never breastfed. This was a dose-response relationship: the longer women lactated, the lower their cardiovascular risk. The authors noted that lactation improves glucose tolerance, lipid metabolism and C-reactive protein. Another study found that breastfeeding was related to lower C-reactive protein, another inflammatory marker for cardiovascular and other chronic diseases, in 26-year-old women who participated in the Dunedin Multidisciplinary Health Study (Williams, *et al.*, 2006).

Since stress is related to the onset of depression, Mezzacappa and Endicott (2007) examined the impact of parity and whether it mediated the effect of feeding method on maternal stress. This study compared primiparae who were breast- or bottle-feeding and multiparae who were breast- or bottle-feeding. The authors found that oxytocin was greater in multiparae than in primiparae. Further, breastfeeding had greater stress-reducing effects on multiparae than it did on primiparae. In this study, among the primiparous women, 35% of those bottle feeding and 16% of those breastfeeding were depressed. Among multiparous women, 37% of those bottle feeding and 12% of those breastfeeding were depressed. After controlling for confounding variables, breastfeeding by multiparous women was associated with significantly decreased odds of having depression compared with women who bottle fed. The authors indicated that parity was a critical factor mediating the effect of lactation on depression (Mezzacappa and Endicott, 2007), and suggested that previously contradictory findings be re-examined with this framework in mind.

## Nighttime breastfeeding and maternal mental health

Another issue related to depression and breastfeeding is nighttime feeding. If mothers want to continue breastfeeding, they are frequently told to eliminate nighttime breastfeeding so they can get more sleep. This advice is more and more common in postpartum depression treatment programs and books written for new mothers. But is this good advice? At first glance, it may seem to be. Since breast milk is lower in fat and protein than formula, we might assume that breastfeeding mothers sleep less than their formula-feeding counterparts. However, recent research has revealed the opposite: that breastfeeding mothers actually get more sleep – particularly when the baby was in proximity to the mother.

## Breastfeeding and maternal fatigue

In a study of 33 mothers at four weeks postpartum, Quillin and Glenn (2004) found that mothers who were breastfeeding slept more than mothers who were bottle feeding. Data were collected via a questionnaire that recorded five days of mother's and newborn's sleep. When comparing whether bedsharing made a difference in total sleep, the researchers found that bedsharing, breastfeeding mothers got the most sleep and breastfeeding mothers who were not bedsharing got the least amount of sleep. Mothers who were bottle feeding got the same amount of sleep whether their babies were with them or in another room.

Sleep patterns of 72 couples were compared from pregnancy to the first month postpartum via sleep diaries and wrist actigraphy (Gay, *et al.*, 2004). Most of the mothers were at least partially breastfeeding (94%) and 80% were exclusively breastfeeding. Most of the babies slept in their parents' room and 51% regularly slept in their parents' beds. Sleep and fatigue outcomes were not associated with type of birth, parent-infant bedsharing, or baby's age. Mothers who were exclusively breastfeeding had a greater number of nighttime wakings (30 vs. 24) compared with mothers who were not breastfeeding exclusively. The exclusively breastfeeding mothers slept approximately 20 minutes longer than mothers not exclusively breastfeeding.

A study from France compared fatigue levels in exclusively breastfeeding (N=129) and exclusively formula-feeding mothers (N=114) at two to four days, six and twelve weeks postpartum (Callahan, *et al.*, 2006). The study found no significant difference between the groups at any time point on the measure of maternal fatigue. The authors suggested that all mothers experience postpartum fatigue, independent of feeding method, and informing mothers ahead of time that breastfeeding is not likely to be the cause of their fatigue may help them persist.

In a study of mothers and fathers at three months postpartum, data were collected via wrist actigraphy and using sleep diaries (Doan, *et al.*, 2007). The study compared sleep of exclusively breastfed infants with those supplemented with formula. In this sample, 67% were fed exclusively with breast milk, 23% were fed a combination of breast milk and formula, and 10% were exclusively formula fed. Mothers who exclusively breastfed slept an average of 40 minutes longer than mothers who supplemented. Parents of infants who were breastfed during the night slept an average of 40 to 45 minutes more than parents of infants given formula. Parents of formula-fed infants had more sleep disturbances. The researchers concluded that parents who are supplementing with formula under the assumption that they are going to get more sleep should be encouraged to breastfeed so they will get an extra 30 minutes of sleep per night.

Another sleep study compared 12 exclusively breastfeeding women, 12 age-matched control women, and 7 women who were exclusively bottle feeding (Blyton, *et al.*, 2002). They found that total sleep time and REM sleep time were similar in the three groups of women. The marked difference between the groups was in the amount of slow-wave sleep (SWS). The breastfeeding mothers got an average of 182 minutes of SWS. Women in the control group had an average of 86 minutes. And the exclusively bottle-feeding women had an average of 63 minutes. Among the breastfeeding women, there was a compensatory reduction in light, non-REM sleep.

## Depression and breastfeeding cessation

Depression also has a role in breastfeeding cessation, with depressed mothers being more likely to quit. Forty women (20 depressed, 20 non-depressed) were recruited into a study at 21 weeks' gestation (Field, *et al.*, 2002b). At eight months postpartum, the researchers found that depressed mothers often breastfed less, stopped breastfeeding significantly earlier, and scored lower on the Breastfeeding Confidence Scale than their non-depressed counterparts.

A study of 226 women from Barbados also showed a relationship between breastfeeding and maternal depression (Galler, *et al.*, 2006). This study assessed women's feeding practices and attitudes in the first six months postpartum. Women's belief that breastfeeding was bet-ter than bottle feeding was associated with lower postpartum depression at seven weeks and six months postpartum. Mothers with depressive symptoms were less likely to believe that breastfeeding was better for infants and more likely to believe that breastfeeding was private and restrictive. Even after controlling for maternal feeding attitude, maternal mood at seven weeks was still significantly associated with infant feeding practices at six months.

In a study from England (Bick, *et al.*, 1998), 906 women were interviewed 45 weeks after delivery. In this sample, 63% had breastfed, but 40% of these had stopped within three months. The predictors of early cessation included depression, return to work within three months, and regular childcare from female relatives. A study from Turkey showed similar results (Akman, *et al.*, 2008). In this study, 60 mothers of newborns were enrolled prospectively. Mothers and babies were assessed at one and four months postpartum. The percentage of mothers exclusively breastfeeding was high: 91% at one month and 68% at four months. Mothers with higher EPDS scores at Time 1 were less likely to be breastfeeding at Time 2.

A study from Pakistan produced results that were consistent with those of the other studies (Taj and Sikander, 2003). In this sample were 100 women with breastfeeding-age children ranging from 2 months to 2 years. Thirty-eight percent of these women had stopped breast-feeding, and their average scores on the Urdu version of the Hospital Anxiety and Depression Scale (HADS) were 19.66, compared with 3.27 for the breastfeeding women. Of the women who had stopped breastfeeding, 36.8% reported that their depression had preceded breast-feeding cessation. The authors concluded that maternal depression causes mothers to stop breastfeeding.

In a sample of 209 women from Oklahoma, researchers examined risk factors associated with a score of over 13 on the EPDS (McCoy, *et al.*, 2006). The risk factors they identi-fied included formula feeding (OR=2.04), a history of depression (OR=1.87), and cigarette smoking (OR=1.58). Breastfeeding is associated with a significantly lower occurrence of postpartum depression. Approximately 39% of this sample had an EPDS score indicating pos-sible depression. This high incidence of postpartum depression could be due to the relatively high percentage of low-income women in this sample.

Women were assessed for depression with the EPDS at six and twelve weeks postpartum (N=185) (Hatton, *et al.*, 2005). At six weeks, depressive symptoms were related to lower rates of breastfeeding. This relationship persisted even after controlling for prior history of depression, life stress, and current antidepressant use. There was not a relationship between breastfeeding and depressive symptoms at twelve weeks postpartum. The authors concluded that depressive symptoms in early postpartum may lead to early breastfeeding cessation. They offered several possible explanations for their findings including that depressed women may not have initiated breastfeeding, or that perhaps early depression impacted milk production or let-down. They also noted that stressful life events can have a negative impact on breastfeed-ing, and are also predisposing factors for postpartum depression.

A study from Canada had similar results (Dennis and McQueen, 2007). This sample included 594 community women who were surveyed at one, four, and eight weeks postpar-tum. The women were surveyed about their feeding method and depressive symptoms on the EPDS. The researchers found no relationship between maternal mental health and feeding at one week postpartum. However, mothers with an EPDS score of 12 or greater at one week postpartum were significantly less likely to be breastfeeding at four and eight weeks. They were also more likely to have been unsatisfied with their infant feeding method; to have expe-rienced serious breastfeeding problems, and to have reported lower levels of breastfeeding self-efficacy. Mothers who thought breastfeeding was progressing terribly at Week 1 were more likely to develop depressive symptoms. But when depression was removed from this analysis, the effects disappeared. The authors felt these findings reflected depressed mothers' moods and cognitions rather than objective problems. They concluded that early identification of mothers with depressive symptoms can both halt morbidity associated with depression and increase breastfeeding duration.

Postpartum anxiety can also impact breastfeeding initiation and duration (Britton, 2007). In a study of mothers at discharge and one month postpartum, predischarge anxiety was inversely related to breastfeeding confidence. Mothers who were high in post-discharge anxiety were less likely to be fully or exclusively breastfeeding and were more likely to have stopped breastfeeding at one month.

A study of 852 pregnant women in Brazil (Rondo and Souza, 2007) found that distress and worry about breastfeeding, concern about body changes, and work outside the home were negatively related to intention to breastfeed. However, depression and anxiety scores were not related to intention to breastfeed.

One hundred twenty-two depressed women described their breastfeeding experiences (McCarter-Spaulding and Horowitz, 2007). The researchers collected data during three home visits. They noted that in this sample, severity of depression was not related to breastfeeding, but older maternal age, living with a partner, and higher income were. Maternal education was the most important predictor of exclusive breastfeeding and combination feeding. Depression was most severe at the four- to six-week assessment, dropping off after that. By 14 to 18 weeks postpartum, 78% had EPDS scores below the cut-off. All of the women were encouraged to seek outside care for their depression, but only 11% to 12% had gone to psychotherapy, and 3% to 6% had used medications. In terms of breastfeeding patterns, by 14 to 18 weeks, exclusive breastfeeding had dropped from 34% to 22%. At 14 to 18 weeks, 33% were using a combination of feeding methods and 45% were exclusively formula feeding. McCarter-Spaulding and Horowitz (2007) noted that their findings of high rates of breastfeeding, despite severity of the mothers' postpartum depressive symptoms, are consistent with previous research that suggests a link between depression and early weaning. What depression seemed to affect was exclusive breastfeeding, which was lower than in the larger sample from which the respondents were drawn.

In a qualitative review of 49 articles that specifically examined the link between depression and breastfeeding, Dennis and McQueen (2009) found that depressive symptoms in early postpartum may be related to decreased breastfeeding duration, increased breastfeeding difficulties, and decreased levels of breastfeeding self-efficacy. Further, depressed women may be less likely to initiate breastfeeding and to breastfeed exclusively. Mothers with depressive symptoms were more likely to discontinue breastfeeding earlier than non-depressed mothers. Depressive symptomatology was related to lower breastfeeding self-efficacy, demonstrating that depressed mothers were less confident in their ability to breastfeed.

## Implications

1   Since depression is a major risk factor for breastfeeding cessation, lactation specialists should screen for it.
2   Maternal stress and fatigue reduce prolactin levels and may lead to breastfeeding cessation. High levels of cortisol can delay lactogenesis II.
3   Breastfeeding difficulties, especially nipple pain, can lead to depression and need to be addressed promptly (see Chapter 5).
4   Breastfeeding mothers actually get more sleep than their formula-feeding counterparts.

When mothers try supplementing with formula at night to get more sleep, they may encounter the opposite effect.

5 Depressed mothers should be encouraged to continue breastfeeding since it protects infants from the harmful effects of maternal depression (see Chapter 7).

Regarding the role of healthcare providers caring for women who are breastfeeding and depressed, McCarter-Spaulding and Horowitz (2007:10) noted the following.

Nurses caring for women who are at risk or struggling with PPD also may feel that breastfeeding is perhaps an unnecessary burden that should be discontinued.

Although nurses might expect that mothers with depression may not want to continue or may not be able to maintain breastfeeding, such assumptions may not be accurate.

# 4   Assessment of postpartum depression

Postpartum depression is often suffered privately. Because clinicians identify fewer than half of the women with this mood disorder, routine, periodic screening for one year after delivery is imperative.

(Beck, 2006: 47)

Healthcare providers often fail to detect depression in new mothers because they are not familiar with it or do not know what to look for. In addition, mothers themselves may hide their depression (Beck, 2006). In a study of 1,102 new mothers (MacLennan, *et al.*, 1996), only 49% of women with serious depression sought help for it. In another study, almost half of the depressed mothers were not identified by healthcare providers. These mothers made an average of 14 healthcare visits each (Hearn, *et al.*, 1998).

Because of depression's serious consequences, screening for it is necessary; depression is much more common than conditions that occur during pregnancy that are routinely screened for (Beck, 2006). For example, in one recent study, 15% of women had depressive symptoms. In contrast, 2.4% had gestational diabetes, 5.5% had pregnancy-associated hypertension, and 10% had a preterm birth (McGarry, *et al.*, 2009).

## Challenges to assessing postpartum depression

One reason that postpartum depression is often missed is that mothers do not tend to seek care for it, and may, in fact, actively conceal it (Beck and Gable, 2001a). An analysis of data from 1,970 patients from the Utah PRAMS study indicated that 60% of women with depressive symptoms did not seek help (McGarry, *et al.*, 2009). A review of 40 studies (Dennis and Chung-Lee, 2006) indicated that women's inability to disclose their feelings was a common help-seeking barrier. The authors noted that women did not proactively seek help, and this was often reinforced by family members and health professionals. Other women viewed depression as a matter of course in becoming a mother. Mothers also feared losing their babies. Still others did not want to bear the stigma and shame of depression. Another barrier was when care providers offered medications as the only treatment alternative. The combination of a lack of knowledge of postpartum depression and the acceptance of myths regarding depression were significant barriers to seeking help.

In a qualitative study of 18 women's barriers to seeking care, Sword and colleagues (2008) examined individual-, social network-, and health system-related factors that facilitated or hindered care seeking. The women were eight weeks postpartum when the data were collected. Among the hindering factors were women's beliefs that depressive symptoms were just a normal part of motherhood. In addition, their limited understanding of postpartum depression, waiting for symptom improvement, discomfort discussing mental health concerns, and fears of being judged or having their children taken away were also barriers to care.

Factors that facilitated care seeking included being aware that they were depressed and not feeling like themselves. Friends, family, and healthcare providers sometimes hindered care because they also normalized or failed to understand symptoms. Some barriers in the health-care system included healthcare providers telling mothers that their symptoms were normal, or offering women treatments that they found unacceptable. Care seeking was facilitated by supportive relationships, outreach and follow-up, legitimization of postpartum depression, and timeliness of care (Sword, *et al.*, 2008).

In a survey of 94 mental health providers in Rochester, New York, Springate and Chaudron (2006) found that 80% were not experienced with perinatal mood disorders. These clinicians offered several types of psychotherapy including interpersonal (90%), supportive (86%), and cognitive-behavioral (76%). Only 16% offered direct medication management. While most providers accepted private insurance, only a small percentage took government insurance (e.g. only 12% accepted Medicaid). The authors indicated that their findings highlighted several barriers for women receiving perinatal mental health care, such as limited access to care for women on government insurance and a long waiting period to see a psychiatrist.

## Use of healthcare services

One possible indication of maternal depression is increased use of healthcare services. In an Australian study (Webster, *et al.*, 2001), depressed mothers made more visits to pediatricians or their primary care providers. They were also significantly more likely to visit a psychiatrist or social worker, to seek the assistance from a postpartum depression support group, and to contact the Nursing Mothers' Association of Australia, and significantly less satisfied with those services than were non-depressed mothers. The depressed women felt that their providers did not listen, and that they received poor-quality information. Webster and colleagues (2001) speculated that the mothers could be unhappy because the real reason for their visit (i.e. depression) was not identified. They also found that women rarely raised the issue of depression themselves, but provided "hints" to their providers about the way they were feeling. The authors recommended the use of screening questions to help identify mothers with depression.

A Canadian study also found higher rates of healthcare utilization among women with postpartum depression (Dennis, 2004a). A cohort of 594 women in British Columbia completed questionnaires at one, four, and eight weeks postpartum. At four weeks, women with depressive symptoms had a higher number of contacts with family practice physicians and public health nurses, and were twice as likely to be classified as a high-utilizer of healthcare services at both four and eight weeks. In addition, depressed women were more likely to perceive their health as poor. The author emphasized the importance of family care physicians in the identification and treatment of new mothers and recommended that women with high-utilization patterns should be screened for possible depression.

Another large study of women at three to eight weeks postpartum (N=7,794), found that healthcare use predicted depression. Mothers were significantly more likely to be depressed if their infants had more than one problem-oriented visit to the infant's primary provider, or if they made even one visit to the emergency department. The number of problem-oriented visits in the first month was positively associated with increased rates of depressive symptoms. This was also true in months two through five, but the relationship was weaker. Well-child visits were not associated with maternal depression (Mandl, *et al.*, 1999). The authors speculated on possible reasons for their findings. They felt that depression may color a mother's perceptions of the wellness of her infant. Mothers may also seek care for their infant as an indirect way to get care for themselves. Seeing a primary provider may seem less stigmatizing than seeking help for depression. Conversely, mothers may be depressed because their infants are actually ill. Care providers must be careful not to attribute all of a mother's concerns regarding their infants to depression.

Increased use of healthcare services come at a substantial cost. In the Ontario Mother and Infant Survey (Roberts, *et al.*, 2001), mothers who were depressed and mothers who made less than $20,000 per year had the highest healthcare costs. The total health and social service costs were almost double for both groups (calculated separately) compared with the rest of the sample. Other variables that predicted higher healthcare costs included mothers' perception of their own health as poor, perception of inadequate help and support at home, and a postpartum hospital stay of less than 48 hours.

Not every study has found an increase in healthcare utilization among depressed mothers. A study of 665 Canadian mothers of infants aged 2 to 12 months found no increase in the use of any type of healthcare services for mothers with either depression or anxiety (Anderson, *et al.*, 2008). The main outcome variable was use of services over a six-month period, including visits to the primary care provider, Emergency Department, and walk-in clinics for the baby. Anderson and colleagues (2008) identified that 11% of the women had postpartum depressive symptoms and 8.8% had postpartum anxiety.

## Screening for depression

As indicated above, women may provide hints that they are depressed. But active screening is much more likely to identify mothers who are depressed. One way to screen is to ask mothers if they have any of the known risk factors for depression. In an Australian study, 2,118 women were screened during pregnancy (Webster, *et al.*, 2000a). Of these women, 33% had one or more risk factors for depression during pregnancy. At four months, 26% of women with one or more risk factors were depressed, compared with only 11% of women with no risk factors. The risk of depression increased with the number of risk factors. Forty-eight percent of the women with five risk factors were depressed. The authors felt they could have improved predictions by adding questions about infant behavior, severe blues, and a history of childhood abuse. They acknowledged that many of the women in their local postpartum support group were sexual abuse survivors, and adding this variable, in particular, would have improved detection rates.

Another study found that depression at week one postpartum predicted depression at four and eight weeks (Dennis, 2004b). This study included 594 women from British Columbia. Using an EPDS cut-off score of greater than 9, Dennis found a rate of 29.5% of depressive symptoms at Week 1, and rates of 23% and 20.5% at four and eight weeks, respectively. Mothers with a score greater than 9 at Week 1 were 30.3 times more likely at four weeks and 19.1 times more likely at eight weeks to have postpartum symptoms.

Non-response can also indicate depression. In a study of obsessive-compulsive disorder during pregnancy, George and Elliot (2004) made a surprise discovery. They found that failure to respond to the antenatal questionnaire predicted higher rates of depression postpartum than the screening questionnaire itself. They concluded that non-response to a questionnaire conveys as much information as actually completing one, and urged clinicians to follow up on non-response.

### Screening in obstetric settings

Morris-Rush and Bernstein (2002) indicated that screening for depression during the postpartum visit is often helpful and is standard of care. In a survey and chart-review study, obstetric providers charted EPDS score in 39% of the visits and counseled their patients in 35% of the visits (Delatte, *et al.*, 2009). All respondents to the survey of 47 providers agreed that they are responsible for screening for depression and 94% were confident that they could diagnose it. Far fewer were actually doing it. There was a significant difference in referral rates depending on the provider type. Residents had the lowest rates (17%), followed by attendings (42%), certified nurse midwives (67%) and nurse practitioners (94%). This study was designed to evaluate the effectiveness of a policy of universal screening at a local medical center. The researchers noted that their results highlight the gap between what providers know should be done and what is actually being done at postpartum visits.

### Screening in pediatric settings

Because of the high number of visits to the pediatrician during the first year postpartum, pediatric visits are considered by many to be the perfect setting to screen for maternal depression (Currie and Rademacher, 2004; Heneghan, *et al.*, 2007). Pediatricians should use a screening tool to assess depression rather than relying on their observation alone as observation misses a substantial number of cases. Currie and Rademacher (2004) consider screening, making referrals, providing a list of resources to mothers, and encouraging them to see their own doctors to be well within the pediatricians' scope of practice. But how effective is it to screen for depression in pediatric settings?

A study of screening in well-baby clinics included 96 mothers at eight weeks postpartum in Arizona (Freeman, *et al.*, 2005). Of the mothers screened, 14.6% had a score of 12 or greater on the EPDS. Higher scores were associated with smoking and a family history of psychiatric disorders or substance abuse. Interestingly, a number of factors that are traditional risk factors for postpartum depression did not predict depression. These included mother's age and ethnicity, marital status, employment, lifestyle habits, medical complications during pregnancy, labor or delivery, reproductive history, and perceived help with the baby. The sample included a high percentage of Hispanic women. Freeman and colleagues (2005) noted that pediatricians are in an ideal and unique position to improve detection of PPD. Depressed mothers, particularly those with severe depression, may neglect self-care and so may not go to the doctor's for themselves. Therefore, screening in a pediatric setting is even more important. The authors noted that screening appeared feasible and was relatively well accepted by participants.

Similarly, Heneghan and colleagues (2007) noted that pediatricians see infants approximately seven times in the first year for well-baby checks, making it quite feasible to identify maternal depression. They surveyed 662 pediatricians with the goal of exploring which characteristics of pediatricians are associated with identification and management of maternal depression. They found that 77% reported that they had "ever" identified maternal depression, and 82% of these referred the mother to services. The authors found that the following characteristics were associated with routinely identifying depression: practicing in the Midwest; using more than one method to address maternal depression; working in a practice that provides child mental health services; thinking that maternal mental health has a substantial impact on child health, and having attitudes that inclined the pediatricians to identify and manage maternal depression.

Pediatricians' attitudes about maternal depression were also measured in another study (Park, *et al.*, 2007). In a survey of 651 practicing, non-trainee pediatricians, the authors used an exploratory principal components analysis to examine interrelationships among attitudinal measures. The analysis indicated three subscales: acknowledging maternal depression (confidence in their ability to identify and treat depression; belief that advice from a pediatrician is the best way to help mothers seek treatment for depression); perception of mothers' beliefs (that mothers don't want pediatricians to investigate their depression; mothers are fearful of losing their children if they disclose depression; pediatricians feel that they are invading mothers' privacy); and treating maternal depression (confident to treat maternal depression with medications or brief counseling; pediatricians can be effective in treating maternal depression; mothers want pediatricians to treat their depression). The authors felt that one possible target for future education efforts was use of screening instruments to identify depression as only about 25% of those surveyed felt confident in their ability to identify depression. Most relied on observation, rather than using screening instruments, which tends to result in lower rates of detection.

A study in Turkey screened for depression at well-child visits (Orhon, *et al.*, 2007). The researchers found that 34% of mothers were in the clinical range on the EPDS. Eighty percent of these mothers were identified at the one-month visit. Mothers with depressive symptoms were more likely to have more negative perceptions of their infants and to report more fussing, crying, sleep and temperament problems. When the depression was treated, these symptoms improved, especially poor quality of mothers' sleep, infant cry-fuss problems, and mothers' perceptions of infant temperament. But there was a 59% dropout rate for treatment. Maternal depression was associated with mothers' report of infant sleep problems and their own poor or inadequate sleep. Interestingly, depressed mothers were more likely to complain of insufficient milk supply during the first two months, but infant feeding pattern was not associated with depressive symptoms. Further, the rate of breastfeeding initiation was 100%, with high continuation rates among the depressed mothers.

Head and colleagues (2008) also found that pediatricians were in an ideal position to detect maternal depression. They surveyed 1,600 members of the American Academy of Pediatrics regarding knowledge of perceived barriers to addressing maternal depression. The pediatricians they surveyed fell into three groups: those in practice for five or more years; those in practice less than five years, and pediatric residents. Residents were more likely to have attended a course on maternal depression in the past two years than the other two groups; although only approximately 20% had done so. The researchers found that those in practice five or more years reported more barriers to addressing maternal depression than pediatric residents. Some of these barriers included lack of training in adult mental health and lack of interest in maternal depression. However, even with residency reforms, 81% of current residents reported no training in adult mental health issues. The authors concluded that education for pediatricians during their residency appears to be helpful when it is present. But a large percentage still haven't had training on the topic.

An earlier study by Tam, *et al.* (2002) indicated that screening may be problematic in well-baby settings. In this study, the researchers screened women via telephone. The women were then asked to pick up packets that contained depression assessment screening scales. Out of 160 packets distributed, only seven were completed. The author concluded that there was reluctance to participate in the study. Five of these women were in the clinical range. All refused to participate in phase 2 of the study, a clinical interview, but they all accepted referrals to a psychiatrist. Provider barriers included lack of confidence in their ability to handle the situation if a mother cried or had suicidal thoughts. They indicated that it would be like "opening Pandora's box," and reiterated the belief that pediatricians were the ideal professionals to screen for depression and recommended finding a way to screen in a non-threatening way. They also suggested offering a range of treatment options for patients.

With this in mind, Wisner, *et al.* (2008) described a Web-based education program for physicians and other primary healthcare providers as these providers have the most ongoing contact with postpartum women – the URL for the website is: http://www.MedEdPPD.com. This site was designed to provide tools: CME modules; current literature and classic papers; a comprehensive slide library, and other resources. As at March, 2008, the site had had 17,000 unique visitors. Nurses made up the largest percentage (34%) of these visitors, followed by mothers (27%) and social workers (18%). Clinical psychologists (7%) and physicians (5%) were still represented in small numbers. Wisner and colleagues (2008) concluded that the site provides numerous training opportunities and is flexible, cost-effective, and meets the needs of healthcare providers.

## Assessment scales

Fortunately, there are screening scales for depression, including two designed specifically for postpartum women. These are described below.

### *Patient Health Questionnaire-2 (PHQ-2)*

The Two-item Patient Health Questionnaire (PHQ-2) is a reliable initial health screening that can be used in all healthcare settings. The PHQ-2 includes the following two questions, and assesses frequency of anhedonia (little interest or pleasure in doing things) and depressed mood (feeling down, depressed, or hopeless) during the past two weeks.

> Over the past two weeks, how often have you been bothered by any of the following problems?

- little interest or pleasure in doing things;
- feeling down, depressed, or hopeless.

The response categories include "Not at All," "Several Days," "More than Half the Days," and "Nearly Every Day" and are scored from 0 to 3. The higher the number, the higher the risk of depression.

A study examined the accuracy of the Patient Health Questionnaire-2 (PHQ-2) particularly for identifying depression in low-income women (Cutler, *et al.*, 2007). Ninety-four women participated in this study from an inner-city well-child clinic. The children ranged in age from 3 days to 5 years. The agreement between the PHQ-2 and EPDS was moderate. The sensitivity of the PHQ-2 was 43.5% and specificity 92.7%. The sensitivity was higher for mothers with higher levels of education. The authors concluded that the PHQ-2 is not an effective screen in the case of low-income, ethnically diverse women.

The PHQ-2 is designed to screen for depression in general, and can be used as a quick screen. But results are likely to be more accurate with one of the two measures designed specifically for new mothers.

### The Edinburgh Postnatal Depression Scale (EPDS)

The Edinburgh Postnatal Depression Scale (EPDS) is the most commonly used screening tool for postpartum depression in the world. The EPDS is a 10-item self-report questionnaire that can be completed in five minutes (Cox, *et al.*, 1987). It was designed to give primary-care providers and other healthcare workers a simple tool for screening in the postpartum period.

Women are asked to report how they have felt in the past week, and the items are scored from 0 to 3. The standard cut-off is 12, but higher and lower cut-offs have been used. EPDS has been used in numerous research studies, in populations all over the world, and it is available free of charge. The authors have granted use of their questionnaire without charge or the need to request permission, as long as the source of the scale is listed, and the copyright is respected. A summary of some of the studies that have used the EPDS is given in Table 4.1.

*Scale cut-offs*

The cut-off used on the EPDS can vary depending on its purpose and whether it is used for broad screening, or more specifically to identify only women with more serious depressions. Dennis (2004b) used 9 or higher as the cut-off for depressive symptomatology, which increases the scale's sensitivity and makes it more appropriate for community screening (Dennis, 2004b). She argued that a lower cut-off has higher sensitivity and leads to fewer false negatives. In contrast, a higher cut-off has more specificity, but might miss some depressed women. In her sample of 594 women, a cut-off of 12/13 at Week 1 failed to detect depression in 42.9% of mothers at four weeks and 53% of mothers with depression at eight weeks.

Moses-Kolko and Roth (2004) make the following recommendations regarding scores on the EPDS. If a woman scores above 9, she is likely to be depressed and they recommend a full psychiatric evaluation. This evaluation includes assessment of whether she is thinking of harming herself or her baby. The full assessment includes psychiatric history of herself and her family members; gravid history; psychosocial history; routine lab results (including thyroid-stimulating hormone), and screening for bipolar disorder. If symptoms have persisted for more than two weeks, she should be referred for treatment that can include psychotherapy, support, and possibly medications. If a woman scores between 5 and 9 on the EPDS, she may be at risk for depression within the next 6 to 12 months. Clinicians can give women copies of the EPDS and instruct them to seek care if they score above 9. If the mother indicates that she intends harm to herself or her baby, she should be seen immediately (Moses-Kolko and Roth, 2005). A woman with a EPDS score lower than 5 is unlikely to be depressed and needs no further follow-up.

*Advantages and disadvantages of the EPDS*

The EPDS offers a number of advantages. It is easy to complete and score. Mothers can answer all the questions in a few minutes. It is specifically written for new mothers. Indeed, it was because of the limitations of the more generic depression measures that the EPDS was developed.

Although widely used, there are some disadvantages to the EPDS. The scale is written in British rather than in American English. American mothers sometimes find the wording of some the questions confusing, or a little odd. Lappin (2001) cautions that the EPDS is designed to be used in the early postpartum period, and has only been validated for that use. It should

*Table 4.1* Studies using the Edinburgh Postnatal Depression Scale (EPDS)

| Study population | Authors | Conclusions |
| --- | --- | --- |
| 101 low-income, rural women in Ethiopia | Hanlon, *et al.*, 2008 | EPDS had poor validity. It was poorly understood, showed inadequate discrimination between cases and non-cases, and had unacceptably low internal consistency. Items 1 to 3 frequently had to be repeated and items 4, 5, and 9 were often misunderstood. |
| 48 Bangladeshi women (EPDS translated to Syhleti/Bengali) | Fuggle, *et al.*, 2002 | The EPDS worked well with this sample. Some difficulty translating item 1. Compared results with the General Health Questionnaire. |
| 88 Japanese mothers (assessed early postpartum disturbance) | Yamashita, *et al.*, 2000 | Compared EPDS with other instruments. EPDS identified all depressed mothers at one month postpartum. |
| 892 women from 9 countries (U.S., Guyana, Italy, Sweden, Finland, Korea, Taiwan, India, and Australia) | Affonso, *et al.*, 2000 | Moderate concordance between Beck Depression Inventory and EPDS. Authors concluded that both are useful for screening and assessment. Also useful with a diverse, international population. |
| 100 Nepalese women, two to three months postpartum; 40 control women | Regmi, *et al.*, 2002 | EPDS is a reliable and easy-to-use tool for PPD screening. |
| 145 Chinese women at six weeks postpartum | Lee, *et al.*, 2000 | Compared EPDS and General Health Questionnaire. Substantial improvement in screening when both instruments are used instead of using either form alone. |
| Low-income American sample (two conditions: 35 routine clinical evaluation, 37 using EPDS) | Fergerson, *et al.*, 2002 | The EPDS was significantly better than routine evaluations for identifying depression; 30% in EPDS group identified as "at risk" for depression; 0% in the clinical assessment group. |
| 208 fathers (EPDS scores compared with those of Diagnostic Interview Schedule) | Matthey, *et al.*, 2001 | Authors conclude that the EPDS is a reliable and valid measure of depression and anxiety in mothers, but should have a cut-off 2 points lower for fathers than for mothers. |
| 134 women at six weeks postpartum; 199 women at three months postpartum (EPDS and Present State Examination) | Leverton and Elliott, 2000 | With a cut-off of 12/13, EPDS sensitivity=70%; specificity=93%. With a cut-off of 9/10, sensitivity=90%; specificity=84%. Home visitor description of women as depressed or "fed up" at six weeks was a better predictor than EPDS. |
| 56 Norwegian women at six weeks postpartum | Eberhard-Gran, *et al.*, 2001 | Cut-off ≥10 identified all women with major depression (100% sensitivity, 87% specificity), but wide confidence intervals. Authors concluded that EPDS is a valid screening instrument for postpartum depression. |
| 224 low-income Canadian mothers (22nd and 35th days postpartum) | Des Rivières-Pigeon, *et al.*, 2000 | Used a confirmatory factor analysis. Good construct validity for EPDS. Cronbach α=.82 |

not be used for screening for depression in pregnancy, or to diagnose depression beyond the postpartum period. However, it is often used in both of these situations. Lappin (2001) also cautions against interpreting one- to two-point differences as indicating increased severity. This instrument performs best in predicting depression if the cut-off is 12 points. Similarly, Elliot and Leverton (2000) note that the EPDS is a reliable and valid screening tool, but that it has been misused. They emphasize the importance of ongoing training and quality control to ensure that it is used properly.

Another caution comes from Guedeney and colleagues (2000). They provided a case report of three false negatives on the EPDS with women with major depressive disorder (according to the Research Diagnostic Criteria). They noted that the EPDS seems better able to identify depressed postpartum women with anhedonic and anxious symptoms than depressed women with psychomotor retardation.

### Variations of the EPDS with better predictability

A sample of 299 women completed the EPDS at two to three days and four to six weeks postpartum (Chabrol and Teissedre, 2004). The authors used exploratory factor analysis to predict EPDS scores at four to six weeks. The three factors they extracted were anxiety, depressive mood, and anhedonia. Of these, anxiety was the main predictor of higher EPDS scores at four to six weeks. It was the only significant predictor of postpartum depression. The items included under anxiety were self-blame (item 3), anxiety (item 4), scare or panic (item 5), inability to cope (item 6), and difficulty in sleeping (item 7).

Another study specifically used three items of the EPDS, the anxiety subscale, and compared them with the accuracy of the full 10-item scale and the ultrabrief 2-item screener (Kabir, *et al.*, 2008). Their sample was 199 participants aged 14 to 26 years, in a adolescent-oriented maternity program. A total of 21% of the mothers met the criteria for depression (EPDS greater than 10). Of the scales that were compared, the EPDS-3 had the best performance, with a sensitivity of 95% and a negative predictive value at 98%. It identified 16% more mothers as depressed than the full EPDS did. The EPDS 2-item scale was markedly inferior and did not identify mothers who were depressed as well. The 3-item screener included the following questions:

- I have blamed myself unnecessarily when things went wrong;
- I have felt scared and panicky for no very good reason;
- I have been anxious or worried for no good reason.

In contrast, the 2-item screen resembles the PHQ-2 and was much less effective, with a sensitivity of 48% and a negative predictive value of 80%. The two items were:

- I have looked forward with enjoyment to things;
- I have felt sad or miserable.

Kabir and colleagues (2008) suggested that the EPDS-3 is brief enough to be incorporated into well-baby checks and that it identified a higher percentage of women as possibly depressed than the full EPDS.

## The Postpartum Depression Screening Scale

Another tool designed specifically for new mothers is the Postpartum Depression Screening Scale (PDSS). The PDSS is a 35-item Likert-scale self-report instrument. It measures functioning on seven dimensions: sleeping/eating disturbances, anxiety/insecurity, emotional lability, cognitive impairment, loss of self, guilt/shame, and contemplating harming oneself. It takes 5 to 10 minutes to complete, and is available for a small fee from Western Psychological Services (http://www.wpspublish.com).

Like the EPDS, the PDSS is useful for screening mothers for depression. In addition, the subscales can provide information for clinicians in treating mothers by highlighting specific areas of difficulty. In developing this scale, Beck and Gable (2000) attempted to address the limitations of the EPDS. For example, they noted that the EPDS did not measure postpartum feelings, such as loss of control, loneliness, irritability, fear of going crazy, obsessive thinking, concentration difficulty, and loss of self. In a study of 525 new mothers, confirmatory factor analysis supported the seven dimensions of the PDSS. The internal consistencies on the seven dimensions ranged from 0.83 (sleeping/eating disturbances) to 0.94 (loss of self). A panel of experts also established the content validity of the scale, and item-response theory techniques provided further construct validity (Beck and Gable, 2000).

In another study (Beck and Gable, 2001a, 2001b), 150 mothers who were 12 weeks postpartum completed the PDSS, EPDS and the Beck Depression Inventory-II (BDI-II). Following completion of these questionnaires, each woman was interviewed by a nurse/psychotherapist using the Structural Clinical Interview for DSM-IV Axis I disorders. The results of the PDSS correlated with the EPDS ($r=0.79$) and the BDI-II ($r=0.81$). The authors then performed a hierarchical regression to ascertain the level of variance that the PDSS accounted for above and beyond the other two measures. The results indicated that the PDSS accounted for an additional 9% of the variance in the diagnosis of depression. A cut-off score of 80 for major depression has a sensitivity of 94% and a specificity of 98%. A cut-off of 60 can be used for both major and minor depression, and has a sensitivity of 91%, and a specificity of 72%. The PDSS was superior in this sample in identifying major depression partly because it included items on sleep and cognitive impairment (Beck and Gable, 2001b).

## Additional factors to assess

Once you have determined that a mother is depressed, you must make some additional assessments to help guide her to the right level of help and support. These additional factors include the severity of the current episode, and whether she is abusing substances, at risk for suicide, or requires hospitalization.

### Severity of current episode

If a mother is depressed, the severity of her depression must be evaluated. In attempting to evaluate severity of the current episode, there are three factors to consider: duration of symptoms, intensity of symptoms, and level of impairment. Symptoms must be present for two weeks for a diagnosis of major depression. Intensity of the symptoms and level of impairment can also indicate whether aggressive treatment is warranted. Indications of severe impairment can include when patients suddenly stop paying attention to personal grooming, cannot manage their households, or have days when they cannot get out of bed.

### Assessing active substance abuse

Another consideration is whether patients are actively abusing alcohol or drugs. Substance abuse can be co-morbid with depression or PTSD. Since active substance abuse complicates treatment for depression, if it is detected, patients should be referred to a substance-abuse treatment program. Below are some screening questions for possible substance abuse (Institute for Clinical Systems Improvement, 2000).

Have you ever:

- felt you ought to cut down on your drinking or drug use?
- had people annoy you by criticizing your drinking or drug use?
- felt bad or guilty about your drinking or drug use?
- had a drink or used drugs first thing in the morning to steady your nerves, get rid of a hangover or to get the day started?

If a patient says "yes" to two or more of these questions, make a referral to a substance abuse program for further evaluation.

### Assessing suicide risk

Suicide risk is always an important consideration when working with depressed mothers. Although it is rare, the consequences are so serious that it is useful to screen all mothers who are depressed. The Institute for Clinical Systems Improvement (2000) lists some specific signs that may indicate increased suicide risk. These are listed below. Even with these signs, it is still difficult to predict suicide. Be sure to chart your assessment of suicide risk. The risk factors are as follows:

1   previous history of suicide attempts
2   suicidal ideation, particularly with specific suicide plans
3   substance abuse or dependency
4   personality disorder
5   family history of suicide
6   single marital status
7   recent death of a loved one
8   recent divorce or separation
9   insomnia
10   panic attacks
11   diminished concentration
12   severe anhedonia or hopelessness.

Even if only one of these risk factors is present, this may call for a more specialized consult. According to Remick (2002), detailed suicide plans, social isolation, previous suicide attempts, substance abuse, and a family history of suicide all increase risk. These patients should be closely monitored through frequent visits, encouraging the mother to reside with family or friends, or by being hospitalized. Contact your local suicide-prevention hotline for information about how best to proceed and for referrals of people who can help.

### Assessing the need for psychiatric hospitalization

Finally, hospitalization may be necessary when severe symptoms are present. Particularly troubling are signs that mothers plan to harm themselves or their babies. When making a decision about whether psychiatric hospitalization is necessary, there are a few considerations (Institute for Clinical Systems Improvement, 2000).

- Does the patient have suicidal thoughts or plans?
- Do you fear for the patient's safety?
- Does the patient have plans to assault or kill another person, including the baby?
- Is there psychotic thinking?
- Has the patient lost the ability to care for him- or herself?

Hospitalization can be voluntary or involuntary. If at all possible, try to find a hospital where mothers are allowed to have their babies stay with them. Some hospitals have mother/baby units that are designed with the needs of postpartum women in mind. Failing that, try to find a situation were mothers can see their babies frequently.

If mothers are hospitalized while still breastfeeding and they want to continue, try to make arrangements to protect their milk supply, or to help them wean gradually as sudden weaning increases their risk of infection. These mothers need access to a hospital-grade electric pump. For mothers who chose to continue breastfeeding, a regular schedule of pumping can ensure that their milk supply is maintained. It also gives mothers a vision of life beyond the hospital.

## Conclusion

Mothers are often not forthcoming about their depression. They may not even realize that they are depressed. But they often know that *something* is wrong, which may prompt them to seek health care – often for themselves and for their babies.

You can screen for depression by using some general questions about their level of fatigue and stress. You can also use one of the screening measures designed specifically for new mothers. Screening can also help you determine whether a mother is suicidal, needs to be hospitalized, or needs a referral for other assistance.

Once depression has been identified, mothers need to be treated. There are a wide range of treatments available for depressed new mothers. These are described in Chapters 9 through 13.

# Part II

# Causes

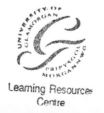

# 5 The psychoneuroimmunology of postpartum depression

Some of the most exciting developments in postpartum depression research comes from the field of psychoneuroimmunology (PNI). PNI research examines the role of the immune system in stress and depression. Of particular interest is the role of proinflammatory cytokines in the etiology of depression (Corwin and Pajer, 2008; Kendall-Tackett, 2007). Proinflammatory cytokines are messenger molecules of the immune system. They have the adaptive function of healing wounds and protecting us from infection. But when they are systemic and chronically elevated, they increase the risk of depression and a number of serious diseases.

Maes and colleagues (2000) were the first to document that women with postpartum depression and anxiety had elevated levels of proinflammatory cytokines. When describing the relationship between depression and inflammation over a decade ago, Maes and Smith (1998) noted that there are a number of plausible explanations for why inflammation might increase the risk for depression. First, when inflammation levels are high, people experience classic symptoms of depression, such as fatigue, lethargy, and social withdrawal. Researchers discovered this connection when using inflammatory cytokines as treatments for conditions such as cancer or hepatitis. When patients are treated with cytokines, depression increases in a predictable and dose-response way: the greater the dosage of cytokines, the more depressed the patients (Konsman, et al., 2002). Second, inflammation activates the hypothalamic-pituitary-adrenal (HPA) axis, dysregulating levels of cortisol. Cortisol generally keeps inflammation in check. However, depression dysregulates cortisol and fails to restrain the inflammatory response (Dhabhar and McEwen, 2001). Finally, inflammation decreases serotonin by lowering levels of its precursor, tryptophan.

To further understand the role of inflammation in depression, it's helpful to first review the human stress response – the normal physiologic response to a perceived threat. Inflammation is part of the three-part stress response.

## How humans respond to a perceived threat

When faced with a threat, human bodies have a number of interdependent mechanisms designed to preserve our lives. This physiologic response is the same for both physical and psychological threats.

The sympathetic nervous system responds first by releasing catecholamines (norepinephrine, epinephrine, and dopamine). This is the fight-or-flight response, and it occurs instantly.

The HPA-axis also responds to threat with a cascade of stress hormones within 20 to 30 minutes after threat exposure. The hypothalamus releases corticotropin-releasing hormone (CRH), which causes the pituitary to release adrenocorticotropin hormone (ACTH), which causes the adrenal cortex to release cortisol, a glucocorticoid. The HPA-axis has far-reaching effects on immunity, metabolism, and reproduction. This system returns to baseline a few hours after stress exposure. If stress continues, however, it becomes dysregulated, and patterns of either hyperactivity or hypoactivity appear (Corwin and Pajer, 2008).

The regulation of the HPA-axis changes markedly during pregnancy. CRH is also produced by the placenta during pregnancy, and not solely by the hypothalamus as it is in a non-pregnant state. Cortisol stimulates CRH in the placenta rather than downregulating it, as it does when it originates in the hypothalamus. One recent study found that elevated corticotropin-releasing hormone in pregnancy is a strong predictor of postpartum depression (Yim, *et al.*, 2009). In this study, serum samples from 100 pregnant women were assessed at 15, 19, 25, 31, and 37 weeks' gestation. Serum samples were assayed for CRH, ACTH, and cortisol. Depression was assessed at four points antenatally and at one time postpartum. Elevated CRH at 25 weeks' gestation predicted postpartum depression.

The final component of the stress response is the immune system, which responds to threat by releasing proinflammatory cytokines (Corwin and Pajer, 2008; Kendall-Tackett, 2007). Researchers generally assess inflammation by measuring serum levels of proinflammatory cytokines (Miller, *et al.*, 2002). The proinflammatory cytokines identified most often in depression research are interleukin-1β (IL-1β), interleukin-6 (IL-6), and tumor necrosis factor-α (TNF-α). Researchers sometimes include other measures of inflammation in their studies. These include interferon-γ (IFN-γ), intercellular adhesion molecule (ICAM), fibrinogen, or C-reactive protein (CRP). Maes (2001: 193) described the stress-depression-inflammation connection as follows.

> The discovery that psychological stress can induce the production of proinflammatory cytokines has important implications for human psychopathology and, in particular, for the aetiology of major depression. Psychological stressors, such as negative life events, are emphasized in the aetiology of depression. Thus psychosocial and environmental stressors play a role as direct precipitants of major depression or they function as vulnerability factors which predispose humans to develop major depression. Major depression is accompanied by activation of the inflammatory response system (IRS) with, among other things, an increased production of proinflammatory cytokines, such as IL-1β, IL-6, TNF-α and IFN-γ, signs of monocytic- and T-cell activation and an acute-phase response.

One of the original studies that established the link between chronic stress, inflammation, and premature mortality was not a postpartum sample, but a sample of elderly men and women (average age=70 years), approximately half of whom were caring for a spouse with Alzheimer's (Kiecolt-Glaser, *et al.*, 2003). This study particularly focused on the proinflammatory cytokine IL-6, which has been linked to a number of chronic diseases, including cardiovascular disease, type-2 diabetes, cancer, and overall functional decline. The impact of caregiving was such that IL-6 levels were four times higher in the caregivers than in age-matched non-caregivers. These levels remained elevated even after the spouse had died. At the end of the six-year follow-up, 78 of the 119 caregivers had died. These researchers concluded that chronic stress accelerated the risk of disease by prematurely aging the immune response.

The three systems illustrated in Figure 5.1 are interrelated, with a series of checks and balances – when the system is working normally. Inflammation influences levels of serotonin and catecholamines, and impacts the HPA-axis, which secretes cortisol. But if the system is overwhelmed, it fails.

Proinflammatory Cytokines

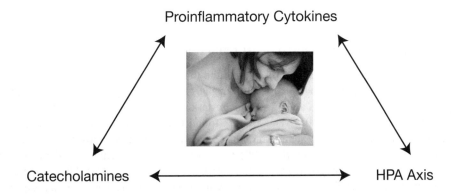

Catecholamines ⟷ HPA Axis

*Figure 5.1* Three components of the stress response

Depression is one state where the normal checks and balances fail. In a normally functioning system, once inflammation starts, it triggers the HPA-axis to release cortisol to keep it under control. Specifically, cortisol downregulates IL-1, IL-2, TNF-$\alpha$ and IFN-$\gamma$ (Corwin and Pajer, 2008; McEwen, 2003). However, depressed people either have abnormally low levels of cortisol or they become cortisol resistant. In either case, cortisol fails to restrain the inflammatory response (Schiepers, *et al.*, 2005). For example, Groer and Morgan (2007), in their study of 200 postpartum women, noted a downregulation of the HPA-axis and abnormally low levels of cortisol in depressed women at four to six weeks postpartum.

Another study of 72 women had similar findings (Miller, *et al.*, 2005). Depressed and non-depressed women were exposed to a stressor in the form of a mock job interview. Researchers then drew blood to assess levels of proinflammatory cytokines. They found that stress increased monocytes, neutrophils, C-reactive protein, IL-6 and TNF-$\alpha$ for all the women in the study. However, the depressed women had a blunted cortisol response to stress and increased resistance to the molecules that normally terminate the inflammatory response. The researchers hypothesized that depression created a long-term decrease in sensitivity to cortisol, which allowed inflammation to continue unchecked. These same researchers had similar findings in a sample of parents caring for children with cancer (Miller, *et al.*, 2002). This study compared parents of healthy children with parents of ill children. They found that parents of ill children had a blunted response to cortisol, which did not restrain inflammation.

The net result of these findings is that our bodies "translate" physical and psychological stress into inflammation, and it underlies all the other risk factors for depression. Inflammation is not simply *a* risk factor; it is *the* risk factor for depression, the one that ties the others together (Kendall-Tackett, 2007).

## Why inflammation is particularly relevant to depression in new mothers

Pregnant and postpartum women are particularly vulnerable to this effect because their inflammation levels normally rise during the last trimester of pregnancy – a time when they are also at highest risk for depression (Kendall-Tackett, 2007). Indeed, the pattern of elevated cytokine levels in the last trimester matches the pattern of perinatal depression more accurately than the pattern of other biological markers, such as the rise and fall of reproductive hormones.

The findings on women's increased risk of depression during pregnancy vs. postpartum are summarized below.

## Depression risk is highest during last trimester of pregnancy

Several studies of perinatal depression have found that a higher percentage of women were depressed during pregnancy than postpartum. In a large study of pregnant women (N=9,028), depression was measured at 18 and 32 weeks' gestation, and at eight weeks and eight months postpartum (Evans, *et al.*, 2001). The authors found that depression rates were highest at 32 weeks' gestation and lowest at eight months postpartum. Similarly, Hobfoll and colleagues (Hobfoll, *et al.*, 1995; Ritter, *et al.*, 2000) found the highest percentage of depression in women occurred during pregnancy (28% and 25%), not postpartum (23%). Their sample was 192 low-income women from the inner city. Fifty-three percent of the women with postpartum depression were also depressed during pregnancy.

In a study conducted in India (Patel, *et al.*, 2002), 23% of mothers had postpartum depression (N=252). Seventy-eight percent were also depressed during pregnancy, and only 21% of these developed depression for the first time postpartum. Moreover, 59% of women depressed at six weeks were still depressed at six months postpartum.

In a sample of 80 women, 25% experienced depression during pregnancy, and 16% experienced depression at four to five weeks postpartum (Da Costa, *et al.*, 2000). Women who were depressed postpartum reported more emotional coping, and higher state and trait anxiety during pregnancy. Depressed mood during pregnancy best predicted postpartum depressed mood. In a low-income, ethnic-minority sample (N=802), 37% of the women had depressive symptoms, and 6.5% to 8.5% had major depression at three to five weeks postpartum. Fifty percent of these women were also depressed during pregnancy (Yonkers, *et al.*, 2001).

Not all studies have found increased depression during pregnancy, however. Among 4,398 women whose pregnancies ended in live births, 15% were identified as being depressed either before, during or after their pregnancies (Dietz, *et al.*, 2007). This sample was drawn from a large health-maintenance organization in Oregon and Washington State. Nine percent had depression diagnosed before their pregnancies, 6.9% during their pregnancies, and 10.4% after their pregnancies. Of the women who were depressed before pregnancy, 56.4% were also depressed during their pregnancies. Among women depressed postpartum, 54% were also identified as depressed before or during their pregnancies. The study collected data via chart review, so that only women with diagnoses of depression in their medical charts were included in the depressed group. This methodology may have underestimated the true incidence of depression.

## Immune markers remain elevated in postpartum women

Proinflammatory cytokine levels are generally elevated in women after giving birth. One study found that postpartum women are generally higher in the cytokines IL-6, IL-6R, and IL-1RA than they were before delivery (Maes, *et al.*, 2000). Another study compared anxiety scores of primiparous with those of multiparous women and found higher levels of anxiety in primiparae (Maes, *et al.*, 2004). Noting that depression and anxiety are associated with activation of the inflammatory response system, the researchers found that primiparae had higher levels of anxiety than did multiparae at days 1 and 3 postpartum. They also found higher serum IL-1RA and lower sCD8. Another marker of the inflammatory response system is prolyl endopeptidase (PEP). This was also elevated in the primiparae but not in the multiparae after delivery. Maes and colleagues (2004) noted that since monocytic cytokines, such as IL-1, IL-6 and TNF-α, may induce depression and anxiety, it is reasonable to hypothesize that increased monocytic activity in the puerperium in primiparae may have caused higher anxiety levels. PEP also appears to have a role. One possible explanation is that PEP plays pivotal role in the final degradation and processing of behaviorally active hormones and neuropeptides, such as thyrotropin-releasing hormone (TRH), Substance P, neurotensin, oxytocin, and AVP. All of these have key roles in anxiety, emotion, stress responsivity, and social interactions.

Maes and colleagues (2002) also examined the impact of inflammation in the early puerperium by IL-6, IL-8 and kynurenine, a major tryptophan catabolite. They found that in the postpartum period there was a significant increase in kynurenine and the K/T quotient. The increases in plasma kynurenine were significantly more pronounced in women with elevated depression and anxiety scores. These changes were significantly related to the immune markers. The researchers concluded that increased K/T quotient at the end of pregnancy and early postpartum indicates inflammation-induced degradation of tryptophan along the kynurenine pathway. Depressive and anxiety symptoms are causally related to an increased catabolism of tryptophan in kynurenine, most likely due to immune activation.

## Physical and psychological stressors that increase inflammation and risk of depression

As described in the previous section, human bodies are designed to respond in a certain way when they are threatened. Whether these threats are physical or psychological, the body's response is the same. Moreover, some types of stressors have both physical and psychological elements. Three stressors – fatigue, pain, and trauma – are particularly relevant to new mothers. Studies that examine fatigue and pain with regard to inflammation are described below. Trauma will be further described in Chapters 6 through 8.

### *Fatigue and sleep deprivation*

Fatigue's role in postpartum depression is often overlooked because almost *all* new mothers are tired (Bozoky and Corwin, 2002). However, it can be debilitating and can decrease women's abilities to care for their babies, decrease their enjoyment of motherhood, and dramatically increase their risk of depression (Corwin and Arbour, 2007). For example, one large Australian study found that 60% of new mothers reported exhaustion or extreme tiredness, and 30% reported lack of sleep or a baby crying in the first eight weeks (Thompson, *et al.*, 2002). These problems eventually resolved, but 49% still reported exhaustion, and 15% reported lack of sleep at 24 weeks. Mothers who had cesarean sections were more likely to report exhaustion than mothers who had had assisted or unassisted vaginal deliveries.

In a sample of 109 women who were hospitalized in a mother-baby psychiatric unit, 91% of the women were clinically fatigued (Fisher, *et al.*, 2002b). These mothers also felt overwhelmed (76%) and anxious (75%). Some things that distinguished hospitalized women from postpartum women in general were a greater number of obstetric and reproductive problems, poor postpartum hospital care, lack of social connections, partners who worked long hours, inadequate practical assistance, and the presence of other stressful life events.

Fatigue may also be the way that depression presents. This is especially true in developing countries, or in subcultures in the U.S., where having a physical problem may be more culturally acceptable than saying you are depressed (Patel, *et al.*, 2001).

*Sleep disturbances and depression*

Fatigue can be both a symptom of depression and a cause. When describing the relationship between fatigue and depression, we are often left a with chicken-and-egg type of question, not knowing which came first. But fatigue can be a clue that something is amiss, particularly when women cannot sleep even when their babies are sleeping. Depression and sleep problems are mutually maintaining: poor sleep quality is a risk factor for major depression and depression is a risk factor for the onset of poor sleep quality. Severe fatigue also predicts future depression (Posmontier, 2008).

One study recruited 38 healthy new mothers, who had had uncomplicated births, in the first day postpartum (Bozoky and Corwin, 2002). The authors assessed fatigue on days 0, 7, 14, and 28 postpartum, and depression at day 28. They found that fatigue at day 7 predicted depression at day 28. Indeed, fatigue on day 7 accounted for 21% of the variance in depressive symptoms. Fatigue was not related to marital status, presence of other children at home, breast- or bottle-feeding, or hemoglobin concentration. Similarly, a study of 465 postpartum women also found that sleep problems predicted depression (Chaudron, *et al.*, 2001). In this sample, 27 women became clinically depressed. At one month postpartum, there were four factors that predicted depression at four months: trouble falling asleep, maternal age, depression during pregnancy, and thoughts of death and dying.

*Characteristics of depressed sleep*

Ross and colleagues (2005) noted that several factors suggest a relationship between sleep problems and depression in postpartum women. These are as follows:

1    Insomnia is a significant risk for new-onset depression.
2    Sleep disturbances are common in most psychiatric disorders.
3    Treatments that manipulate sleep and circadian rhythms can be used to treat mood disorders.

In a review of polysomnographic studies of postpartum women, Ross, *et al.* (2005) noted that there are differences in REM latency for women at risk for postpartum depression or who have current postpartum depression – reduced REM latency, increased total sleep time during pregnancy, and decreased total sleep time postpartum. REM latency refers to the time during the night when REM sleep becomes the predominant pattern. A pattern of reduced REM latency means that REM occurs earlier in the nightly sleep cycle, and is a symptom of depression. As a result of these sleep disturbances, women are more fatigued during the day. The authors noted that these changes may represent an underlying vulnerability to depression as they do with non-postpartum populations. They also noted that women with a history of affective disorders may be more sensitive to the normal physiologic changes of pregnancy.

Mothers (N=425) with postpartum major depression reported substantially poorer sleep than their non-depressed counterparts at four to eight weeks postpartum (Dennis and Ross, 2005). The mothers were assessed for depression at one week postpartum and women who were depressed at that time point were excluded from the study to eliminate pre-existing depression as a cause of sleep problems. Mothers with an EPDS score of greater than 13 at one week were more likely to report that their baby cried often, that they were woken three or more times a night, and that they received less than 6 hours' sleep in a 24-hour period. Further, they were more likely to report that their baby did not sleep well and that their baby's sleep pattern did not allow them to get a reasonable amount of sleep. Infant temperament mediated the relationship between infant sleep and maternal fatigue, with fussy babies sleeping less. One methodologic issue to consider in interpreting these findings is that it relies solely on mothers' reports, not actual sleep measures.

A Taiwanese study of 163 first-time mothers found that 50% were depressed at 13 to 20 weeks postpartum (Huang, *et al.*, 2004). Depressed mothers had poorer sleep than non-depressed mothers. Half reported that their sleep quality was either fairly bad or bad. The average time it took for mothers to fall asleep was 26 minutes vs. 20 minutes for non-depressed mothers. Depressed mothers had overall poorer sleep quality, took more time to fall asleep, had a shorter sleep duration, and reported more daytime dysfunctions.

In a study of 46 mothers at 6 to 26 weeks postpartum, data were collected via wrist actigraphy for seven days, and by questionnaire (Postmontier, 2008). Half of the mothers were depressed. Postpartum depression was measured via the Postpartum Depression Screening Scale (PDSS). The author found that women with postpartum depression had substantially poorer sleep quality than non-depressed women, and that as depression symptoms increased, so did the sleep problems. Women with postpartum depression took longer to go to sleep (sleep latency), were more likely to wake after sleep onset, and had poorer sleep efficiency. She concluded that for women with postpartum depression, nighttime breastfeeding demands, high-needs infants, and little nighttime support may negatively impact sleep quality and further exacerbate depressive symptoms. This was true even though the non-depressed group was breastfeeding and had fewer nighttime wakings than the depressed group.

A longitudinal study of 124 primiparous women collected data during the last trimester, and at one, two, and three months postpartum (Goyal, *et al.*, 2007). At Time 1, 26% had clinically high depressive symptoms. Depressed women had more sleep disturbance, more trouble falling asleep, more daytime sleepiness and early awakening than women who were not depressed. The mothers who had the highest depression scores reported the most difficulty falling asleep. The authors concluded that delayed sleep onset may be the most relevant clinical screening question to assess risk of postpartum depression.

*Sleep disturbances and depression in non-postpartum samples*

Sleep disturbances are related to depression in the general population. In a large Japanese study (N=24,686), respondents who slept less than six or more than eight hours per night were more likely to be depressed on the Center for Epidemiologic Studies Depression Scale (Kaneita, *et al.*, 2006). In this study, those with a sleep duration of six to eight hours per night had the lowest rates of depression.

A Canadian survey of three indigenous groups living in northwest British Columbia (N=430) found that the prevalence of sleep complaints was high: 17% reported insomnia; 18% restless leg syndrome, and 8% sleep apnea. Twenty-eight percent had moderate to severe depression. All types of sleep disturbance were independently associated with depression (Froese, *et al.*, 2008).

In a study of 253 pregnant women, depressed women had more sleep disturbances and higher depression, anxiety, and anger scores during the second and third trimester (Field, *et al.*, 2007). The newborns of depressed mothers also had more sleep disturbance. They spent less time in deep sleep, and more time in disorganized sleep. The babies of depressed mothers also spent significantly more time fussing and crying.

Sleep disturbances can occur in depressed mothers even when the baby is absent. A study of mothers and fathers of infants in a neonatal intensive care unit (NICU) found that sleep was disturbed for both (Lee, *et al.*, 2007). Sleep disturbance was high for both mothers and fathers: 93% of mothers and 60% of fathers reported disturbed sleep. Mothers had longer sleep latency, more nighttime wakings, and more subjective fatigue than fathers. Data were collected via wrist actigraphy and sleep diaries. The total minutes of sleep were significantly lower for mothers than for fathers, and mothers reported more morning and daytime fatigue.

### Inflammation and sleep

Sleep disturbances and fatigue are also related to cytokine levels. Interleukin-1β (IL-1β) was related to fatigue in postpartum women (Corwin, *et al.*, 2003). Corwin and colleagues collected measures of fatigue, and urinary excretion of IL-1β, over four weeks postpartum. The authors found that IL-1β is elevated during the postpartum period, and that this elevation has a significant, though delayed, relationship to postpartum fatigue.

In a study of women four to six weeks postpartum, Groer and colleagues (2005) found that mothers' fatigue levels correlated with their levels of stress and depression. They also found that fatigue, stress and depression increased the risk of infection for both mother and baby. Interestingly, this same study also found that mothers who were stressed, depressed, and fatigued had lower levels of prolactin in both their serum and their milk. These same mothers also had higher levels of melatonin, the hormone that regulates circadian rhythms, in their milk (Groer, *et al.*, 2005).

In a more recent study of 200 women at four to six weeks postpartum, Groer and Morgan (2007) found that depressed mothers reported more fatigue and daytime sleepiness than did non-depressed mothers. The depressed mothers had abnormally low levels of cortisol, which may also have caused their fatigue. The authors describe how chronic fatigue syndrome, various chronic pain syndromes, and posttraumatic stress disorder are also associated with low cortisol levels. The depressed mothers also had more health problems since the baby was born and had more health-related events such as sprains, dental pain, and allergies. They had higher levels of perceived stress, anxiety and more negative life events. The serum IL-6 levels were three times higher in the depressed mothers, but this was not a significant difference because of measurement variability.

In summary, sleep disturbances and fatigue are physical stressors that increase the risk of depression. The relationship between sleep problems and proinflammatory cytokines appears to be bidirectional: sleep disturbances increase cytokines and cytokines increase sleep disturbance by delaying sleep onset, increasing daytime fatigue, and perpetuating the cycle of disturbed sleep and inflammation.

### Sleep deprivation and psychosis

Although psychosis is not the main focus of this book, it is important to mention it here, since sleeplessness is a common symptom in puerperal psychosis (Ross, *et al.* 2005). Sleep deprivation has been related to delusional thinking and other psychotic symptoms in men and non-postpartum women. Is it any surprise that it could have this same effect on women who have recently given birth? Personal accounts of postpartum psychosis, and accounts given by women interviewed for this book, indicated that women who developed psychosis had been unable to sleep for two to three days before the onset of their illness. Inability to sleep is a red-flag symptom that requires immediate medical attention. Charlotte describes her experience.

My second postpartum experience was a nightmare. I was exhausted. I decided to wean my baby at two months because I was so exhausted and depressed.

I thought about suicide, institutionalization and separation from my family constantly. That postpartum psychosis exists was such a revelation to me because in April I had experienced a week of near-total insomnia. During these truly sleepless nights, I had no control over my thoughts, as if my brain had been put in a food processor. The first half of a thought would be rational and the second half would be totally unrelated, nonsensical.

The exact mechanism for the sleep-deprivation/psychosis link is unclear at this time. Psychosis could be the result of biochemical changes resulting from lack of sleep. Or the lack of sleep may have been due to an underlying condition, such as bipolar disorder.

In a study that sought to identify a biologic marker for psychotic depression (Stefos, *et al.*, 1998), 44 patients with non-psychotic major depression were compared with 44 patients with psychotic major depression. Sleep-related biological markers were significantly more common in the psychotic depressed patients. These included increased wakefulness, diminished REM latency, hypercortisolism, and blunted thyroid-stimulating hormone response to thyrotropin-releasing hormone stimulation. Shortened REM latency was related to both depression and psychosis.

The sleep–psychosis connection has also been described in case studies. One classic case study of sleep deprivation involved a New York disc jockey named Peter Tripp. In January 1959, Tripp tried to stay awake for 200 hours in a glass booth in Times Square as a fundraiser for the March of Dimes. Below are excerpts from the government report on what happened to him.

> Almost from the first, the desire to sleep was so strong that Tripp was fighting to keep himself awake. After little more than 2 days and 2 nights, he began to have visual illusions; for example, he reported finding cobwebs in his shoes. By about 100 hours the simple daily tests that required only minimal mental agility and attention were a torture for him. He was having trouble remembering things, and his visual illusions were perturbing: he saw the tweed suit of one of the scientists as a suit of fuzzy worms. The daily tests were almost unendurable for Tripp and those who were studying him. "He looked like a blind animal trying to feel his way through a maze." A simple algebraic formula that he had earlier solved with ease now required such superhuman effort that Tripp broke down, frightened at his inability to solve the problem, fighting to perform. Scientists saw the spectacle of a suave New York radio entertainer trying vainly to find his way through the alphabet.
>
> By 170 hours the agony had become almost unbearable to watch. At times Tripp was no longer sure he was himself, and frequently tried to gain proof of his identity. Although he behaved as if he were awake, his brain wave patterns resembled those of sleep. In his psychotic delusions he was convinced that the doctors were in a conspiracy against him to send him to jail. At the end of the 200 sleepless hours, nightmare hallucination and reality had merged, and he felt he was the victim of a sadistic conspiracy among the doctors.
>
> (Luce, 1966: 19–20)

Tripp recovered fairly quickly after he slept for about 13 hours, but he complained of depression for three months afterwards. There were a number of similarities in his experience to those of the women suffering from postpartum psychosis, including delusions, hallucinations, and paranoia. It is interesting, too, that this case study was conducted on a man who would not be subject to the same hormonal influences common in postpartum or menstruating women, yet he manifested symptoms similar to women suffering from postpartum psychosis. However, it is important to note that not everyone who is sleep deprived develops symptoms of psychosis. Nonetheless, sleep deprivation could be a catalyst for women who are already vulnerable. Judy, a labor and delivery nurse, describes how sleeplessness preceded her bout with postpartum psychosis. She was initially diagnosed with schizophrenia. Her diagnosis was later changed to bipolar disorder. She was hospitalized for 28 days.

> In the months after her birth I often was easily overwhelmed. Fatigue did not vanish. Fears of losing her, my boys, and/or [my husband] grasped me frequently. Exhaustion came, but I did not submit. After [my daughter] was asleep, thoughts bombarded me for hours only to awake alert at 4 or 5 a.m. The week after the [childbirth education] seminar, sleeplessness continued. A whimper or sneeze from one of my children would jar me into a state of alertness. Racing thoughts about the deficits of the maternity care system in the U.S. or my childhood bombarded my mind. I'd enter their room … hoping one of the three would be awake. Usually they weren't so I spent hours formulating and recording plans and ideas.
>
> As the week progressed, I became less functional. We delayed leaving for a camping trip Thursday night since I was unable to accomplish packing. [My husband] received phone calls from relatives telling him of the strange content of the lengthy long-distance calls I'd placed. He forbid me to use the phone. I continued, though, because I sensed a great urgency of my thoughts.

*Summary*

Fatigue and sleep deprivation can be important signs of – or even triggers for – postpartum depression and psychosis. While most new mothers are tired, those who seem exceptionally tired and unable to cope may be depressed or are at risk of depression. Sleeplessness not related to baby care can be a particularly ominous sign that requires close monitoring.

### *Hypothyroidism*

Sleep deprivation is the most obvious source of fatigue, but there are also other causes. Another line of research examines the role of thyroid function in postpartum depression. Thyroid is a hormone that regulates metabolism. Low thyroid levels can cause a wide range of depression-like symptoms, including an inability to concentrate, tiredness, and forgetfulness. Low thyroid can also cause intolerance to cold, persistently low body temperature, low blood pressure, weight gain, puffy face and eyes, constipation, and dry hair and skin. In mothers who are very tired, evaluating them for postpartum hypothyroidism is often prudent.

A study of 31 women examined the relationship between thyroid in late pregnancy and postpartum and the development of postpartum depression (Pedersen, *et al.*, 2007). Thyroid was measured at 32 to 35, 36, and 37 weeks' gestation. All of the women had normal thyroid levels. They also rated their mood every other week between 2 and 24 weeks postpartum. Mean antenatal thyroxine concentrations and free thyroxine indices correlated significantly and negatively with mean depression scores during each the postpartum assessment points. Women with lower total and free thyroxine concentrations had significantly higher depression scores, via EPDS and Beck Depression Inventory, at all three postpartum assessment points. The researchers concluded that women with thyroxine levels in the euthyroid range may be at greater risk of developing postpartum depressive symptoms.

Another study, however, has failed to find a link between postpartum depression and postpartum thyroid dysfunction (Lucas, *et al.*, 2001). This study recruited 641 women during their 36th week of pregnancy, and followed them through the first year postpartum (N=444 at the 12-month assessment). The authors found that 56 women (11%) developed postpartum thyroid disorder. None of these women were diagnosed with postpartum depression (using the Beck Depression Inventory). Their sample's rate of postpartum depression was abnormally low (1.7%). The researchers did find that women with a history of postpartum depression were significantly more likely to become depressed again.

The rate of postpartum thyroid dysfunction is approximately 2.5% (Corwin and Arbour, 2007). Although screening all mothers may not be necessary, it is a low-risk test that can be helpful when working with mothers with severe fatigue. Risk factors for postpartum hypothyroidism include diabetes mellitus and a personal or family history of hypothyroidism. But some mothers will have no risk factors at all. Screening tests include TSH levels and free or total T4. The American Association of Clinical Endocrinologists recommends that hypothyroidism be considered and assessed in all patients with depression (cited in Corwin and Arbour, 2007).

## Pain

Pain is another risk factor for postpartum mental disorders that can stem from both biological and psychosocial causes. Manning (2002) notes that pain and depression may share a common monoamine synaptic pathway in the central nervous system. The neurotransmitters serotonin and norepinephrine appear to be important in both. These substances are often low in depressed individuals, and both modulate pain sensitivity via the descending pain pathway. The involvement of both neurotransmitters could also explain why tricyclic antidepressants, or others that address both serotonin and norepinephrine, are often more effective in treating chronic pain than ones that address only serotonin levels (e.g. selective serotonin reuptake inhibitors).

After childbirth, women may experience pain from a variety of sources: abdominal incisions, uterine contractions, swollen or engorged breasts, cracked nipples, episiotomies and/or perineal lacerations, back pains and headaches from spinal or epidural anesthesia, and muscle aches and pains. This pain, although transitory, can be severe and frightening. In a large sample of mothers at eight weeks postpartum, 53% reported backache, 37% reported bowel problems, 30% reported hemorrhoids, 22% reported perineal pain, and 15% reported mastitis (Thompson, *et al.*, 2002). Unfortunately, postpartum pain is often under-medicated, as a study on analgesia for women who had had forceps deliveries found (Peter, *et al.*, 2001).

In an Australian study, 48 lactating women with nipple pain were compared with 65 lactating women without nipple pain (Amir, *et al.*, 1996). Thirty-eight percent of women in the pain group scored above the threshold for depression compared with 14% in the control group. In addition, women in the pain group had significantly higher scores on all mood factors on the Profile of Mood States. Once the pain resolved, the scores on these scales dropped to normal levels.

Unfortunately, according to two recent studies, nipple pain appears to be common. The first sample was from Minneapolis, Minnesota. In this sample, an astonishing 50% of women had nipple pain at five weeks (McGovern, *et al.*, 2006). Another study from Toronto, Canada had similar results. In this study, 52% of mothers reported cracked or sore nipples at two months postpartum (Ansara, *et al.*, 2005).

In the study of 109 women hospitalized in a private mother-baby unit (Fisher, *et al.*,

2002), pain was also an issue. In this sample, 41% reported that their postpartum pain was inadequately controlled and 41% described nipple pain that persisted longer than one week. Twenty-nine percent of these mothers had experienced at least one episode of mastitis. A high degree of postpartum pain was also associated with depression at eight months postpartum in another study of primiparous women (Rowe-Murray and Fisher, 2001).

In a study of 465 women, Chaudron and colleagues (2001) found that women who reported ten or more somatic complaints were nearly three times more likely to develop depression than women who reported nine or fewer symptoms. They also found a linear relationship between postpartum depression and an increasing number of physical or somatic complaints. Women in pain were more likely to be depressed and anxious.

Another possible link between pain and depression is the impact of pain on sleep. Sayar and colleagues (2002) compared 40 patients with chronic pain with 40 healthy control subjects on sleep quality, depression and anxiety. As predicted, the chronic pain patients had significantly poorer sleep quality, more depression and more anxiety. Pain intensity, anxiety and depression correlated significantly to poorer sleep quality. However, in a multivariate analysis, depression was the only factor that was significantly correlated to sleep – explaining 34% of the variance.

*Pain and inflammation*

Depression and pain are also related to inflammation, and the relationship between pain and inflammation appears to be bidirectional. When a woman experiences pain, stress hormones and levels of proinflammatory cytokines increase. High levels of proinflammatory cytokines, in turn, increase pain. Cytokines (especially IL-1) are stimulated by Substance P. Substance P is the neuropeptide that is high in patients with pain. High levels of Substance P increase proinflammatory cytokines, which increase prostaglandin synthesis, which increases pain (Geracioti, *et al.*, 2006).

In one study, patients with major depression or posttraumatic stress disorder were compared with healthy controls (N=101). The patients with depression or PTSD had significantly elevated levels of Substance P in their cerebrospinal fluid. Moreover, the levels of Substance P rose significantly when the patients were presented with a laboratory-induced stressor. The authors concluded that Substance P was related to both depression and PTSD and responded to acute stress (Geracioti, *et al.*, 2006).

In a study of non-postpartum post-operative pain, three methods of pain relief were included in the trial (Beilin, *et al.*, 2003). All the patients were having elective lower abdominal surgery. The first type of pain relief was opiates on demand. The second was patient-controlled analgesia. The third was patient-controlled epidural analgesia, an approach that combines opiates with local anesthesia, which is opiate sparing. The local anesthesia is anti-inflammatory, which may contribute to its pain-reducing effects. The researchers described the post-operative period as a time associated with neuroendocrine, metabolic, and immune alterations. They found that pain intensity was lowest in the epidural group. There were higher levels of IL-1β and IL-6 in the on-demand opiates and patient-controlled analgesia groups than in the epidural group. The authors argued that proinflammatory cytokines mediate hyperalgesia, including the upregulation of Cox-2 and increased production of Substance P and nerve growth factor. Nociception and proinflammatory cytokines are mutually upregulatory; because of the feedback cascade between nociception and proinflammatory cytokines, pain increases inflammation and inflammation increases pain. Under certain circumstances, central pain sensitization can lead to the development of chronic or neuropathic pain.

In summary, postpartum pain is a common experience among women who have recently given birth (Ansara, *et al.*, 2005). Addressing pain promptly, and providing mothers with the means to cope with their pain can halt the cascade of stress hormones and proinflammatory cytokines, decreasing their risk of depression. Postpartum pain will also be described more fully in Chapter 6.

## Hormonal influences

The hormonal theory of postpartum depression is the oldest, and best-known, of the physiological theories of postpartum depression. At present, we know that women undergo substantial changes in hormone levels in the immediate postpartum period. The bone of contention, however, is whether these changes are related to depression. As I indicated in Chapter 1, research has produced mixed results, with little support for the reproductive hormonal etiology of depression.

### Reproductive hormones

Estrogen and progesterone, and their metabolites, are the best-studied hormones in relation to postpartum depression. Depression is hypothesized as being most likely to occur if estrogen and progesterone levels are low. And there is a large drop in the levels of these hormones immediately after birth. Alternatively, there might be increased sensitivity to these changes for women at risk of depression (Meltzer-Brody, *et al.*, 2008). None of these explanations, however, has held up particularly well when examined empirically.

Hormonal research has proceeded along several lines: by studying the day-five peak; by comparing the hormone levels of depressed and non-depressed women, and by treating depressed women with hormones. A brief summary of these studies is found below.

### The day-five peak

The 'day-five peak' refers to the time in the immediate postpartum period when women are tearful, irritable, have difficulty concentrating, and are sleepless. These changes are said to correspond to the dramatic drop in progesterone, estradiol, and cortisol, with the most dramatic change around the fourth or fifth day postpartum. Studies in search of the day-five peak have had mixed results.

In a prospective study of 120 women (Harris, *et al.*, 1994), the maternity blues were associated with high antenatal progesterone the day before delivery, and lower levels of progesterone from the day of delivery to the day of peak blues. Women who had had cesarean sections were excluded from the study. The authors described their findings as a "weak but significant" association between progesterone and the blues. They concluded that progesterone levels immediately following delivery are responsible for maternal mood, and they recommended possible treatment of mothers with progesterone .

However, at least one study found that there is a similar pattern following surgery. Levy (1987) compared emotional reactions of puerperal women (N=37), women who had had major surgery (N=28), and women who had had minor surgery (N=22). The surgeries were not reproductively related. Her results revealed a similar pattern of distress for the puerperal women and for women who had had major surgery. In fact, there was *more* dysphoria following major surgery than after childbirth. Further, crying and depression peaked in the same way in the post-operative women as it did in the puerperal women, with many post-operative patients commenting that the blues occurred suddenly and unexpectedly around the fourth post-operative day. These findings suggest an alternate mechanism than shifts in reproductive hormones.

There are a number of factors that argue against a wholly hormonal explanation for the day-five peak. For example, not every mother experiences these emotions, which we would expect since all mothers experience hormonal shifts postpartum. Further, in some cultures, the majority of women do not experience the day-five peak, suggesting that a woman's environment can modify a biological process (Stern and Kruckman, 1983). In addition, fathers and women who adopt children often experience a day-five peak and depression, but do not experience hormonal adjustments.

### *Hormone levels in depressed and non-depressed women*

In a carefully controlled study, O'Hara and colleagues (1991) analyzed blood and urine samples from approximately 173 women (number of participants varied slightly from assessment to assessment) at 34, 36, and 38 weeks' gestation, and at days one, two, three, four, six, and eight postpartum. The authors studied levels of estradiol, free estriol, progesterone, prolactin, total cortisol, and urinary free cortisol. The depressed subjects in their sample (N=18) showed significantly lower levels of estradiol at 36 weeks' gestation and at day two postpartum, but there were no other significant differences. Specifically, there were no significant differences in levels of free estriol, total estriol, progesterone, prolactin, total plasma cortisol, or urinary free cortisol between depressed and non-depressed subjects at any of the other assessment periods. Further, there were no significant differences between depressed and non-depressed subjects for ratios of prolactin to estradiol or progesterone for any of the assessments. The authors concluded that there was little evidence of a hormonal influence in postpartum depression. O'Hara came to a similar conclusion in his review of the literature.

> In spite of a large sample size and accurate estimations of hormone levels, there was *weak support* for the hormonal hypothesis. In fact, on at least two postpartum days, in direct contrast to our prediction, measures of free and total estriol levels were significantly *higher* in women experiencing the blues than in women not experiencing the blues.
>
> (O'Hara, 1995: 134, emphasis added)

Researchers continue to study this phenomenon. In a more recent study, the authors were able to induce a postpartum-depression-like syndrome in the laboratory. Bloch and colleagues (2000) recruited two groups of eight women: women with previous postpartum depression and women with no history of postpartum depression. They simulated the high hormone levels of pregnancy with gonadotropin-releasing hormone agonist leuprolide acetate, and added back supraphysiologic dose of estradiol and progesterone for eight weeks. They then withdrew the steroids under double-blind conditions. During withdrawal, 62.5% of the women with a history of postpartum depression developed significant mood symptoms when the steroids were withdrawn. None of the comparison women were affected. The authors concluded that their findings constituted direct support for the involvement of reproductive hormones in the development of postpartum depression *in a subgroup of women*. They noted that women with a history of postpartum depression may be differentially sensitive to changes in these hormone levels, and respond with negative mood states.

*Treatment for postpartum conditions using hormones*

The final strategy for studying postpartum hormonal influences involves treating women who are at risk of postpartum depression with hormones. In a well-known study, Dalton (1985) gave progesterone prophylactically to 100 women who had had previous episodes of postpartum depression, and compared them with 221 women who had also had prior postpartum depression but did not receive progesterone. There was a 10% recurrence rate in women who received progesterone, compared with a recurrence rate of 68% among those who received no progesterone. These findings are striking, but the study had one major limitation – it was not double-blinded. The women and their doctors knew they were being treated. The findings could be due to the placebo effect. Moreover, women in the non-treatment group received nothing. The human contact, rather than the progesterone, could have been responsible for the finding.

Another group of researchers (van der Meer, *et al.*, 1984) did conduct a double-blind placebo-controlled trial comparing progesterone suppositories with a placebo on ten women suffering from postpartum depression. There was no significant difference between the effect of the progesterone and that of the placebo. Indeed, when comparing subjective effects, three of the women preferred the placebo.

More recently, Ahokas and colleagues (2000, 2001) have used 17β-Estradiol to treat severe postpartum depression and postpartum psychosis. In the study of depression (Ahokas, *et al.*, 2001), 23 women with postpartum major depression were recruited from a psychiatric emergency unit. They were all severely depressed and had low serum estradiol concentrations. Within a week of treatment with estradiol, the depressive symptoms had substantially diminished, and by the end of the second week, when estradiol levels were comparable to the follicular phase, the scores on the depression measure were comparable to clinical recovery. The study of psychosis was similar (Ahokas, *et al.*, 2000). There were 10 women with postpartum psychosis who all had very low levels of serum estradiol. Within a week of sublingual 17β-Estradiol, symptoms were significantly improved. By the second week, when levels were almost normal, the women were almost completely free of psychiatric symptoms.

These studies are promising, but there are limitations. First, the trials were open label, which means everyone was aware of being treated. Was it the estradiol or the placebo effect? These studies raise some other questions, such as what are the normal levels of estradiol for postpartum women? Presumably, almost every woman is low in estradiol postpartum. How is it that only some become depressed or psychotic? Is there a certain level where we start to see psychiatric symptoms? Why are some women more vulnerable to these changes?

*Summary*

Despite the popularity of the hormonal explanation for postpartum depression, it has only limited scientific support. Future studies may find that reproductive hormones are indirectly related to depression because of their influence on stress hormones, immune markers, or sleep quality. In the meantime, there is not sufficient evidence to support treatment of postpartum depression with reproductive hormones – especially given some of the risks associated with their use.

## Conclusions

Research on the biological underpinnings of depression in general, and postpartum depression in particular, has exploded since the first edition of this book was released. In the original edition, I had to draw from other literatures to make statements about the impact of sleep deprivation, fatigue, and pain on postpartum women. Now, there are many excellent studies on how these physiological phenomena affect the mental well-being of mothers.

Researchers to date have not established that puerperal hormonal changes are related to postpartum depression. The good news is that our models of the biological influences in depression have grown much more sophisticated, due in part to greatly increased research efforts in neuroscience and psychoneuroimmunology. I suspect we are only in the early stages of understanding the complex interplay between the immune system, sleep, neurotransmitters, and hormones. Future research promises to bring us to an even better understanding of how physiological factors can shape mood.

In the next chapter, I describe another major risk factor for postpartum depression – negative birth experiences.

# 6 Negative birth experiences

> The birth of a child, especially a first child, represents a landmark event in the lives of all involved. For the mother particularly, childbirth exerts a profound physical, mental, emotional, and social effect. No other event involves pain, emotional stress, vulnerability, possible physical injury or death, permanent role change, and includes responsibility for a dependent, helpless human being. Moreover, it generally all takes place within a single day. It is not surprising that women tend to remember their first birth experiences vividly and with deep emotion.
>
> (Simkin, 1992: 64)

In Penny Simkin's landmark study (1991, 1992), she documented that women accurately remember details of their births 15 to 20 years later. Not surprisingly, birth experiences had a lasting impact on how women feel about themselves as women and as mothers.

Quality of birth experiences covers a whole range. Some women have wonderful experiences, while others have dreadful ones. Unfortunately, negative birth experiences are more common than we'd like to believe. Some mothers feel they've failed. Others feel betrayed by their partners, doctors, or their own bodies. Still others liken their births to a sexual assault.

How common are negative reactions? One national study has addressed this question (Genevie and Margolies, 1987). Subjects in this study were a nationally representative sample of 1,100 mothers, of ages 18 to 80. Sixty percent of the mothers described their births in predominantly positive terms. This group also included mothers who described their experiences in terms such as "tough, but worth it." However, 40% of mothers in this sample described their births in predominantly negative terms. More concerning, 14% described their births as "peak negative experiences" – one of the worst experiences of their lives. The depth of feeling about their births was expressed in their narratives as well. Several of these women explained that their births had been so difficult that they had elected not to have any more children.

In a more recent study of 60 women who had a cesarean birth, 37% described their experiences as entirely positive (Karlstrom, et al., 2007). In contrast, 63% reported having a mixed or entirely negative experience. Women who had emergency cesareans were twice as likely to describe their experiences as negative than women who had planned cesareans.

In an Australian study of women admitted to a private mother-baby unit for psychiatric care, 53% had had operative births (Fisher, et al., 2002a, 2002b). Thirty-six percent of mothers were disappointed with their births, but this percentage varied by type of birth (66% for cesarean birth, 45% for assisted vaginal, and 20% for unassisted vaginal). Moreover, 52% reported that their postpartum obstetric care was not adequate (Fisher, et al., 2002a).

A study from Italy examined the birth experiences of 160 women who had had normal vaginal births (Cigoli, et al., 2006). The women were assessed at 48 hours and at three to six months postpartum. The researchers found that 1.25% had clinically relevant posttramatic stress disorder (PTSD) following birth, and 29% had symptoms in at least one PTSD subscale. Factors related to traumatic stress reactions included first delivery, perceived low levels of support from family members and medical personnel, anxiety, and previous depression. Cigoli and colleagues (2006) noted that women often perceived delivery as a violent event, in which the fear of destroying the baby and the fear of being destroyed by him/her are both present: "such a link between life and death triggers profound ambivalence, emotional upheaval, and contradictory feelings and behaviors" (91).

## Characteristics of negative birth experiences

Why do some women feel so badly about their births? Researchers who've examined the objective characteristics of births have repeatedly found that type of birth was not related to postpartum emotional response. For example, a recent study examined the objective characteristics of births to determine whether they were related to postpartum depression, maternal functional status, and infant care at two weeks postpartum (Hunker, *et al.*, 2009). Data were collected from OB charts and collected via the Peripartum Events Scale (PES). The categories included precipitous labor; traumatic or life-threatening events; cesarean section due to a medical emergency; midforceps or vaginal breech delivery; significant lacerations; abnormal fetal heart rate, and several other variables related to length of labor or abnormal fetal monitoring results. In this study, 46% were identified as having an adverse unplanned event at their births. Depression rates were also high: 26% were depressed during pregnancy and 21% were depressed at two weeks postpartum. The findings of this study indicated that women with adverse, unplanned events during labor or delivery had varying outcomes regarding depression, functional status, and infant care at two weeks postpartum. The authors concluded that it is plausible to consider that there is not an association between adverse birth events and postpartum depression, even after controlling for depression during pregnancy, antidepressant use at delivery, education, age, and parity.

When listening to women's stories about their births, findings such as the above-cited do not tend to ring true, most likely because they focus on the objective characteristics of the birth. In contrast, Simkin (1991) describes how the subjective aspects of birth are often the most salient. Women who were most satisfied with their births felt that they had accomplished something important, that they were in control, and that birth had significantly contributed to their sense of self-esteem and self-confidence. Women whose births were not satisfying felt as if birth had undermined their confidence, and they vividly recalled things that doctors or nurses said or did that were negative. In this next section, I highlight some of the subjective aspects of birth that have been related to negative reactions.

### Sense of control

Women's subjective sense of control is one of the most consistent predictors of positive feelings after birth. But this sense of control can be difficult to achieve in a hospital setting (Rothman, 1982; Wertz and Wertz, 1989). Hospital deliveries have many aspects that take away women's sense of control. Women are stripped of their clothing and surrounded by strangers. Other people control their most basic functions including when and what they eat and drink, whether they receive pain medication, and whether they can have a support person with them. They are likely to be subjected to a series of internal examinations and may be afraid to object for fear of being labeled a "bad patient." Decisions about obstetric interventions are usually made without their input, and they often have little say about when they leave the hospital.

Simkin (1991) noted that being "in control" included two specific elements. The first was "self-control," which included feeling as though they conducted themselves with discipline and dignity. The second aspect was feeling that they had control over what was happening to them. Some of the women in her studies were still quite angry and disappointed by what doctors and nurses did to them. Indeed, Simkin (1991: 210) noted: "the way a woman is treated by the professionals on whom she depends may largely determine how she feels about the experience for the rest of her life."

### Supportive environment

Another subjective factor is mother's perceived level of care. In a study of 790 women at eight to nine months postpartum, Astbury and colleagues (1994) found that women were at increased risk of depression if they had had a cesarean or assisted vaginal birth; were dissatisfied with their antenatal care; had had an epidural or general anesthesia during delivery, or felt that pain control during labor had been inadequate. The interpersonal aspects of care were also important. Women who described their caregivers as unkind, or who had had unwanted people present during their births, were at increased risk of depression.

In this same sample, intrapartum care was also rated (Brown and Lumley, 1994). Women were more likely to be dissatisfied with their care when they were not involved in decision making, had insufficient information during labor, had a high degree of intervention, and perceived that their caregivers were not helpful. The magnitude of these relationships was also of interest. Lack of information was related to a four- to six-fold increase in dissatisfaction. Perceiving caregivers as unkind was associated with a three-fold increase, and perceiving caregivers as unhelpful was associated with a two- to eight-fold increase in dissatisfaction.

Another study compared the experiences of 203 primiparous women who had either vaginal, assisted vaginal, or cesarean births (Rowe-Murray and Fisher, 2001). The authors found three variables related to postpartum depression at eight months: a high degree of postpartum pain; a perceived lack of support during labor and birth, and a less-than-optimal first contact with their babies. These factors accounted for 35% of the variance in depression.

Elizabeth describes how the social environment of the hospital contributed to her psychic distress and physical pain. In a chart, this birth probably appears "fine," but the mother's subjective experience of it was quite different.

> I had 25 hours of labor. It was long and hard. I was in a city hospital. It was a dirty, unfriendly, and hostile environment. There was urine on the floor of the bathroom in the labor room. There were 100 babies born that day. I had to wait 8 hours to get into a hospital room post-delivery. There were 10–15 women in the post-delivery room waiting for a hospital room, all moaning, with our beds being bumped into each other by the nursing staff. I was taking Demerol for the pain. I had a major episiotomy. I was overwhelmed by it all and in a lot of pain. I couldn't urinate. They kept catheterizing me. My fifth catheterization was really painful. I had lots of swelling and anxiety because I couldn't urinate. My wedding ring was stuck on my finger from my swelling. The night nurse said she'd had patients that had body swelling due to not urinating and their organs had "exploded." Therefore, she catheterized me again. They left the catheter in for an hour and a half. There was lots of pain. My bladder was empty but they wouldn't believe me. I went to sleep and woke up in a panic attack. I couldn't breathe and I couldn't understand what had happened.

In Elizabeth's story, we see themes of helplessness, pain, and dissociation. This birth was still vivid when she described it to me, even though several years had elapsed since it occurred, and she had had a subsequent positive birth after this experience. This birth also occurred in a well-known hospital, where the medical care is purported to be top-notch.

## Pain

Women's pain postpartum can also influence their perceptions of their births. Sixty women undergoing cesarean births reported on their postpartum pain levels (Karlstrom, *et al.*, 2007). Seventy-eight percent of the women reported that their pain was a 4 or higher on the Visual Analog Scale (VAS), which indicated that their pain was inadequately controlled. There was no difference in pain level between women who had planned cesarians and those who had elective cesareans. However, the risk of a negative birth experience was 80% higher for women who had emergency cesareans, and post-operative pain had a negative effect on both breastfeeding and infant care. The authors described how adequate pain relief was essential to facilitate a swift recovery from surgery and emotional bonding with the baby. Women who expected high levels of pain before birth scored higher on the VAS after birth. Sixty-two percent reported that their pain interfered with baby care in the first 24 hours, and one-third indicated that it influenced breastfeeding. In a logistic regression, the two predictors of a negative birth experience were emergency cesarean and experiencing a higher level of pain than they expected.

In another study of post-birth pain, Eisenach and colleagues (2008) found that severity of post-birth pain, but not mode of delivery, predicted postpartum depression. This study was a prospective, longitudinal study of 1,288 women who were hospitalized for either a vaginal or a cesarean delivery. Acute pain increased the risk of persistent pain by 2.5 times, and caused a three-fold increase in postpartum depression. Persistent pain at eight weeks was also related to postpartum depression. The authors indicated that pain is often under-medicated because of limited nursing staff and a hesitancy to use adequate pain medication in breastfeeding women. They noted that opioids and non-steroidal anti-inflammatory drugs (NSAIDs), long the mainstays of acute pain treatment, have warnings about their use during breastfeeding. But these warnings are probably unnecessary (Hale, 2008). Eisenach and colleagues (2008) found higher pain scores for mothers who had had surgical or instrumental vaginal births with perineal lacerations. Ten percent of women who had cesarean births had persistent pain at eight weeks.

Another study examined the relationship between maternal fear prior to delivery, partner's level of fear, and level of postoperative pain for 65 women having planned cesareans (Keogh, *et al.*, 2006). Within this sample, mothers who had negative expectations before birth, and who were fearful before delivery, had higher levels of postoperative pain. Partners' fear and anxiety also influenced maternal postoperative pain. In regression analyses, mother's fear was related to partner's fear, and when mother's and partner's fear were both entered into the equation, partner's fear exacerbated mother's pain. Interestingly, mother's fear was not related to mother's pain.

Pain catastrophizing also increased pain intensity during labor and at two days postpartum in a sample of 82 Israeli women (Ferber, *et al.*, 2005). In this study, pain catastrophizing had three elements: rumination (focusing on increasing pain), magnification (a tendency to exaggerate the consequences of the pain), and helplessness. At six weeks postpartum, pain catastrophizing was related both to postpartum depression, measured by the EPDS, and to social functioning. A high pain score was not related to either variable.

## Prior characteristics of the mother

The mother's previous experiences may also influence how she felt about her birth, and be related to postpartum depression. These include prior traumatic events or prior episodes of depression. In a study from Finland (Saisto, *et al.*, 2001), researchers examined the relationship between disappointment with delivery and personality characteristics, socioeconomic status, prior depression, and fear of labor. They found that pain in labor and emergency cesareans were the strongest predictors of disappointment with delivery. But personality traits, such as anxiety and neuroticism, and depression during pregnancy were the strongest predictors of postpartum depression. Women who had been depressed during their pregnancies were significantly more likely to be disappointed with their deliveries and to develop postpartum depression.

Obstetric complications during pregnancy also predicted depression in a French study of 441 pregnant women (Verdoux, *et al.*, 2002). In contrast, a study from Australia (Johnstone, *et al.*, 2001) found no relation between obstetric complications and postpartum depression. The researchers did find a relationship between postpartum depression and psychosocial risk factors including demographic characteristics, personality characteristics, psychiatric history, and current life-stressors.

Depression and PTSD in late pregnancy can increase the risk of obstetric and neonatal complications, increasing the risk of postpartum depression. In a prospective study of 959 women in Hong Kong, depression in the third trimester was associated with increased use of epidural anesthesia, higher rates of cesarean and instrumental vaginal deliveries, and higher rates of infant admissions to neonatal intensive care units (NICUs) (Chung, *et al.*, 2001). These effects were still present even after the authors controlled for pregnancy complications.

PTSD can also lead to pregnancy complications. In a study of 455 women with PTSD, and 638 comparison women, Seng and colleagues (2001) found that PTSD increased the risk of complications during pregnancy. The women with PTSD had significantly higher rates of ectopic pregnancy, spontaneous abortion, hyperemesis, preterm contractions, and excessive fetal growth. The researchers found no relationship between PTSD and labor variables.

Prior trauma may also influence how pregnancy is experienced, and how many symptoms a mother develops. For example, a case control study of 82 women with low-birth-weight infants, and 91 women with normal-weight babies, assessed women for a history of child sexual abuse. The sexually abused women were not more likely to have a low-birth-weight baby. However, they were more likely to smoke during pregnancy. They also had more health complaints during pregnancy and used more antenatal healthcare services. They did not have more obstetric complications (Grimstad and Schei, 1999).

A prospective study of 298 women attempting vaginal births found that prenatal stress was associated with cesarean delivery (Saunders, *et al.*, 2006). Highly stressed women were more likely to receive analgesia, which increased the risk of surgical delivery. Women who received both meperidine and an epidural had the highest rates of cesarean delivery. One possible explanation has to do with the role of stress in prolonging pain, lowering pain tolerance, and exacerbating physical reactions to acute pain. Data analysis controlled for previous cesarean, diabetes, primiparity, advanced maternal age, morbid obesity, medical induction, pre-eclampsia, and meconium staining – all potential confounds.

In contrast, a Dutch study of 354 healthy nulliparous pregnant women found that no psychosocial risk factors predicted instrumental deliveries or cesarean births (van de Pol, *et al.*, 2006). Specifically, the researchers found that social support during pregnancy, lack of depressive symptoms, and specific pregnancy traits are not protective against instrumental and cesarean delivery. In contrast, characteristics of the labor itself were: higher fetal weight, non-occiput anterior presentation and advance gestational age, and fetal distress. They found no independent contributions of personality characteristics or depression on mode of delivery. Oddly, they found that if the women had a better relationship with their partners, this was predictive of higher rates of instrumental and cesarean deliveries. The researcher had no explanation for this finding.

The above discussion has been about birth experiences in general. It is now time to turn our discussion to a form of birth that has been the focus of the majority of research on negative birth experiences: cesarean sections.

## Cesarean sections: are they always negative?

For 25 years, there has been concern about the high rate of cesarean sections in industrialized nations. In 1985, the World Health Organization (WHO) stated that 15% was the highest acceptable limit for national cesarean rates. It based this number on findings from countries with the world's lowest rates of perinatal mortality (WHO cited in Belizan, *et al.*, 1999).

In many developed countries, the number of cesarean sections carried out is well above the recommended WHO rate. There is not enough space here to debate the subject of whether cesareans are usually justified. The issue of concern is the psychological impact of this procedure. The dominant paradigm for studying the impact of birth on women's emotional health has used cesarean sections as the prototype of the "negative" experience, while the vaginal birth is more commonly the "positive" one. As I described above, the issue is more complex than this simple distinction. However, there have been some consistent findings about the impact of cesareans on women. These studies are described below.

In a prospective study of 272 Australian women, Fisher and colleagues (1997) assessed the psychological outcomes of various types of birth. They found that the total number of obstetric interventions made little difference, but that there were significant differences based on the type of delivery. Women who had cesareans were significantly more likely to have negative moods and low self-esteem, whereas women who had spontaneous vaginal deliveries had the most positive moods. Women with assisted vaginal deliveries were somewhere between the two groups.

Fisher, *et al.* (1997) noted several negative factors related to cesarean births. Women who had cesareans were significantly less likely to have their partners present, to see their babies in the first five minutes after birth, or hold them after delivery. Indeed, 31% did not get to hold their babies within the first eight hours after birth. These infants were not more likely to be admitted to the NICU, suggesting that there was routine separation of mothers and babies following cesarean sections. Moreover, women who had cesarean births were significantly more likely to require narcotic pain medication, and to develop postpartum physical complications.

Personal control also varied by type of delivery in this study (Fisher, *et al.*, 1997). Fifty-six percent of women who had had unassisted vaginal deliveries felt that they had personal control over their deliveries compared with 19% of the women who had had cesarean sections. There was no significant difference in the reactions of those who had emergency vs. planned cesarean sections. The authors concluded that operative childbirth carries "significant psychological risks rendering those who experience these procedures vulnerable to a grief reaction or to posttraumatic distress and depression" (Fisher, *et al.*, 1997: 728). The prospective design allowed them to draw causal inferences, and to find that the reactions of the women could not be attributed to pre-existing symptoms.

Durik and colleagues (2000) had contrasting findings. They compared women who had vaginal deliveries (N=74), women who had planned cesareans (N=37), and women who had unplanned cesareans (N=56). The women were assessed at one, four, and twelve months postpartum. As predicted, women with unplanned cesareans appraised their deliveries more negatively than women with planned cesareans or vaginal deliveries at one and four months. But there were no differences by delivery type for postpartum depression or self-esteem.

Another large study (N=1,596) of planned cesarean sections vs. vaginal deliveries for breech presentation had similar findings. The authors found no significant difference in rates of postpartum depression between the two groups (Hannah, *et al.*, 2002). Both groups had a rate of approximately 10%. Breastfeeding rates were also high in both groups and not significantly different. Also, 78% of women found it "easy" or "very easy" to care for their infants, and approximately 82% of the total sample found adjusting to motherhood "easy" or "very easy."

There were some differences in how women perceived their experiences, and what they liked or disliked about them. For example, women in the planned-cesarean group liked the fact that they were able to schedule their delivery, that their experience was not painful, and that they felt reassured about the health of their babies. Women in the planned-vaginal group indicated that they liked the fact that their births were natural, that they were able to actively participate in their births, and that recovery from childbirth was not difficult. Both groups felt reassured about their own health (Hannah, *et al.*, 2002).

Another study compared 40 women who had had four types of birth: spontaneous vaginal, induced vaginal, instrumental vaginal, and emergency cesarean (Maclean, *et al.*, 2000). They found that women who had had the instrumental delivery with episiotomy rated their birth as more distressing, and were less satisfied with the efficacy of pain relief during labor than women in the other three groups. In contrast, women with emergency cesareans reported little distress, lower perceived risk of injury, and significantly greater satisfaction with pain relief. There was no significant difference between the groups in terms of depressive symptoms.

A recent review that specifically examined the relationship between cesarean birth and postpartum depression indicated that the most methodologically sound studies found either no association or mixed results (Carter, *et al.*, 2006). The authors reviewed 24 studies and found that 5 showed an adverse relationship, 15 showed no significant association, and 4 had mixed reactions. They noted that the methodologically superior studies showed no difference and concluded that the link between cesarean delivery and postpartum depression has not been established.

Cesarean delivery impacted women's responsiveness to their babies in another study (Swain, *et al.*, 2008). This study used functional magnetic resonance imaging to view mothers' responses to the crying of their own babies. Mothers needed to differentiate between their babies' cries and cries of other babies. The researchers compared six mothers who had had cesareans and six mothers who had had vaginal deliveries. They found that women who had vaginal deliveries were more responsive in the relevant areas of their brains (e.g. hypothalamus, frontal cortex, hypothalamus, and basal ganglia) than women who had cesareans at two to four weeks postpartum. They also found that independent of mode of delivery, parental worries and mood were related to specific brain activations in response to their own baby's cry.

In summary, the results of the above-cited studies indicate that cesarean births can cause negative reactions for women who experience them. Women who received ample support following their cesareans and who had input in the decision-making process, however, were significantly less likely to have negative reactions. These variations in responses also indicate that it is not the procedure of cesarean delivery *per se* that causes negative reactions.

Therefore, cesarean sections are not always negative if they are medically necessary and women are provided with support and reassurance, and are involved in decisions that concern them.

## Negative vs. traumatic birth

In the prior section, I described some of the factors that led to women having negative birth experiences. Many of these experiences can result in depression, without necessarily producing psychological trauma. However, birth can also produce traumatic-stress reactions, and can lead to an additional diagnosis of PTSD. Even women who do not meet full criteria for PTSD may have some trauma symptoms, such as intrusive thoughts or flashbacks, and these can be troublesome (O'Leary, 2005). According to the review by Alder and colleagues (2006), 1.3% to 6% of women met full criteria for PTSD after birth, with approximately 24% to 30% having posttraumatic symptoms. PTSD after childbirth may result in social isolation, sleep difficulties, and hypervigilance in relation to signs and symptoms in the baby. PTSD is not restricted to women who have had cesareans; women who have had vaginal deliveries can be traumatized too, particularly if they felt they or their infants were in danger (O'Leary, 2005). In fact, as Alder, *et al.* (2006) described, the majority of women who develop PTSD after birth have normal vaginal deliveries, supporting the view that women's subjective experiences of labor are important in determining their reaction to it.

### Diagnostic criteria for PTSD

According to *DSM IV TR* Criteria (American Psychiatric Association, 2000), a traumatic event is one in which the person felt that death or serious injury was possible for themselves or a loved one, and the person responded with fear, helplessness, or horror. In addition, there must be symptoms in each of these clusters: (1) re-experiencing: frequent re-experiencing of the event via nightmares or intrusive thoughts; (2) avoidance: numbing or lack of responsiveness to or avoidance of places that remind patients of their trauma, and (3) hyperarousal: persistent symptoms of increased arousal including jumpiness, sleep disturbances or poor concentration. PTSD is acute if the symptoms have been present for less than three months, and chronic if the symptoms have been present for three months or more. The onset of PTSD is considered "delayed" if it occurs six months or more after the initial stressor.

### Birth as a traumatizing experience

Below is a summary of studies that have shown that some women will meet full criteria for birth-related PTSD. In one study, 289 women were followed prospectively, and they were assessed at thirty-six weeks' gestation, and six weeks and six months postpartum. Women with pre-existing PTSD or depression were not included in the analyses. The authors found that at six weeks, 2.8% of women met full criteria for PTSD. At six months postpartum, 1.5% still met criteria and had developed chronic PTSD (Ayers and Pickering, 2001).

Another study assessed 264 women with unassisted vaginal births assessed at seventy-two hours and six weeks postpartum (Czarnocka and Slade, 2000). Three percent of the women met full criteria for PTSD and had clinically significant levels of intrusion, avoidance, and hyperarousal. Further, 24% had at least one symptom. The factors that predicted traumatic-stress symptoms were similar to those that predicted depression. They included a low level of partner or staff support, and low perceived control during labor.

In a study of 64 couples nine weeks after giving birth, Ayers and colleagues (2007) found that 5% of men and women had severe symptoms of PTSD (avoidance and re-experiencing). The couples who experienced PTSD symptoms had complications, but both groups had had normal vaginal deliveries. The symptoms were strongly associated within couples, and the PTSD symptoms affected neither the parent–infant bond nor the couple's relationship. They concluded that men and women have comparable levels of PTSD after birth, and that PTSD symptoms had little short-term impact on the couple's relationship and parent–infant bonding. The long-term effects are unknown.

The percentage of women who meet full criteria for PTSD may, at first, seem small. But the percentage is similar to that for people who experience other types of trauma. For example, in the weeks following the September 11, 2001 terrorist attacks on New York City, the rate of PTSD in lower Manhattan was 7.5% (Galea, *et al.*, 2003). This percentage is not significantly larger than the up to 6% that other studies have found following birth. The fact that there are *any* women who meet full criteria for PTSD should alert us that something is seriously amiss. And that 24% to 30% had some symptoms is quite concerning. As a culture, we probably need to rethink how we handle women in labor – especially those who are already vulnerable because of prior traumatic events.

## A model for a trauma-producing experience

A model I've found helpful in understanding birth-related trauma is Charles Figley's conceptualization of characteristics of a trauma-producing event. According to Figley (1986), events are troubling to the extent that they are sudden, dangerous, and overwhelming. These three characteristics have a great deal of relevance to birth, and can explain why mothers might be bothered by their experiences. Suddenness occurs when an event strikes and there is not time to prepare, devise an escape plan, or prevent the event. This certainly occurs when women are in labor; change can happen in seconds and there may be little time to react.

The dangerousness of the situation is the second element. Many women perceive that their labor is life-threatening for themselves or their babies (Figley, 1986). In terms of PTSD, it is the mother's perception that matters, not whether her perceptions are medically "true." The situation is similar to that of a crime victim who believes that she will be killed – even if the criminal had no intention of killing her. What she believes is much more relevant to her subsequent reaction than the actual facts associated with the event.

The final element is the extent to which the situation is overwhelming. Some women describe being swept away by their birth experiences and the hospital routines. Being overwhelmed leads to a sense of temporary helplessness and of being out of control. They are overwhelmed by what is happening and cut off from important information. The same can be true for her partner. Sally's emergency cesarean had all three aspects that are likely to put women at risk for traumatic-stress reactions. Her baby was born within 15 minutes of when the cord prolapsed after Sally had been in labor for 23 hours. Her delivery was by cesarean section under general anesthesia.

> They had me on the bed, rear end in the air. My head was down between the headboard and the mattress. The nurse had to hold the baby off the cord. All I kept hearing was "OB emergency, OB emergency" over the loudspeaker, while the nurse kept saying in my ear that the baby would be fine. Everything happened so quickly, I didn't have time to react.

## Possible interventions for negative birth experiences

If you are concerned that a mother has had a traumatic birth, you may want to ask her some questions about it. Alder, *et al.* (2006) recommended screening women for PTSD and PTSD symptoms in the first three weeks after birth. Some possible questions that can be asked about the birth itself and the presence of post-traumatic symptoms are listed below (Alder, *et al.*, 2006). Regarding the birth:

- What was your experience of pain during labor and was your pain adequately addressed?
- Did you feel involved in the decisions that were made regarding your care? Did you have support from your partner or health care team?
- Did you feel that you or your baby might die during the birth?

Regarding trauma symptoms, questions could include:

- Do you avoid thinking about your birth?
- Have you had negative dreams about your birth?
- Do you find yourself thinking about your birth without meaning to?
- Are you having any problems falling or staying asleep?
- Have you been more tense, nervous, irritable, or anxious?
- Are you avoiding people and places that remind you of your birth?

### *Interventions that allow women to talk about their birth*

For women who have had emotionally difficult births, follow-up has been helpful. In one study, parents were interviewed regarding their distress following childbirth (Adler, *et al.*, 2006). If they were distressed, they were randomized into intervention and normal-care groups. The intervention was a 40- to 60-minute counseling session at three days, and a follow-up telephone call at four to six weeks postpartum. At three months, women in the intervention group had lower PTSD total symptom scores than the normal-care group. The intervention group also had lower depression levels, lower self-blame, and higher confidence scores about having another baby. The authors recommended that interventions include counseling about subsequent pregnancies and birth options, and strategies that help lower patient anxiety. A final component was relaxation training including muscle relaxation and guided imagery.

A similar type of intervention is debriefing. Debriefing occurs when a midwife or other healthcare provider talks to women about their births, and allows them to ask questions and discuss any of their feelings of sadness, guilt, anger, or confusion. The results have been mixed as to whether debriefing is helpful to mothers. In one randomized trial, mothers in England were randomly assigned to a debriefing (N=56) or to a standard-care (N=58) condition (Lavender and Walkinshaw, 1998). Midwives provided debriefing that included listening, support, counseling, understanding, and explanation of treatment. At three weeks postpartum, those who received the intervention were significantly less likely to be anxious or depressed.

In contrast, an Australian study of 917 women who had had either cesarean sections, or vaginal births using forceps or vacuum extraction, found that a slightly *higher* percentage of debriefed women were depressed and in poorer health at six months postpartum than women assigned to standard care. These differences between the groups were not significant, however.

Indeed, the overall percentages of depressed women were small (17% vs. 14% for debriefed vs. standard care, respectively) (Small, *et al.*, 2000). Interestingly, these results occurred even though mothers reported that the intervention had been helpful to them. A higher percentage also reported that depression had been a problem for them since the birth (28% vs. 22%). The authors concluded that debriefing was ineffective, and expressed some caution.

In discussing this study, Boyce and Condon (2001) noted some methodological points that temper these findings. First, they noted that debriefing is for the prevention of PTSD, not of depression. Given that, it is not surprising that this intervention did not have an impact on depression. They also noted that women who had had elective vs. emergency procedures were grouped together, and that may have obscured the findings. Finally, they questioned the usefulness of having a midwife debrief who had not been present at the birth. They wondered how she could answer women's questions when she had not been there. The authors also pointed out that even though this particular intervention was not effective, women need to have the opportunity to discuss their experiences.

A review (Gamble, *et al.*, 2002) of midwife-led debriefing found there was insufficient evidence as to the effectiveness of debriefing. The methodological issues Gamble and colleagues (2002) raised included a lack of a standardized debriefing intervention, a lack of comprehensive outcome variables including the non-inclusion of trauma symptoms, and lack of inclusion of the woman's partner in the debriefing. The authors concluded that a single-session intervention would probably be insufficient to deal with the problem. However, they acknowledged that there may have been some benefit to the women of being able to talk with a person about their births. On the other hand, women who had been most deeply traumatized by their births may have been so numb from the experience, or may have desired so strongly to "just get back to normal," that any intervention immediately after the experience would have been pointless.

Astbury, *et al.* (1994) also explained how women may re-evaluate their births after the initial danger has passed, and the crisis of the first few months has resolved. Particularly in the case of a birth where there is a high amount of intervention, the initial reaction may be to just be happy that they survived the experience. Only later may they allow themselves to question some of what was done in the hospital. This could create a delayed response, where, in subsequent months, the birth is viewed more negatively.

Simkin (1992) echoes this possible explanation. In exploring the nature of memory changes over time, she noted that there is often a halo that occurs shortly after birth, where women will gloss over negative parts of their experiences in their initial euphoria. With time, the halo fades and aspects of birth are looked at more realistically. Because of this delay, caregivers are usually blithely unaware of the impact of their actions on the women they serve. Many providers do not realize that women are often quite upset by their births, and that these negative feelings can last for years.

## Conclusion

Women who have had traumatic or difficult birth experiences must acknowledge their trauma if they are ever to move past it. Trying to "just forget it" is not an effective strategy, and trauma that is not acknowledged and dealt with can manifest itself in a variety of destructive and negative behaviors. Women who have not processed their birth experience may manifest symptoms such as depression, blunted affect, and inability to empathize with others (including their infants), helplessness, self-destructive behaviors, somatic complaints, sexual dysfunctions, marital difficulties, anger, and hostility. They may also become pregnant again before they are physically and emotionally ready to do so in order to do things differently "this time." Working through trauma is difficult, but it is the only route to healing.

As a result of working through trauma, a woman has acknowledged and given herself permission to feel pain and anger following her experience. She may need a period of time to grieve over her experience. As trauma and grief are reclaimed, she can give meaning to the events and move forward. She may even come to value her experience and try to do something to help other people.

In conclusion, the research literature on recovery from traumatic events contains a message of hope: people can and do recover from traumatic events. The most important components of any intervention focus on helping women acknowledge and accept their experiences, and helping them regain a sense of efficacy. More specific information on trauma-related treatment is to be found in Chapter 12.

# 7 Infant characteristics and depression in their mothers

Developmental psychologists once believed that mothers influenced their babies, but that the reverse was not true. Eventually, researchers discovered what now seems glaringly obvious; that babies bring quite a lot to the interaction, and could indeed be a major influence on their mothers' emotional state. There are two infant characteristics in particular that influence mothers: infant temperament and infant health status. These are described below.

## Infant temperament

Babies bring their own personalities to their relationships with their mothers. Babies' personalities include how much they cry; how shy they are; how distractible, irritable, soothable, and active. Infant personality is more commonly known as infant temperament. Broadly defined, temperament is a behavioral style and characteristic way of responding to people and the environment.

The most commonly cited work on infant temperament is that of Chess and Thomas (Chess and Thomas, 1977; McGrath, *et al.*, 2008; Thomas and Chess, 1987). Chess and Thomas described infant temperament as falling into three basic types: easy, difficult, and slow-to-warm-up. In their longitudinal study, Chess and Thomas (1977) classified 40% of the children as "easy," 10% as "difficult," and 15% as "slow-to-warm-up." The remaining 35% were somewhere between these three categories. Thomas and Chess (1987) conceptualized temperament as a stable characteristic of newborns that is later shaped and modified by the child's experiences, including how well their personalities match those of their mother's. If the mother and baby's temperaments are in synchrony, there is said to be "goodness of fit." If mothers and babies don't seem to fit together, there is said to be asynchrony between mother and child (McGrath, *et al.*, 2008).

The child with a difficult temperament is central to the topic of the infant's impact on postpartum depression. Difficult infants have strong emotional reactions; cry for long periods of time; are hard to comfort; slow to accept new people, foods, or routines; and less easy to predict or regulate in their eating, sleeping, or elimination schedules. Mothers might describe these babies as "colicky" (Canivet, *et al.*, 2002; Cutrona and Troutman, 1986).

Babies with difficult temperaments can be challenging to care for. They are often unadaptable and irritable, and can make mothers' efforts to soothe them seem ineffective. In a diary study of mothers of newborns (Canivet, *et al.*, 2002), the rate of infant colic was 9.4%, similar to the percentage of babies identified as "difficult" by Chess and Thomas (1977). When babies have difficult temperaments, mothers may conclude that they are not effective or competent (Beck, 1996b), and begin to resent their babies. In addition, they are often afraid to share their feelings with others, as this mother describes.

> My first baby screamed from the day he was born. He screamed all the time, even in the hospital. He reacted oddly to all kinds of different things. The pediatrician said he was a "difficult" child. Even now, he has to have things always the same. When I went back for a check up at two weeks, a nurse asked me how the baby was. She said "aren't they wonderful?" I didn't know what to say. I thought he was the pits.

Cutrona and Troutman (1986) causally linked infant temperament to postpartum depression. They assessed 55 married women during pregnancy and at three months postpartum. The authors found that caring for a difficult infant gradually eroded a mother's feelings of competence as a parent and her overall sense of well-being. When a direct link between infant temperament and maternal depression was examined, infant difficulty alone accounted for 30% of the variance in depression. Prolonged exposure to such infants may make their mothers feel ambivalent toward them, resulting in guilt and self-hatred. When mothers feel this way, they often withdraw from others. A temperamentally difficult infant may disrupt several aspects of a woman's life, as Barbara describes.

> When the baby started throwing up, I felt terrible. I wouldn't go any place with her because I didn't want people to see her screaming. I wanted to be the perfect mother. My mother-in-law said "you've got to relax. She's picking up on your cues." The baby had a difficult temperament. Even now, she's very stubborn and strong-willed. The control issue is big for me. I'm a perfectionist and always have been. I don't want the baby to experiment with food, even though I know it's normal. I don't want her to do it. I wanted this baby so bad. When she came, I hated her. I thought of throwing her out the window. I just wanted her to die. I spanked her when she was three or four weeks old, and I'm still dealing with the guilt of it. I'd yell at her, right in her face "I hate you. I wish you would die."

In a longitudinal study of 139 women, data were collected at eight months' gestation and at two and six months postpartum (McGrath, *et al.*, 2008). Depressed mothers reported that their infants had more difficult temperament at both measurement points. These differences were still apparent even after controlling for mothers' history of abuse or anxiety disorders (both more common among the depressed mothers). There was no difference between the depressed and non-depressed mothers for childcare stress or perceived support. The author recommended interventions that increased goodness of fit between mothers and babies.

A study of 74 first-time mothers and 58 first-time fathers in Switzerland examined the relationship between stress, depression, psychopathology, and child difficulty during pregnancy and at 1, 3, 12, and 18 months postpartum (Perren, *et al.*, 2005). Psychopathology was assessed on the German version of the Revised Symptom Checklist and included measures of somatization, depression, paranoid ideation, obsessive-compulsion, and psychoticism. They found that child difficulty was associated with increased stress, but only for some parents. Surprisingly, child difficulty had a greater effect on fathers than it did on mothers. Contrary to prediction, child difficulty was not associated with increased depressive symptoms. Depressive symptoms decreased in both fathers and mothers from pregnancy to 18 months postpartum. Unlike depression, stress did not decrease across assessment points.

### Infant crying and colic

Infant crying is the most salient behavior in babies with difficult temperaments. Crying can be very challenging for new parents to cope with, and is one of the most common reasons for pediatric visits in the first three months. Colic is usually diagnosed using the "Wessel" criteria: crying or fussing that lasts more than three hours a day, occurring on more than three days in any week, for three weeks or longer (Pauli-Pott, *et al.*, 2000). There is some evidence that colic, or persistent infant crying, can persist even past the first three months (Wolke, *et al.*, 2002).

Kitzinger (1990) gathered a sample of 1,400 women from England, New Zealand and Australia. Out of these, she drew a sample of 100 women whose babies cried the most (more than six hours a day) and 100 women whose babies cried the least (less than two hours a day). Not surprisingly, she found striking differences between the two groups. Eighty percent of mothers of babies who cried the most were depressed (compared with 33% of mothers whose babies cried the least); 57% described a desperate need to escape (compared with 22%); 50% were "itching" to smack the baby (compared with 20%), and 33% made negative comments about their partners (compared with 4%). Common themes included feeling trapped; that they couldn't get away; that they felt guilty, useless, exhausted, inadequate, and bewildered.

The study by Bond and colleagues (2001) of 116 mothers of colicky babies found high levels of psychological distress and anxiety. The mothers reported low self-efficacy, low levels of attachment to the baby, and were less satisfied with their lives since having their babies. Social support did not ameliorate the effects. More recently, infant colic was present in 22% of babies in a prospective, longitudinal study (Akman, *et al.*, 2006). Of the mothers whose babies had colic, 13% had an EPDS score of greater than 13. The mean EPDS score for mothers of babies with colic was significantly higher than it was for mothers whose babies didn't have colic. Moreover, 63% of mothers of babies with colic had an insecure attachment style compared with 31% of mothers whose babies did not. The authors concluded that infant colic was associated with both depressive symptoms and insecure attachment style.

Similarly, Pauli-Pott, *et al.* (2000) found that even when babies did not meet Wessel criteria, mothers were significantly more likely to feel angry and nervous, and to believe that babies cried because they were dissatisfied with their mothers. Mothers in this study appeared to have great difficulty tolerating their babies' crying and handling their babies. These mothers often felt rejected by their babies, and the mothers reacted with anger and disappointment.

Infant crying can also put the infants at risk for being abused. In a study of 84 parents, 32 were considered to be at high risk for physically abusing their children (Crouch, *et al.*, 2008). High-risk and low-risk parents were asked to watch a video of an infant crying. As expected, high-risk parents rated the crying infant more negatively and had more hostile feelings after they had watched the video than did low-risk parents.

Persistent crying in infancy may also be related to problems later on. In a prospective study of 64 infants referred for persistent crying, Wolke, *et al.* (2002) followed-up with them at 8 to 10 years of age, and compared them with a matched sample of 64 classmates. At follow-up, 19% of the children referred for persistent crying had hyperactivity problems compared with only 2% of the control children. Parents, and the children themselves, reported more conduct problems. Parents of the persistent criers rated their children's temperaments as more negative, difficult, and demanding. The academic achievement of persistent criers was significantly lower than that of the control children. This was especially true for those with hyperactivity. There was no difference in current depression for mothers.

### Depression-related distortions

An issue that frequently arises in the study of infant temperament is whether the difficulties are real, or simply a matter of depressed mothers seeing their children in a more negative light

(Najman, *et al.*, 2000). Mothers' mental representations of their infants can influence how they interpret their infants' behaviors, and in turn, their response to their infants. And this can influence how settled their babies are. In one study (Rosenblum, *et al.*, 2002), mothers' beliefs about their infants had an impact on infant affect regulation over and above the impact of maternal depression. In addition, Rosenblum and colleagues (2002) found that mothers with distorted representations of their infants were more likely also to report depressive symptoms.

A study from Sweden (Canivet, *et al.*, 2002) found a sub-group of infants who were genuinely colicky by objective measure. Interestingly, women who indicated, during late pregnancy, that there was a risk of spoiling a baby with too much contact were more likely to have a colicky baby. Infants of these mothers were more distressed, even when given the same amount of physical contact as other babies.

## Mothers' perceptions of older children

The effects of depression on mothers' perception of their children lasts well past infancy. Maternal depression led to negative biases in reporting children's symptoms of attention-deficit hyperactivity disorder (ADHD), general behavior problems, and their own negative parenting styles, compared with laboratory assessment, in a sample of 96 children aged 6 to 10 years old (Chi and Hinshaw, 2002).

Mothers who were depressed or anxious were also more likely to report behavior problems in their children at 14 years of age (Najman, *et al.*, 2000). There was a systematic difference in the way mothers reported on the behavior of their children. Since there was no outside verification of the children's behavior in this study (such as teacher or friend report), the authors had no way of knowing whether the children actually did have more behavior problems. The authors suggested that mothers who are depressed may have more difficulties in coping with their children's behaviors, and may perceive them as more negative across the board.

## The impact of maternal depression and elevated cortisol

There is some debate in the field about whether mothers' depression and/or stress can physiologically alter babies' temperament, either prenatally or via breastfeeding. A study of 247 full-term infants assessed mothers at 18 to 20, 24 to 26, and 30 to 32 weeks' gestation and 2 months postpartum (Davis, *et al.*, 2007). Infant temperament was assessed at 2 months postpartum via the fear subscale of the Infant Temperament Questionnaire. They noted that elevated maternal cortisol levels at 30 to 32 weeks' gestation was related to infant negative reactivity. This was not true for elevated cortisol earlier in the pregnancy. Moreover, the researchers found an association between prenatal anxiety and depression and infant temperament. Maternal cortisol was highest at 30 to 32 weeks' gestation and lowest at the postpartum assessment. The findings were independent of sex of the infant, mode of delivery, parity, or feeding method.

In a study of 253 two-month olds, breastfeeding mothers with higher cortisol levels had babies who showed higher levels of fear behaviors (Glynn, *et al.*, 2007). This relationship was not observed among the formula-feeding mothers. Glucocorticoids easily pass the blood-brain barrier and can be passed to infants via breast milk. The limbic regions of the brain are highly sensitive to their effects. The mothers in the breastfeeding and formula-feeding groups were similar in terms of mean cortisol levels and distributions. Cortisol was not directly assessed in the milk, but was assessed in maternal plasma. The findings were based on maternal reports of infant temperament, so this variable could be more accurately called "maternal perception of infant fear." The authors concluded that breast milk is a potential avenue by which mothers' fear can be communicated to their infants.

In contrast to these findings, breastfeeding has also been shown to increase babies' resilience to psychosocial stress (Montgomery, *et al.*, 2006). These data were part of a longitudinal birth cohort from the U.K. The researchers found that babies who were breastfed were less susceptible to stress following their parents' divorce than babies who were not breastfed. The outcome variable was children's anxiety level at age 10. This effect held even after controlling for possible confounding factors. Although this study is intriguing, the measure of breastfeeding was pretty poor and it does not appear that the amount of breastfeeding was responsible for the effect. The authors themselves felt that breastfeeding may simply be a marker for other resilience factors in women's lives. They also felt that breastfeeding may have had this effect because it downregulated the HPA-axis and probably prevented maternal depression, which would have improved the mother–infant bond.

In summary, if infants have difficult temperaments, this can have a negative impact on their mothers' emotional state. But a mother's depression can also influence how she sees her child's behavior. As described in Chapter 2, interventions that both address depression and give mothers tools to cope with the behavior of their children are more likely to be effective.

## Infant health issues

> My first child was premature. He was born at 35 weeks with severe Hyaline Membrane Disease. He was in the hospital for five months; in the NICU for four months and in intermediate care for one month. The depression started around the time he was three or four weeks old. Up until that time, everything had been so urgent. He had had a couple of arrests. It was overwhelming. Suddenly my son was doing better. Why was I feeling so bad? I had difficulties going to sleep. I was up several times during the night. It was difficult to wake up in the morning. I didn't want to do anything during the day except sleep and call the NICU to check in. I started not to eat well. I felt an impending sense of doom. The depression lasted about a month.
>
> About a month after he came home, I felt physically depressed, same as in the initial postpartum period. I brought home a very sick baby. I think it was a delayed reaction, reliving the early part. [Patricia]

Infants with health problems can also influence their mothers' emotional state. Yet postpartum depression is often overlooked in women whose babies are not healthy. It is important that we don't overlook depression because feelings from the postpartum period can have a long-term impact on how a mother copes, how she sees her child, and her level of attachment. I first describe prematurity, then illness and disability.

### *Prematurity*

The birth of a premature infant precipitates a psychological crisis. Women who give birth prematurely must face the reality of an infant who may be sickly or fragile when they themselves are psychologically and physically depleted. Mothers may experience guilt for an early delivery, or anxiety regarding the viability and morbidity of their infants. The babies may also be born following a history of infertility, difficult pregnancy, and/or an emergency delivery.

Some of the aspects associated with medical care of a premature or sick newborn may contribute to the mother's grief and depression. Jan, who had a very difficult pregnancy and delivery, described her feelings after the birth of her daughter. Her daughter was delivered six weeks premature, via emergency cesarean section, after Jan developed eclampsia.

> They took her away right after delivery. I never got to hold her, after all that [the difficult pregnancy and delivery]. They brought her back, but my arms were tied to the delivery table. I wish they had released at least one arm. It was really hard. Leaving the hospital without the baby was really bad. I left early because I didn't want to leave at 11 am with all the other moms and babies. I shouldn't complain because she only had a few preemie problems. Others in the nursery were so sick. But it was very stressful. It was awful to see them putting the feeding tube down her throat, hearing her gagging and crying. It makes me cry now just to think about it.

Depression can take place at many different times throughout an infant's illness. Mothers may be particularly at risk immediately following their deliveries, after any medical crisis, when the mother must leave the hospital without the baby, when the baby is about to be discharged, or after the baby is home. A mother's risk of depression is further increased if the baby is transferred to another hospital, particularly if the hospital is in another city. If mothers follow their babies to these other hospitals, they may be cut off from their normal support systems, including their partners.

In some cases, especially with babies who are very sick, mothers may experience anticipatory grieving, and begin to mourn the loss of their infants. In this process, they may distance themselves from their babies in order to prepare themselves for their babies' eventual death. When babies recover, this process of mourning is interrupted, and mothers have to readjust.

*Severity of illness*

Severity of illness or degree of prematurity can also influence maternal mental health. The range of illnesses or problems of premature infants varies from very low birth weight (<1,500 g) to those who might have some minor complications. Some babies are hospitalized for only a few days, while others may be in intensive care for several weeks or months.

A study of 40 parents of babies in the NICU found that 44% of the mothers met full criteria for acute stress disorder, while none of the fathers did (Shaw, *et al.*, 2006). Acute stress disorder is the precursor syndrome to PTSD, and was also associated with alternations in the parental role, family cohesiveness, and emotional restraint. Alterations in the parental role included not being able to help, hold or care for the infant, protect the infant from pain, or share the infant with other family members. The subjective appraisal of the seriousness of the illness was more predictive of mothers' reactions than the objective disease characteristics – consistent with PTSD related to other medical conditions. Family environment and parental coping style were significantly associated with trauma symptoms. The authors recommended that care providers help with parental feelings of helplessness and inadequacy, even with severely ill infants.

A longitudinal study of 30 preterm, very low-birth-weight babies examined the relationship between medical complications and developmental outcomes at 36 months (Miceli, *et al.*, 2000). Birth status and medical complications were recorded during the baby's hospital stay. Social support data were collected at 4 months, and developmental measures were taken at 4 and 13 months corrected age, and 36 months chronological age. Medical complications only mediated the relationship at 4 and 13 months, but not at 36 months. Maternal social support and maternal distress were not related to infant outcomes at 4 and 13 months. In the early months, medical complications heightened the risk of depression and accounted for a substantial amount of the variance in developmental outcomes. However, at 36 months maternal distress was related to both the child's internalizing and externalizing behaviors. Maternal social support was related to child linguistic function and internalizing behaviors, but not externalizing, at 36 months. These effects were mediated by the medical condition of the child, accounting for a substantial amount of the variance.

In a study of 30 mothers of premature babies, ways of coping, knowledge of infant development, and ways mothers used to gain information were all related to depressive symptoms (Veddovi, *et al.*, 2001). Mothers who used informal ways of gaining information about infants (e.g. via other mothers), who used more avoidance coping, and who had less accurate information about infant development were significantly more likely to become depressed. These three variables accounted for 48% of the variance in maternal depression.

Mandated bedrest during pregnancy can also make mothers feel that their babies are at high risk (Maloni, *et al.*, 2002). In a study or 63 women who were admitted to hospitals for antepartum bedrest, dysphoria was related to obstetric risk. Women whose pregnancies had the highest risk scores had the highest levels of dysphoria. Gestational age and health of the baby at birth were significantly correlated with postpartum dysphoria.

Women are at risk for depression after using assisted reproductive technologies (ART) as well (Monti, *et al.*, 2009). In this Italian study, a sample of 48 parents (25 mothers, 23 fathers) who used assisted technology was compared with 39 non-ART mothers at 30 to 32 weeks' gestation, and at 1 week and 3 months postpartum. The researchers found that the ART mothers were more depressed at all assessment points than the non-ART women, with the highest rate during pregnancy. Interestingly, the men in ART couples were not depressed at the first two assessment points, but were at month 3. Monti and colleagues (2009) concluded that women using ART are more vulnerable to depression that may persist until after delivery, and suggested ongoing monitoring for this possibility.

## Prior infant loss

Mothers who have premature babies may also have a history of infertility, miscarriage or fetal loss, and this can also increase their risk for depression and anxiety with subsequent pregnancies (Geller, 2004). Janssen and colleagues (1996) compared 227 women whose babies had died with 213 who gave birth to live babies. Six months later, women whose babies had died showed greater depression, anxiety, and somatization than women who had given birth to live babies. At one year, the mental health symptoms had subsided, and the women who lost babies appeared comparable to those who had not lost babies. However, the authors noted that pregnancy loss is a stressful life event that can lead to a marked deterioration in a women's mental state, particularly in the first six months.

Hughes, *et al.* (1999) compared women who had had a previous stillbirth with a group of matched controls (N=82). Women who had a stillbirth had more depression and anxiety in their third trimesters, and more depression postpartum. The results were strongest for women who were most recently bereaved. Not surprisingly, depression during pregnancy was highly predictive of postpartum depression. In the year following delivery, 8% of the control group and 19% of the bereaved women scored high for depression.

Mothers can also experience trauma during an ultrasound following a previous perinatal loss (O'Leary, 2005). Parents who have previously lost a baby may experience ultrasound as a harbinger for more bad news rather than a reassuring diagnostic test. A descriptive phenomenologic study of 21 parents (12 mothers, 9 fathers) explored mothers' and fathers' experiences of ultrasound. All had lost babies in the previous year. Most of the parents indicated that the current ultrasound reminded them of when they had seen their babies die on the previous ultrasound. Many aspects of the experience reminded them of that event: the smells, sights, feelings, and sounds of the ultrasound room. During the ultrasound, some mothers experienced flashbacks to when they lost their previous babies – even when the current baby was healthy. Both the fathers and the mothers showed equal levels of trauma symptoms following the ultrasound. Based on her research, O'Leary (2005) recommended recognizing that parents may be remembering their previous babies when undergoing testing for a current pregnancy. She also recommends preparing parents for possible flashbacks during ultrasound: let them hear the heartbeat first before the ultrasound; acknowledge and validate the parents' concerns while assuring them that the current baby is healthy; and finally, recognize that fathers may be as traumatized as mothers.

A study from Germany examined mothers' feelings of grief after a pregnancy termination for fetal anomalies (Kersting, *et al.*, 2005). This study compared the reactions of 83 women who had undergone a termination 2 to 7 years previously; 60 mothers who had undergone a termination 14 days prior, and 65 women who had had a full-term baby. Contrary to the expectations of the researchers, they found that there was no difference in traumatic symptoms between the two groups who had a termination. Both groups differed significantly from the mothers who had had a full-term baby, and were significantly higher on all three sub-scales of the Impact of Events Scale (hyperarousal, avoidance, and re-experiencing). The events experienced as traumatic were the invasive medical procedures, the wait for labor pains to begin, and delivery of a dead fetus. The authors noted that mothers experienced intense grief reactions in addition to trauma symptoms. They concluded that these terminations had been emotionally traumatic events that led to severe posttraumatic stress responses that persisted for years.

Reproductive loss can be life-threatening for mothers as well. Van Pampus and colleagues (2004) described three case studies where mothers developed trauma symptoms after their experience with HELLP (Hemolytic anemia, Elevated Liver enzymes and Low Platelet count) syndrome. HELLP syndrome is a serious form of pre-eclampsia that includes hemolysis, low platelets, and liver damage. It is also a potential cause of mother and infant mortality and morbidity. Even several years after the event, the women described were still highly fearful and did not want to become pregnant again for fear of what might happen. The researchers noted that women who experience HELLP syndrome may suffer from significant emotional sequelae and should therefore be monitored so that they might receive intervention.

Fathers can also become depressed following infant loss. In a longitudinal study of men one year after birth or a miscarriage, Johnson and Baker (2004) found that none of the pregnancy variables predicted men's stress. Predictors of depression at one year included cognitive approach, avoidance, and depression at birth/miscarriage. The authors concluded that pregnancy, birth, and miscarriage are major life events for men as well as for women, and are often associated with a range of negative affective outcomes. Approach-oriented strategies, such as problem solving, seeking support, and positive reappraisal, are used more often in situations with positive outcomes. Their decrease following a negative outcome is not surprising.

In a review of 17 studies, Badenhorst, *et al.* (2006) also found that fathers were affected by prior loss. The fathers experienced classic grief symptoms, but less guilt than mothers. Fathers also experienced anxiety and depression, but at a lower level than mothers. They may also develop PTSD. The authors concluded that fathers may also be traumatized by stillbirth or neonatal death and may need help in their own right before they can support their partners.

Healthcare providers can provide support for mothers in the wake of infant loss. In a study of women in Sweden who had given birth to live or stillborn babies, 314 had had a stillborn baby (Radestad, *et al.*, 1996). Among these women, 80% had caressed their babies, 90% reported that the medical staff showed respect, and almost 70% reported that the hospital had good routines to support mothers of stillborn children. However, 37% reported that they had been deeply hurt or angered by the behavior of the medical staff. When pictures of their babies were taken, 70% indicated that they were very or quite satisfied. About 16% were not at all satisfied, and much had to do with the lack of care taken when the photo was taken (e.g. the baby was placed on the floor for the photo, or the baby was covered with blood). Twenty-one percent had no token of remembrance of their babies.

## Interventions

### KANGAROO CARE

One technique that can be useful for mothers of premature infants is Kangaroo Care (KC). This involves placing the baby, wearing only a diaper, between the mother's breasts or on one breast, under her clothing. The babies are held in a sling or pouch. Fathers can also do KC. The benefits for babies appear almost immediately. The babies are calmer and their body temperature is stable. They cry less, thereby conserving precious calories. The babies do better physically, and are discharged from the hospital earlier. Mothers also benefit. They feel more confident in caring for their babies, and are more likely to form a secure attachment (Anderson, 1991).

In a study in India, Parmar and colleagues (2009) studied families of 135 babies with an average birth weight of 1,460 g and a gestational age of 30 weeks. Kangaroo Mother Care (KMC) was started in the first week of life. The researchers found that infants in KMC had an improved oxygen saturation levels, that their temperature and respiration stabilized, and that their heart rate was lowered by three to five beats. Ninety-six percent of the mothers, 82% of the fathers, and 84% of other family members accepted KMC as a treatment. In addition, healthcare workers found it an acceptable and conservative treatment for babies in the NICU. The mothers reported that they felt closer to their babies and that KMC elevated their mood, although they were initially frightened about trying it. The mothers also reported increased confidence in handling their babies. Healthcare workers reported that it made mothers feel more confident; increased breastfeeding, and that the babies also cried less and slept more.

A study from Israel showed similar results with a larger sample (Feldman, *et al.*, 2002). This study randomly assigned preterm infants to either KC or standard care. The mothers were matched for birth weight, gestational age, medical severity, and demographics. At 37 weeks' gestation, mothers in the KC group had more positive affect, touch, and adaptation to their infants' cues. The infants showed more alertness and less gaze aversion. The mothers were less likely to be depressed and to report that their infants were abnormal. At three months, mothers and fathers were more sensitive and provided a better home environment (based on their score on the HOME inventory). At six months, the KC mothers were more sensitive to their babies' cues, and their infants scored significantly higher on the Bayley Mental Developmental Index and the Psychomotor Developmental Index. The authors speculated that KC influenced infant development directly by having a positive impact on infants' perceptual-cognitive and motor development. There may have also been an indirect impact because KC improved maternal mood, perceptions of their infants, and their interactive behavior. In another study, KC was related to successful lactation in mothers of very low-birth-weight infants, even after controlling for maternal age, race, marital status, and education beyond high school (Furman, *et al.*, 2002).

In a case study, Dombrowski and colleagues (2001) found that KC was helpful for a mother at very high risk for depression. She was 22 years old, single, and had given up a previous baby for adoption. She and her younger brother were removed from their home when she was five because of repeated physical and sexual abuse by her father. She and her brother were adopted at age 9 after four years in multiple foster homes. She had an active history of substance abuse. Immediately after her baby's premature birth, she was severely depressed. However, within 24 hours of starting KC, she was no longer depressed. She was assessed at six weeks, three months, and seven months, and was neither depressed, nor abusing substances at any of these assessments. In describing her experience, she noted the following:

> It was important to both of us for bonding. It made me feel closer than I felt holding her regular, you know, wrapped. It calmed her down a lot more and made her more secure. It made me close to her and I was scared to be a mother but it gave me a sense of peace that I could do it (take care of the baby). It made me less stressed and able to relax – a "time out" together kind of thing. I was able to forget everything else. It worked well for both of us on stress. I felt like I needed something and being a recovering drug addict I needed this to help.
>
> (Cited in Dombrowski, *et al.*, 2002: 215)

KC was also helpful for full-term babies in another study from Iran (Kashaninia, *et al.*, 2008). In this study, 100 healthy neonates were assigned to either the KC group or the control group. The infants in the KC group were held in KC 10 minutes before an injection and during the procedure. The KC infants had a significantly lower score on the Neonatal Infant Pain Scale than did infants in the control group. This scale measured facial expression, crying, breathing pattern, arm and leg movements, and state of arousal. The control-group infants' scores were significantly higher on all measures, including duration of crying, than babies in the KC group.

SOCIAL SUPPORT INTERVENTIONS

In addition to KC, providing specific social support improved outcomes for mothers of premature babies (Jotzo and Poets, 2005). Mothers were randomly assigned to a crisis intervention offered at five days after birth, or they received usual care. The intervention took place in the NICU twice a week, for 5 to 15 minutes. Elements of the crisis intervention included helping mothers reconstruct the events before and after their births, teaching them relaxation techniques, explaining stress and trauma responses, discussing with them personal resources and current support, providing them with support during "emotional outbursts," and offering them possible solutions for concrete problems. At discharge, mothers in the intervention group had significantly lower trauma symptoms than mothers who received standard care.

Prematurity is only one type of health issue that can influence mothers. Infants' long-term health problems, such as disability and chronic illness, can also affect mothers. Studies on this topic are described below.

### Infant disability or chronic illness

Disabilities also vary considerably in their impairment of a child's functioning and how they impact mothers. In a sample from India, infant hospital admission was significantly associated with postpartum depression (Patel, *et al.*, 2002). Similarly, serious infant health problems were a risk factor for Turkish women at six months postpartum (Danaci, *et al.*, 2002). Even relatively minor problems can lead to mothers being separated from their babies, increasing the risk of depression.

Low birth weight and prematurity can also lead to other problems in children, including ongoing health problems and chronic conditions. In one study, low birth weight was related to the development of ADHD. In this study (Mick, *et al.*, 2002), 252 children with ADHD were compared with 231 children without ADHD. The results indicated that children with ADHD were three times more likely to have been born low birth weight than the comparison children. These findings held even after controlling for prenatal exposure to alcohol and ciga-rettes, parental ADHD, social class, and comorbid disruptive behavior of family members. Low birth weight appears to be an independent risk factor for ADHD, but children with low birth weight are a relatively small percentage of children with ADHD.

### Longer-term effects of infant/child illness

Chronic health problems in children can influence mothers' emotional health, as found in a study of mothers of children with epilepsy (Mu, *et al.*, 2001). The children in this study ranged in age from 1 to 19 years. The authors found that there were three factors associated with maternal depression: boundary ambiguity, uncertainty, and mothers' age, with younger moth-ers having more difficulty coping with their children's illness. These three factors accounted for 21% of the variance in maternal depression. Uncertainty refers to inadequate ability to structure or categorize an event due to lack of sufficient cues. Epilepsy, by its unpredictable nature, makes it difficult to predict. Boundary ambiguity refers to an uncertain role of the child in the family. Because of the child's illness, parents are unsure what role their children can fulfill. For example, should the child be assigned household chores? Caretakers may be either inadequately or excessively involved.

Similarly, mothers' feelings that they could not manage their children's asthma increased the likelihood of hospitalization of their children for asthma (Chen, *et al.*, 2003). In this study, 115 children (aged 4 to 18) were followed for a year. All the children had had at least one hospitalization during the study period. If parents thought there was nothing they could do to manage their children's asthma, or if they felt overwhelmed by caring for their children, their children were more likely to be hospitalized for acute attacks. This effect was found even after controlling for baseline severity of asthma, medications, and child age. Some other characteristics related to increased hospitalization included greater levels of family strain and conflict, and greater financial strain.

### Social support for mothers of infants with health issues

Social support can mediate many of the negative effects of having a baby or child with a health problem. Social support can take many forms including the provision of information, practical assistance, and emotional support. But sometimes "support" is stressful for mothers of babies or children with health problems.

> I found it difficult to speak with my husband and family about being depressed, and about my constant concern and worry. They kept trying to be positive, saying what they would do with him when he got well. I don't know if my medical knowledge made it worse. I knew how serious it was. It made me more depressed when my family was upbeat and

tried to deny how serious it was. I had to deal with their denial and I felt they were heaping expectations on me.

I got lots of support from a couple we're friends with. She's a NICU nurse. They would offer to sit at the hospital for us so we could go out. They also made meals for us. They were people who understood the medical issues. They didn't say everything would be OK. They realized it could be fatal. [Patricia]

*Why social support is sometimes stressful*

When considering whether a woman is receiving adequate support, it is easy to be fooled by appearances. We might assume that a woman who knows a lot of people, or is receiving functional assistance, is experiencing social support. But this is not always the case. People in a woman's social network might not offer to help. And even if they help, the woman may not *perceive* it as support. Unwanted help can undermine a woman's confidence in her mothering abilities, threaten her self-esteem, and engender dependency on the person providing the help. Even when a woman is grateful for the assistance, she may be uncomfortable accepting it if she is an independent or private person and is used to doing things for herself (Affleck, *et al.*, 1989). Christine describes how having her mother and her in-laws come to help after the baby was born made her uncomfortable.

Everyone was really helping with the baby but me. They were too supportive. I know my husband wouldn't want to think that. I felt like they were taking over everything, that I had to be able to do it all. I kept trying to be the perfect wife. I'm a very private person. I felt like everything was exposed.

One study found that formal social support for mothers of high-risk babies is only effective if the mothers perceive a need for support (Affleck, *et al.*, 1989). When the mothers thought they needed support, the program (consisting of support and information from in-home nurse consultants) improved mothers' sense of perceived control, competence, and responsiveness. The program had a negative effect on mothers who had a low-perceived need for support, by actually making them feel less competent and more anxious. This was a surprising finding. To explain it, the authors took a closer look at the interaction between the home visitors and mothers in this group. They found that since these mothers didn't feel they needed services, the home visitors were trying to convince them that they did. Not surprisingly, the mothers felt more anxious after receiving this type of "support."

## Summary

Both mothers and at-risk babies bring special challenges to the mother–infant relationship. Mothers may be in the process of grieving when they are forced to deal with babies who are different from what they expected, and who may be difficult to handle. In spite of these difficulties, attachment can develop between mother and baby, especially if the mother is given adequate support, and it is something she perceives as support. You can do much to facilitate these types of positive reaction. Helping mothers feel competent in caring for their at-risk babies is vital for reducing risk for postpartum depression and helping mothers to become attached to their babies.

In the next chapter, I describe psychological risk factors for postpartum depression.

# 8    Psychological risk factors

There are a number of psychological factors that increase women's risk of depression. These include a woman's attributional style; her expectations about what it will be like to be a mother; her self-esteem; how competent she feels as a parent; and prior vulnerability factors such as loss, previous psychiatric illness, and a dysfunctional or abusive family history. Each of these increase women's risk of depression, and may co-occur. The first factor described has to do with how mothers see the world.

## Attributional style

People have different ways of looking at the world. They are either "optimists" or "pessimists." A pessimistic attributional style increases vulnerability to depression because people learn to interpret events in a way that makes them more stressful and negative (Abramson, et al., 1978). Specifically, pessimists are more likely to become depressed after a negative event because they maintain internal, global, and stable attributions about why negative events occurred. Internal attributions mean that the cause of the negative event is within the person's control. Negative events can also be attributed to stable ("I am stupid") or unstable ("I was tired") characteristics. Global attributions mean that a person feels that the negative event affects many areas of their life, while persons who make specific attributions realize that the negative event only affects one or two areas. Barbara's story shows characteristics of the pessimistic style.

> I hadn't handled a lot of babies. The nurse was yelling at me saying, "What's the matter, haven't you handled a baby before?" I was offended and hurt. All I could think of was "I'm a bad mother." When [the depression] was really bad, I thought "I'm a bad person. I should have never had a baby, never gotten married. I'm a bad mother. I'm crap." I talked about it all the time until others were sick of hearing about it. At one point, my mom said to me "I don't know what you are worried about. One baby is no work." All I could think was "I'm a failure." [Barbara]

While the research cited above refers to depression in general, attributional style has also been studied in relation to depression in new mothers. An Australian study of 65 primiparous women found that dysfunctional attitudes were related to depression at six weeks postpartum. This was especially true for women with high amounts of postpartum stress or whose babies had difficult temperaments (Grazioli and Terry, 2000). Negative thinking and thoughts of death and dying at one month postpartum predicted depression at four months in another study of 465 postpartum women (Chaudron, et al., 2001). The authors considered thoughts of dying as a prodrome of later depression. Interestingly, although women who breastfed their infants did not differ from women who bottle-fed in the development of depression, women who *worried* about breastfeeding were significantly more likely to become depressed than those who did not worry.

Optimism was found to influence birth outcomes in a medically high-risk sample of 129 women (Lobel, *et al.*, 2000). In this study, prenatal stress and optimism were examined in relation to birth outcomes (birth weight and gestational age), controlling for risk, and ethnicity. Women who were less optimistic had babies who weighed significantly less even after controlling for gestational age. Prenatal stress did not have an effect once optimism was added to the model. Some of this difference may have been behavioral: optimists were more likely to exercise, and exercise lowered the risk of preterm birth.

## Self-esteem, self-efficacy, and expectations

> The truth of the matter is that I'm ashamed. Why is it so hard for me and looks so easy for other mothers? I saw other full-time mothers always doing things better. I felt I couldn't keep up. I used to be able to "run with the guys." Now, I'm in a traditional mommy role, but I'm not relating to this role. So where does this leave me? Not fitting into either role. I'm used to being the best at what I do. But I felt I couldn't [function as a mother]. Especially when I look at other moms. I can't seem to understand why I can't do this. I was depending on other people's expectations. Maybe even my own expectations were too high. This led to feeling down, out of control. That's when the depression really started. Doubting I could do it. It got to where I was scared to death, nervous, chest tightness, crying, not wanting to eat. [Michelle]

Self-esteem, self-efficacy, and expectations are three concepts that refer to a woman's adjustment to her role as a mother, what she expects of herself, and how competent she feels. These concepts are closely related and tend to interact. In a meta-analysis of 84 studies, Beck (2001) found that self-esteem had a moderate effect on postpartum depression. Low self-esteem at one month postpartum predicted depression at four months in another recent study of 465 women (Chaudron, *et al.*, 2001). And a prospective study of 191 low-income, inner-city women found that self-esteem was related to lower levels of depression in both the prenatal and postpartum periods (Ritter, *et al.*, 2000).

In a sample of 53 low-income single mothers, childhood abuse and low self-esteem predicted depressive symptoms, and these symptoms influenced women's reactions to their babies (Lutenbacher, 2002). Everyday stressors, when combined with depression, predicted higher levels of anger in the mothers. In another study, maternal self-efficacy acted as a mediator between infant temperament and postpartum depression in a study of 55 married women. Women who had infants with difficult temperaments felt less competent as mothers and had higher levels of postpartum depression. Social support buffered this effect by increasing self-efficacy and helping the women feel more competent (Cutrona and Troutman, 1986).

In a meta-synthesis of 18 qualitative studies, Beck (2002) found that expectations played a large role in postpartum depression at several different levels. Beck describes how both mothers and professionals who care for them still harbor the belief that motherhood brings total fulfillment to women. However, the expectation of total fulfillment from this role, without acknowledging the difficulties, sets standards that are impossible to meet. Women often try to be "perfect" mothers, and when motherhood turns out to be different from what they expected, they feel that they have failed. These women often do not confide in others because they believe that no one else ever felt that way; that they are abnormal mothers. Beck (2002) noted that first-time mothers were more prone to the myth of the perfect mother, whereas multiparous women's expectations focused on trying to cope with the new addition to their families.

Expectations of self can also be related to the expression of goals. In a Finnish study (Salmela-Aro, *et al.*, 2001), an increase in goals for self ("to grow as a person," "develop myself," or "promote my mental growth") increased depressive symptoms for new mothers. Conversely, family-related goals, such as "take good care of my children" or "take good care of my family," decreased depression. When mothers adjusted their personal goals to the demands of the transition to motherhood, their depression declined. The ability to adapt goals to fit within with current constraints and resources is an important component of mental health. The authors noted that when people cannot adapt their goals, depression is the likely consequence. Women in this study were assessed during early pregnancy, at eight months' gestation, and at three months and two years postpartum.

Women's expectations about their babies can also lead to depression. In a sample of 68 at-risk African American women, those who worried about spoiling their babies reported more depression, and had more inappropriate developmental expectations of their babies than mothers who were less worried about spoiling. These findings suggested that fear of spoiling may influence maternal responsiveness in mothers who are at risk, and may lead to potentially disturbed mother–infant relationships (Smyke, *et al.*, 2002).

In summary, women are more likely to experience postpartum depression if they have unrealistic expectations of themselves as mothers and of their babies. If they have low self-esteem, and feel incompetent as mothers, they are also more likely to be depressed.

## Previous psychiatric history

Women's history of previous depression can increase their risk of postpartum depression. A study in Canada (N=622) found that women with a previous psychiatric history were almost four times more likely to have depressive symptomatology at eight weeks postpartum (Dennis and Ross, 2006a). Family psychiatric history was not a significant risk factor. The factors most predictive of depressive symptoms at eight weeks were maternal antenatal depression, maternal history of postpartum depression, and an EPDS score greater than 9 at eight weeks. This model accounted for 42% of the variance. In this sample, 45% reported a personal psychiatric history and 62% had a close family member who had a psychiatric history.

In an Irish sample, previous treatment for depression was one of four risk factors that strongly predicted depression in this population (Cryan, *et al.*, 2001). Previous psychiatric history of the mother or her spouse also predicted the development of postpartum depression in a sample of 257 women from Turkey at six months postpartum (Danaci, *et al.*, 2002).

Neuroticism has also been found to be related to postpartum depression in a study from the Netherlands (Verkerk, *et al.*, 2005). Introversion and neuroticism were measured at 32 weeks' gestation in 277 pregnant women. Depression was measured at three, six, and twelve months postpartum. A high neuroticism score indicates feelings of tension, emotional liability, and insecurity. A high introversion score indicates inhibition and shyness in social interactions. Only the combination of high neuroticism and high introversion predicted depression across the first year postpartum. In contrast, a personal history of depression was only predictive of clinical depression at three months.

Previous psychiatric history may increase risk of depression because of a heightened inflammatory response to current stressors (Maes, 2001). In a study of 16 women with a history of depression and 50 without depression at one and three days postpartum, IL-6, sIL-6R, and sIL-1R were measured. After delivery, IL-6, sIL-6R, and sIL-1R were elevated in all women. As hypothesized, women with a history of depression had even greater increases in serum IL-6 and sIL-1RA during early postpartum than did women without a history of depression. The authors concluded that major depression sensitized the inflammatory response system, increasing risk of subsequent depressive episodes.

## Depression during pregnancy

Researchers have also found that depression in pregnancy is a strong risk factor for postpartum depression (Beck, 2001). In a large sample (N=9,028), depression rates were highest at 32 weeks' gestation and lowest at eight months postpartum (Evans, *et al.*, 2001). In a low-income minority sample (N=802), 37% of the women had depressive symptoms and 6.5% to 8.5% had major depression at three to five weeks postpartum. Fifty percent of these women were also depressed during pregnancy (Yonkers, *et al.*, 2001).

Hobfoll and colleagues (1995; Ritter, *et al.*, 2000) found the highest percentage of women were depressed during pregnancy. These rates were 28% and 25% antepartum, and 23% postpartum in a sample of 192 low-income women from the inner city. Only 47% of the women with postpartum depression did not have prepartum depression.

In a study of 139 women in their third trimester of pregnancy, 38% of the women had scores greater than 16 on the Center for Epidemiologic Studies Depression Scale (CES-D) (Records and Rice, 2007), a subclinical level of depressive symptoms. In a stepwise linear regression, 46% of the variance was due to brief and intermittent mood states that occurred during the first trimester, lack of marital satisfaction, lack of social support, and gravida. Lifetime abuse did not contribute to depression during the third trimester.

In a sample of 252 mothers from India, 23% had postpartum depression (N=252), but 78% of these women were also depressed during pregnancy. Only 21% developed depression for the first time during the postpartum period, when they were assessed at six weeks postpartum. Fifty-nine percent of women depressed at six weeks were still depressed at six months postpartum (Patel, *et al.*, 2002).

Similarly, in a sample of 80 women, 25% experienced depression during pregnancy, and 16% experienced depression at four to five weeks postpartum (Da Costa, *et al.*, 2000). Women who were depressed postpartum reported more emotional coping, and higher state and trait anxiety during pregnancy. The best predictor of postpartum depressed mood was depressed mood during pregnancy.

In a systematic review (Gaynes, *et al.*, 2005), 14.5% of women had a new episode of major or minor depression during pregnancy and 14.5% had a new episode in the first three months postpartum. For major depression, 7.5% had a new episode during pregnancy and 6.5% had a new episode during the first three years postpartum.

Although previous episodes of depression increase the risk for depression postpartum, it is by no means inevitable. Mothers with previous episodes are at higher risk, so they should alert their caregivers during pregnancy, arrange for follow-up postpartum, and get extra help and support after their babies are born. Depending on the severity of the episode, prospective use of antidepressants may be appropriate as well. Recognizing risk and taking steps to counter it can often prevent a recurrence.

## Violence against women

Violence against women (VAW) is an unfortunate fact of life for millions of women around the world. VAW, too, can increase the risk of depression and other perinatal mood disorders. A recent study of 332 postpartum women in Toronto found that 14% reported a history of child sexual abuse; 7% reported child physical abuse; 13% reported adult sexual abuse; 7% reported adult physical abuse, and 30% reported adult emotional abuse (Ansara, *et al.*, 2005). In a study of 79 pregnant and parenting adolescents (Gilson and Lancaster, 2008), 20% reported either physical or sexual abuse. In this study, there was not a higher rate of depression or anxiety during pregnancy. However, by six weeks postpartum, those who had been physically or physically and sexually abused had higher rates of depression and anxiety (physical abuse only). By six months, there were significantly higher rates of depression and anxiety for those who had been sexually or physically abused, and for those who experienced both, than for their non-abused counterparts (Gilson and Lancaster, 2008).

A study of 44 pregnant women explored the impact of child maltreatment on women's experiences of pregnancy and in the first year postpartum (Lang, *et al.*, 2006). They found that sexual abuse and emotional neglect were related to psychopathology during pregnancy. Physical abuse and neglect predicted poorer maternal outcomes at one year postpartum.

In a study of 559 pregnant women in Israel, 27% reported childhood sexual abuse (CSA) (Lev-Wiesel and Daphna-Tekoa, 2007). Women in the sexual-abuse group also reported more miscarriages than non-victims, and 40% of women in the CSA group had also experienced other types of trauma. The abused women had a significantly higher level of PTSD but not depression. Women who had experienced sexual abuse and other types of additional trauma had a higher level of symptoms than women who experienced sexual abuse alone.

### *How abuse impacts women's birth experience*

A study in the Netherlands examined the impact of past sexual abuse on birth (van der Hulst, *et al.*, 2006). This study included 625 women with low-risk pregnancies. Of these women, 11.2% were abuse survivors. Compared with the non-abused women, the abuse survivors suffered more emotional distress, more internal beliefs about their health, and more pelvic pain. The abused women were more likely to smoke and to have lower incomes. The sexually abused women also reported higher levels of autonomy and, interestingly, had lower rates of episiotomies. Rates of pharmacologic pain relief and cesarean births were similar between the abused and non-abused groups. The authors also found no significant difference in rates of major birth-related obstetric technical interventions, but there were trends towards more assisted deliveries and higher frequencies of augmentation among the abuse survivors.

According to Hobbins (2004), when sexual abuse survivors give birth, they may fall into one of four styles: fighting, taking control, surrendering, and retreating. In fighting, they struggle against their body sensations. It's a combination of maintaining control and a panic response. In taking control, the survivor can be very angry and distrustful, with actions that are intended to intimidate the staff. She may bring an entourage with her to protect her from the staff, or delay transit to the hospital so long that she "accidentally" delivers at home (this pattern may also occur in patients with previous birth or other medical trauma). By their actions, these women have maintained control of their bodies. In surrendering, women completely submit to everyone's rules and become completely submissive and compliant so as not to be labeled a "bad" patient. The fourth pattern, retreating, is when they remove themselves mentally and emotionally from their births. They frequently have flat affect and monotone voice, and can be described as stoic. This may also be a dissociative response.

In her article describing the role of the nurse in caring for women who are CSA survivors, Hobbins (2004) contrasted the medical model of care with the feminist model. In the medical model, the presumption is that the abuse survivor doesn't know what she needs and it's up to the care provider to take care of that. The medical model also does not acknowledge or incorporate the values, philosophies, or cultural healing approaches of other cultures. In contrast, the feminist model focuses on empowerment of patients and believes that patients do indeed know what they need.

### *Depression in abuse survivors*

Depression as a result of violence is a very common finding in non-postpartum samples. For example, in Hulme's (2000) study of women in primary care, 23% reported a history of CSA. The women reported a wide range of physical symptoms and chronic pain syndromes. Those particularly related to risk of depression include breast pain, eating binges and/or vomiting, insomnia, pelvic pain, pregnancy complications, and lifetime history of depression. Further, 52% indicated that they could not sleep at night; 20% reported suicidal ideation in the past two years (compared with 1.9% of the non-abused group); 66% reported low self-esteem, and 52% were not able to trust others.

CSA also increases both depression and experiences of pain in women. In a study of 66 women with major depression and a history of CSA, patients who reported high amounts of pain had more severe depression than those with low pain (Poleshuck, *et al.*, 2009). Even following treatment, patients with high pain still had more depressive symptoms after treatment. The patients were all in treatment for depression, and while all patients' moods improved, those with higher levels of pain showed less improvement.

In another non-postpartum sample of 3,568 women aged 18 to 64, past physical and sexual abuse was related to depression and overall poor health (Bonomi, *et al.*, 2008). In models that adjusted for age and income, women who experienced both types of abuse had increased prevalence of depression, severe depression, physical symptoms, joint pain, nausea and vomiting, and self-rating health as fair or poor. Reported rates of insomnia were 25% for the non-abused group, 33% for the group having suffered physical abuse only, 36% for those having suffered sexual abuse only, and 43% for women who had experienced both.

Adverse childhood experience (ACE) is a broader conceptualization of traumas that occur during childhood. ACEs include childhood physical and sexual abuse, neglect, parental mental illness, parental substance abuse, parental partner violence, or parental criminal activity. These experiences all increase the risk of depression in adults; the more types of ACE people experience, the higher the risk. For example, in a study of 254 adults with major depression or bipolar disorder, 59% of the women had had three or more ACEs. The most common experiences were witnessing domestic violence (67%), sexual abuse (58%), physical abuse (54%), foster or kinship care (42%), parental separation or divorce (36%), parental mental illness (39%), and parental death (10%). In addition to depression, the cumulative exposure to ACEs increased the rate of PTSD, high-risk behaviors, substance abuse, exposure to trauma in adulthood, physical and sexual abuse as adults, medical service utilization, and homelessness (Lu, *et al.*, 2008).

The Christchurch Health and Development study, a cohort 25-year longitudinal study of 1,265 adults in Christchurch, New Zealand, found an increased risk of depression, anxiety disorders, conduct/anti-social personality disorders, substance abuse, suicidal ideation, and suicide attempts during adolescence among those who experienced childhood physical or sexual abuse (Fergusson, *et al.*, 2008). Those who had experienced CSA had 2.4 times higher rates of mental disorders than non-exposed individuals. The authors concluded that CSA, in particular, was related to an increased risk of depression and other mental disorders.

A smaller study showed similar results (Weber, *et al.*, 2008). In this study, 96 patients with diagnoses of major depression, schizophrenia, drug addiction, or personality disorders were compared with individuals without psychiatric diagnoses. The authors found that high rates of ACEs were related to depressive and PTSD symptoms, severity of the disorders, and diagnoses of major depression and personality disorders. The same was not true for trauma experienced as adults.

Adverse life events were also predictive of PTSD symptoms in a sample of college students (Smyth, *et al.*, 2008). In this sample of 6,053 college students, between 56% and 85% reported exposure to adverse life events. These included death of a loved one; divorce or separation of parents; traumatic sexual experience, or upsetting academic upheaval. Of these students, 97 were interviewed in depth, with 9% reporting clinical levels of PTSD, and an additional 11% reporting subclinical levels.

### Abuse survivors in the postpartum period

Not surprisingly, a history of childhood abuse or ACEs increases the risk of depression in the postpartum period. A study of 200 Canadian women at eight to ten weeks postpartum found that women with a history of abuse are more likely to experience both depression and physical health symptoms in the postpartum period (Ansara, *et al.*, 2005).

A three-year follow-up of 45 Australian mothers who were hospitalized for postpartum major depressive disorder found that half had a history of CSA. The sexually abused women had significantly higher depression and anxiety scores and greater life stresses compared with the non-abused depressed women. Moreover, the sexually abused women had less improvement in their symptoms over time (Buist and Janson, 2001). In a review of 17 studies, Ross and Dennis (2009) found that there were high rates of postpartum depression among women who were abusing substances and those who had experiences of past abuse. There was not an increased risk of postpartum depression among the third group they studied: women with chronic illnesses.

Val describes how her past history of sexual abuse related to her postpartum depression, and how it manifested in obsessive thoughts of harming her twin babies.

> My depression started three days after birth. It came on very suddenly. My husband was coming to the hospital. We were going to give the babies a bath. As we were giving [my daughter] a bath, I was suddenly afraid that I might abuse her. I had been sexually abused as a child. I didn't tell anyone until the next day. It started with "Oh my God. I was abused. I could abuse them." Then it was more general. Everything was a danger. Everything could hurt the kids. I can't tell you how surprised I was. I haven't done anything to hurt the kids. I first visualized my son being thrown into the fire. Then it was me throwing him in. I worried about plastic. I'd have thoughts of smothering the kids with pillows. There were certain rooms in the house I couldn't even go in. I couldn't drink coffee. I'd have thoughts of pouring it on the kids. Through all of this I never neglected my children's needs, no matter how difficult. No one ever questioned that I would hurt the kids. I'm the only one. I feel it could be from the sexual abuse. I obsess and worry about things. I've had times and traumatic events that I've worried about before, but it's always been just me. [Val]

## Violence in the perinatal period

Women are also vulnerable to abuse and violence in the perinatal period. Neither pregnancy nor the postpartum period offers protection from abuse, as the results of the studies below indicate, and this too increases mothers' risk of depression.

Three recent large, population-based studies found that many women are beaten during pregnancy and the postpartum period, but no clear pattern emerged about which was the highest-risk time. In a Chinese study that included 32 communities, 8.5% of women were beaten before pregnancy, 3.6% during pregnancy, and 7.4% after pregnancy (Guo, *et al.*, 2004). In North Carolina, 6.9% were beaten before pregnancy, 6.1% during pregnancy, and 3.2% postpartum (N=2,648; Martin, *et al.*, 2001). Finally, in Bristol Avon, U.K. (N=7,591), 5% were beaten during pregnancy and 11% postpartum (Bowen, *et al.*, 2005). In this sample, a number of social adversities reported during pregnancy predicted postpartum victimization. Women who experienced one social adversity during pregnancy were 2.73 times more likely to report physical victimization. Women who reported five or more social adversities were 15 times more likely to report postpartum victimization.

A study of 570 teen mothers showed the continuity between antenatal and postpartum violence. The prevalence of intimate partner violence (IPV) was highest at three months postpartum (21%) and lowest at 24 months (13%). Seventy-five percent of mothers beaten during pregnancy were also beaten during their first two years postpartum. And 78% who experienced IPV at three months postpartum had not reported IPV during their pregnancy (Harrykissoon, *et al.*, 2002).

Lutz (2005) also described the continuity between past and present violence in her qualitative study of 12 women who were survivors of IPV during at least one childbearing cycle. Among these women, depression, posttraumatic stress disorder (PTSD) and anxiety were common. The study participants reported many types of violence during their lives: child physical, emotional, and sexual abuse; neglect; parental IPV and substance abuse; current IPV; adult sexual assault; and community violence. The women experienced each exposure to violence as influencing and flowing into the next. They viewed IPV during childbearing as just part of the continuum of abusive experiences in their lives.

In a sample of rural women, Ellis and colleagues (2008) found that women who were experiencing partner violence sought care for their babies more often in the first six weeks postpartum and had significantly higher levels of stress than non-abused women. There was no difference between the groups in the type of healthcare consultations they sought. Not surprisingly, the abused women were also more depressed and had less support. An important intervention that care providers can offer is screening for partner violence at all prenatal and postpartum visits.

## Abuse and the inflammatory response

The experience of violence increases the inflammatory response, and this can also increase the risk of depression. Previous child maltreatment was related to high C-reactive protein levels when they were assessed 20 years later (Danese, *et al.*, 2007). The participants (N=1,037) were part of the Dunedin Multidisciplinary Health and Development Study, a study of health behavior in a complete birth cohort in New Zealand. Researchers assessed the participants every two to three years throughout childhood, and every five to six years through to age 32. The impact of child maltreatment on inflammation was independent of other factors that could have accounted for the findings, such as co-occurring life stresses in adulthood; early life risks; or adult health or health behavior. The effect was also dose-responsive; the more severe the abuse, the more severe the inflammation.

A similar finding resulted from a study of women abused by intimate partners. In this study, 62 women who had had abusive partners 8 to 11 years previously had significantly higher interferon-gamma (IFN-γ) levels than non-abused women (Woods, *et al.*, 2005). The women also had high rates of depression (52%) and PTSD (39%). Even several years after their abuse had ended, these women were still manifesting significant physical symptomatology. Inflammation was also found to be elevated in a study of 15 women who had been raped, 24 to 72 hours after their assault, compared with 16 women who had not been sexually assaulted. Sexually assaulted women had higher adrenocorticotropic hormone (ACTH), C-reactive protein, IL-6, IL-10, IFN-γ than women in the non-assaulted group (Groer, *et al.*, 2006).

## *Abuse history and parenting difficulties*

Women who have been abused as children or adults may also have problematic relationships with their children, which can add to their life stress and compromise the health of mother and child. In one study, women with a history of CSA were more anxious about the intimate aspects of caring for their own babies, including activities such as diapering. These mothers were more worried that their normal parenting behaviors were inappropriate – or that others would see them that way. Finally, they reported more parenting stress than their non-abused counterparts (Douglas, 2000). This lack of confidence can have an erosive effect on their mental health, also increasing their risk for depression.

Dubowitz and colleagues (2001) found that when mothers had experienced multiple types of abuse, they were more likely to be depressed. They also used harsher discipline and had more problems with their children (N=419). Mothers abused as children and as adults, or who were both physically and sexually abused as children, had worse outcomes than those who suffered only one type of abuse. Mothers' depression and harsh parenting were associated with internalizing and externalizing behavior problems in their children. The authors speculated that mothers who have been victimized may be less attentive to their children, and less emotionally available. These mothers may also have less tolerance for the day-to-day stresses of parenting, and may be more inclined to view their children's behaviors as problematic. The authors concluded that a mother's history of victimization appears to be highly prevalent in high-risk samples. More than half of the mothers in their sample had been physically or sexually victimized at some time, and half of the mothers victimized during childhood or adolescence were revictimized as adults.

A study of primiparae included 107 women with a history of CSA and 156 comparison mothers (Schuetze and Das Eiden, 2005). When the mothers were reinterviewed when their babies were 2 to 4 years of age, CSA was associated with both maternal depression and higher rates of partner violence. CSA women also had higher rates of parenting difficulties, but these disappeared when depression and partner violence were accounted for.

A study comparing 670 non-abusing families with 166 abusive families found similar results (Gracia and Musitu, 2003). The families in this sample were Colombian and Spanish. The authors found that in both cultures abusive parents showed lower levels of community integration, participation in social activities, and use of formal and informal organizations than parents who were providing adequate care for their children. The abusive parents tended to be more socially isolated and negative in their attitudes towards their community and neighborhood.

## Abuse and breastfeeding

Breastfeeding is also an issue for many abuse survivors. So far, there is little empirical information on how past or current abuse influences a woman's desire and ability to breastfeed. Although not specifically related to depression, this issue can become a central concern for women. Surprisingly, abuse survivors are more likely to want to breastfeed than their non-abused counterparts.

Benedict and colleagues (1994) studied 360 primiparous women in the Baltimore area. The sample was a predominantly African American and low-income one. Of these women, 12% were sexual abuse survivors. A higher percentage of sexual abuse survivors (54%) indicated an intention to breastfeed than their non-abused counterparts (41%). There were no significant differences between the abuse survivors and non-abused women on rates of cesarean sections, induction or augmentation of labor, anesthesia during labor or birth, or failure to progress.

Prentice and colleagues (Prentice, *et al.*, 2002) had similar findings with a different population of mothers. This study included a national sample of 1,220 mothers with children younger than age 3. Of these women, 7% were survivors of sexual abuse. As with the previous study, women who had been sexually abused were twice as likely to initiate breastfeeding (OR=2.58).

A study from Hong Kong indicated that IPV during pregnancy and early postpartum depression may influence breastfeeding initiation rates (Lau and Chan, 2007). This study included 1,200 Chinese mothers. Women who had no experience of IPV during pregnancy were significantly more likely to initiate breastfeeding than women who had experienced IPV, even after adjusting for demographic, socioeconomic status (SES) and obstetric variables. Early postpartum depression was not associated with breastfeeding initiation in a logistic regression model.

In a sample of 212 women recruited from a WIC[1] population, Bullock and colleagues (2001) examined the question of whether women with abuse histories, or those currently being abused, would be less likely to breastfeed their infants. The authors found no relationship between past or current abuse and feeding choice for infants. Abuse survivors breastfed their infants in the same proportion as those who were not currently being abused. More than half reported a history of lifetime abuse, and approximately 7% reported being hit while pregnant. The proportion of women who breastfed during current abuse was identical to the proportion who bottle-fed. It should be noted that the sample of women currently experiencing abuse was small, with 10 in the bottle-feeding group and 11 in the breastfeeding group.

## Mothers' experiences of breastfeeding after sexual abuse

The subjective experiences of abuse survivors who breastfeed vary quite a bit. For some, it can be quite healing. For others, it can be extremely difficult. Below are two accounts of women's experiences. In the first account, abuse survivor Beth Dubois (2003) describes how she was nervous about giving birth and breastfeeding her son. The theme of low self-efficacy is evident. But she also describes how breastfeeding was healing and empowering for her.

> As the time of my son's birth approached, my worries about breastfeeding came into sharp focus. I knew the benefits of breastfeeding, and had plenty of book knowledge on the subject. I knew I wanted to breastfeed. I had been sexually abused when I was a child, however, and I was concerned. I worried that I would not be able to maintain the constant physical closeness breastfeeding would require and that breastfeeding might

trigger memories of the abuse. I was especially distraught because I believed that I would be failing my child and myself if I were not able to breastfeed.

(Dubois, 2003)

After describing her experiences of pregnancy, labor and delivery, she describes the positive impact breastfeeding has had on her.

I now see that not only has breastfeeding been possible for me, a survivor of childhood sexual abuse, it has been immensely healing. My desire to have a fulfilling breastfeeding relationship forced me to face emotional territory I would probably have otherwise avoided. One wound left by the abuse is an underlying sense of "I can't do it. It's not even worth trying." Birthing and breastfeeding Theodore has helped to replace this with a very real sense of capability and confidence. Also, the heightened sensitivity to both myself and my son, which I gained through our breastfeeding relationship, serves us in other ways, especially now that Theodore is in the "terrific twos."

(Dubois, 2003: 50–1)

Unfortunately, it would be negligent to only report positive findings regarding breastfeeding after abuse. Some abuse survivors struggle immensely to breastfeed, and may get to the point where they cannot continue. In a detailed case study, Beck (2009) presents the story of a woman with a history of CSA and rape as an adult. During Marilyn's birth, she dissociated and had a flashback to her abuse experience.

A haze of hospital labor room, nakedness, vulnerability, pain. Silence, stretching, breathing, pain terror, and then I found myself 7 years old again, and sitting outside my parents' house in the car of a family acquaintance, being digitally raped … my birth experience did not look traumatic at all – because the trauma physically took place 23 years before and only in my mind the labor room.

(Cited in Beck, 2009: e4 and e5.)

After birth, her milk never came in, possibly due to the trauma of her birth or her pre-eclampsia. She felt that inability to breastfeed only compounded her sense of shame and inadequacy. What she remembered most about her postpartum experience was an incredible feeling of numbness. She felt that she could not connect with her baby, husband, life, or anything. She describes her breastfeeding experience as follows:

Of course, I couldn't tell anyone what was really going on in my head when I tried to breastfeed. When I placed my baby to the breast, I experienced panic attacks, spaced out and dissociated. It triggered flashbacks of the abuse and a sick feeling in my stomach. I hated the physical feeling of breastfeeding. I hated having to offer my body to my child, who felt like a stranger. Whenever I put her to breast, I wanted to scream and vomit at the same time. My body recoiled at the thought of placing my baby to my breast. The thought of breastfeeding made my skin crawl. The very act of breastfeeding, which was sustaining my baby, was forcing me to relive the abuse. I resented her for needing to breastfeed. I did actually experience some relief when I expressed, rather than breastfeeding directly; however, my supply was so poor that for an hour's effort expressing, I'd only have about 10 mm of milk to give my daughter. At the moment I gave myself permission to give up on breastfeeding, things started to look up. I slowly started to feel a sense of connection with my baby, and with my life, and I even began to feel a bit like my old self again.

(Cited in Beck, 2009: e6)

Breastfeeding can be strongly positive or strongly negative for individual abuse survivors. Even the mother in the above case illustration got to the point where she "kind of liked" breastfeeding with a second baby. Some have shared with me that they never got to the point where they liked breastfeeding. But they got to the point where they could tolerate it, and that was an important goal for them. As care providers, it is important that we be open to the whole range of reactions that mothers may have and support them in their decisions to breastfeed, to pump and bottle-feed, or to simply bottle-feed.

### *Summary*

Abuse survivors have a higher lifetime risk for depression than the general population. We should, therefore, not be surprised when they are at increased risk during the postpartum period. As I described in the case of previous psychiatric illness, past abuse is a risk factor for depression. But depression is not inevitable. It can be helpful for mothers to check in with their care providers periodically, as well as any mental health providers that they have seen in the past. You might also want to have a list of referral sources ready for mothers who are dealing with past abuse for the first time in the postpartum period.

## Loss

The final psychological factor I describe is loss. Previous loss can also increase the risk of depression, and take many forms. Childhood illness and childhood abuse can also represent loss of a "normal" childhood. Childbearing loss can also increase the probability of depression during subsequent pregnancies and after a new baby is born. Recent loss of a partner through death or divorce, or loss of a parent, can also predispose a woman to postpartum depression.

One study examined the long-term effects of parental divorce, later depression, and the subjects' subsequent divorce (O'Connor, *et al.*, 1999). There was a long-term correlation between parental divorce in childhood and depression in adulthood. This association was partly mediated by the quality of the parent–child relationship, teenage pregnancy, leaving home before age 18, and the subject's level of educational attainment.

Loss was also a theme in Beck's (2002) metasynthesis of 18 qualitative studies of postpartum depression. She noted, "loss permeated deep into the crevices of depressed mothers' lives. It insidiously seeped into the very fiber of their beings" (Beck, 2002: 466). There were several types of loss that women in these studies described. The first was the loss of self. This consisted of two components: loss of who you are and loss of a former self. Women didn't know who they were after they had had their babies, and described how they had lost their sexuality, power in the family, personal space, intellectual ability and memory, and occupation. Related to this is loss of identity. This was especially an issue for women who had worked outside the home before they had their babies.

Beck (2002) also described loss of relationships. Women agonized over lost relationships with their infants or other children, partners, friends, and family. They felt depression had robbed them of the positive feelings they should have for their babies. Sometimes women described how they resented and became angry with their babies. Loss of relationships also occurred with women's older children. They suddenly became resentful of their older children's needs, and felt that their older children were "suffocating" them. Women's relationships with their partners became strained. Women admitted resenting their partners, and wishing that their partners would take the initiative to help them. On the other hand, many were ashamed that they were struggling because it meant they were inadequate, or failures as mothers. These feelings of inadequacy kept them isolated from other mothers, whom they assumed were doing a much better job than they were.

The final loss described by Beck (2002) was loss of voice. Mothers suffering from depression made a conscious effort to silence their own voices. They feared the reaction of others if they admitted how they had been struggling. They didn't want to burden friends or family, and feared being rejected or misunderstood. One mother described her experience as "imprisoned in my own prison" (Beck, 2002: 468). When they did find their voice, partners or others often did silence or reject them, contributing further to their loss of voice.

### *Pregnancy loss and high-risk pregnancy*

As described in Chapter 7, traumatic experiences can also include a history of childbearing loss. Women may have had previous abortions, ectopic pregnancies, stillbirths, or miscarriages. This may make them feel that they cannot deliver their babies. Sometimes women who have had previous negative birth experiences can only remember their births with sadness, anger, pain, or fear. A highly detailed birth plan may also indicate a trauma history, where a woman felt completely out of control in a previous situation. Her detailed plan may be an attempt to regain some of this lost control.

## Conclusion

The above-cited studies demonstrate that how a woman feels about herself, her general outlook on life, and how her family history can either protect her or make her vulnerable to depression in the puerperium and beyond. Psychological factors such as prior trauma and loss, a negative attributional style, and unrealistic expectations can all contribute to a mother's risk of depression.

Depression in pregnancy also raises some issues about how we conceptualize postpartum depression. It appears, from this research, that depression during pregnancy is at least as likely as postpartum depression. If that is the case, then it is inaccurate to consider postpartum a time of unique vulnerability. On the other hand, it might be useful for us to conceptualize postpartum depression in lifespan perspective – to see vulnerability to depression as occurring over the life of a woman, and that both pregnancy and postpartum are vulnerable times. On a more hopeful note, even with significant risk factors, depression is not inevitable.

It is now time to turn our attention to the other half of psychosocial factors – social factors. These include women's social environments and their relationships with others.

## Note

1   U.S. Women, Infants and Children supplemental feeding program.

# 9 Social risk factors

Women do not become mothers in a vacuum. They live in families, extended families, cultures, and societies. At each of these levels of social connection, mothers can be protected from, or made more vulnerable to depression. The social factors related to depression include the amount of help she has with her baby and other children, the amount of emotional support she receives from her partner and others around her, her socioeconomic status, and her exposure to stressful life events. Research on these social risk factors is described below.

## Stressful life events

If women experience significant life stresses during pregnancy or postpartum, they are more vulnerable to depression. Stressful life events have a causal role in major depression (Alexander, 2007). For example, Chinese women who developed postpartum depression experienced significantly more stressful life events than their non-depressed counterparts (Xu and Lu, 2001). In her meta-analysis, Beck (2001) found that childcare and life stress had a moderate effect on postpartum depression.

Stressful life events were positively correlated with postpartum depression in a sample 191 low-income women (Ritter, *et al.*, 2000). There were eight categories of stressful life events: death of a loved one, problems with their spouses or partners, economic hardships, problems with friends or family, discrimination, stressful life events related to pregnancy, general life difficulties, and events that had caused depression for these women in the past (e.g. death of a parent).

Stressful life events can also take place in the broader community. Donna describes how the events of September 11, 2001 influenced her and made her vulnerable to depression.

> We had a joint baby shower on September 8. September 11 was three days later. My sister was injured, and they couldn't find her for several hours. I was getting bits and pieces of information. I think my depression started then. I didn't get really bad until after delivery. I've been seeing a psychologist, sometimes twice a week. We're dealing with the disappointment with my difficult pregnancy, my birth, the guilt about not being the perfect mother, September 11. My sister had severe eye lacerations, and my dad still works down there.

### Acculturation

One specific type of life stress is acculturation. Acculturation refers to the cultural adaptation people must experience when they immigrate to a new country, often due to fleeing a war or other political situation that makes life in their home country untenable. Not surprisingly, the degree of acculturation is specifically related to mental health. Some aspects of acculturation include the ability to perform adequate skills for the new country (such as learning the language or how to navigate essential systems, such as housing), preservation of the original culture, social integration into the new society, the moral attitudes of the new country, and loss feelings concerning the country of birth and people with the same cultural background (Knipsheer and Kleber, 2006).

A study of acculturation in new mothers interviewed ten immigrant new mothers with a score of 10 or higher on the EPDS at 12 to 18 months postpartum (Ahmed, *et al.*, 2008). Many of the women in this group attributed their depression to social isolation, physical changes, feeling overwhelmed, and financial worries. Some of the barriers these mothers encountered to receiving care included stigma, embarrassment, language, fear of being labeled unfit, and staff attitudes. Some of the factors which aided in their recovery included getting out of the house; getting support from friends, family and community support groups; and personal psychological adjustment.

In a sample of Vietnamese and Hmong women living in the U.S. (N=30), 43% were clinically depressed or anxious. These rates were much higher than in other samples, with less-acculturated mothers having the highest rates. Particularly disturbing was that one-third had contemplated suicide in the past week. On a more hopeful note, the author noted that even with high levels of depression and anxiety, these mothers were still responsive to their babies (Foss, 2001).

In a multi-factorial model, Dennis and colleagues (2004) found that stressful life events, including immigration in the past five years, predicted depressive symptoms at one week post-partum. Stress-related factors included number of life events during the previous 12 months, mothers' dissatisfaction with their jobs, and a high score on the measure of substance abuse and family violence. Other predictors were a history of non-postpartum depression, lack of perceived support, lack of readiness for hospital discharge, dissatisfaction with their infant feeding method, and pregnancy-induced hypertension. The study included 594 mothers in Vancouver, British Columbia. Mothers with an EPDS score of 9 or above were considered to have depressive symptomatology. Their percentages ranged from 29% at one week post-partum to 20% at 8 weeks. Recent immigrants had almost five times the rate of depression (Dennis, *et al.*, 2004).

Not all studies have shown an effect of acculturation, however. In a study of Hispanic mothers, Beck and colleagues (2005) explored the relationship between acculturation and postpartum depressive symptoms among Hispanic subgroups. Data were collected in two loca-tions: Connecticut (N=377) and Texas (N=150), respectively. Puerto Rican mothers showed more acculturation than mothers of Mexican or other Hispanic origin. Beck, *et al.* (2005) found no consistent relationship between acculturation, postpartum depressive symptomatol-ogy, and diagnoses of postpartum depression. The two significant predictors of depression were Puerto Rican ethnicity and cesarean delivery. The Puerto Rican mothers were actually more acculturated, but were also younger, had more children, bottle-fed more, and were more likely to be single. The findings were limited in that language was the main measure of acculturation. Further, the researchers noted that Hispanics are a heterogeneous group and should not be treated as if they were all the same.

## Summary

Life events can act as stressors. They are particularly likely to cause postpartum depression when a mother is already vulnerable. Factors that increase mothers' vulnerability include a negative attributional style, low self-esteem and self-efficacy, lack of social support, or a combination of these factors.

## Maternal age

Research on the relationship between postpartum depression and maternal age has yielded inconsistent results, but mothers on the high and low ends of the age spectrum have the highest risk for depression. One recent prospective study of 901 women found that women under the age of 20 were at high risk for postpartum depression (Webster, *et al.*, 2000a). The high-risk mothers were also significantly more likely to be unmarried and primiparous. Another study of 465 women found that women ages 20 to 24, *or* 30 and older, were significantly more likely to be depressed at four months postpartum (Chaudron, *et al.*, 2001). At nine months postpartum, mothers aged over 34 were at increased risk for depression (Astbury, *et al.*, 1994). In another study, adolescent mothers reported significantly lower self-esteem, more parenting stress, more child-abuse potential, and a poorer quality of home environment than mothers who were not adolescents (Andreozzi, *et al.*, 2002). While this study did not address depression, it does demonstrate that the younger mothers are more prone to risk factors for depression.

In a large study of U.S. adults (N=2,592), Mirowsky and Ross (2002) compared three groups of young adults: non-parents, those who became parents before age 23, and those who became parents after age 23. They found that respondents who were younger than age 23 at first birth reported more depression than non-parents. And non-parents were more depressed than respondents whose first birth was after age 23. Women who had their babies at age 30 had the lowest levels of depression.

### Summary

Mothers at either end of the age spectrum are vulnerable to depression. Young mothers may be more at risk for depression because they have a higher likelihood of single marital status, low socioeconomic status, and possible past abuse (reflected in teen-mother status, and/or earlier age of consensual sexual activity). Older mothers may have been through infertility assessments, high-risk pregnancies, and possible pregnancy losses. They may have had multiples as a result of fertility treatments. In addition, older mothers have often attained a higher education level, and react with shock when mothering is difficult and overwhelming. These mothers often feel that they cannot "complain" since they went to such great lengths to become pregnant.

## Socioeconomic status

Poverty increases the likelihood of depression, and increases the difficulties new mothers experience because it limits support, access to medical care, and access to community resources. Poor mothers often face additional stresses as they deal with uncertain income, dangerous housing or neighborhoods, and the negative effects of being at the bottom of the social strata. The connection between poverty and depression has been found in both American samples and samples from outside the U.S.

### U.S. samples

In a low-income inner-city sample (Hobfoll, *et al.*, 1995) rates of depression range from 23% to 28% – nearly twice that of middle-class samples – during pregnancy and the postpartum period. The researchers considered poverty a significant risk factor for pre- and postpartum depression. In a study of 114 Hispanic and African American women with low-risk pregnancies, 51% were depressed. The women's depression scores correlated to other health-related variables including bodily pain, general health, emotional and physical functioning (McKee, *et al.*, 2001). Yonkers, *et al.* (2001) found that 37% of a low-income minority sample had depressive symptoms, and 6.5% to 8.5% met criteria for major depression.

In the National Maternal Health Survey (N=7,537), a stratified nationally representative sample of births in 1988, 23.8% of the sample were depressed when their babies were approximately 17 months old. This study sampled from 48 states, the District of Columbia, and New York City. Blacks, low and very low-birth-weight babies were oversampled, as were low-income mothers (McLennan and Kotelchuck, 2000; McLennan, *et al.*, 2001). Three years later, 16.6% of the respondents were depressed, and 36% of those with elevated depression scores at Time 1 had elevated depression scores at Time 2 (McLennan, *et al.*, 2001).

Even within the group of poor mothers, there is variation. In a study of 191 low-income women (Ritter, *et al.* 2000), women with a higher relative income, who had social support and higher self-esteem, had lower levels of depression.

### International studies

Low socioeconomic status is a risk factor for depression in other countries as well. Patel, *et al.* (2001) noted how depression is common in developing countries, where there is often a vicious cycle of poverty, depression, and disability for women. In a sample from India, economic deprivation and a poor marital relationship were both important risk factors in the development of postpartum depression, and its continuing on past six months postpartum (Patel, *et al.*, 2002). Other poverty-related variables, such as hunger and low education, were also associated with depression. This entire sample was low-income. Even so, relative poverty made a difference. Similarly, in a sample of 257 Turkish women, living in a shanty was one predictor of depression (Danaci, *et al.*, 2002).

In an Irish sample from a disadvantaged neighborhood, 28% of 377 women were depressed when contacted a year after birth. The four risk factors associated with their depression were lower age; lack of a confidant; previous miscarriage, and previous treatment for depression (Cryan, *et al.*, 2001). In a South African sample of poor women at two months postpartum, Cooper, *et al.* (1999) found that an astonishing 35% met criteria for major depression. The authors found that depression was associated with poor partner support and an unplanned pregnancy.

Debt is one aspect of poverty that has been specifically related to depression. In a longitudinal study of 271 families with young children, worry about debt was the strongest predictor of depression in mothers at the initial and follow-up contacts (Reading and Reynolds, 2001). Indeed, worrying about debt predicted depression six months later. Other economic factors associated with depression included overall family income, not being a homeowner, and lack of access to a car.

### Summary

Although poverty is a risk factor, and depression occurs in low-income communities, we should not assume that all low-income populations have higher levels of depression. Indeed, as I'll describe in subsequent sections, there are populations with much lower incomes that are doing some very important things in terms of protecting new mothers. And even within a low-income population, higher relative income, social support, and high self-esteem buffer the effects of poverty.

## Maternity leave and employment

Maternity leave and decision making about returning to work can also influence depression. In one study, 570 pregnant women were interviewed at five months' gestation, and at one and four months postpartum (Hyde, *et al.*, 1995). At the four-month interview, there was no difference in depression or anger based on return to work. However, full-time workers had more anxiety. Women who took leave of less than six weeks, and had a lot of marital concerns, had the highest depression scores. The authors concluded that short maternity leave, especially when combined with other risk factors, increased the risk for depression in new mothers.

A prospective study of 817 employed mothers in Minnesota studied women at five and eleven weeks postpartum (Dagher, *et al.*, 2009). Using hierarchical linear regression, the researchers found that higher EPDS scores were associated with higher psychological demands, lower schedule autonomy, and lower perceived control over work and family. The prevalence of postpartum depression in this sample was 4.7% at eleven weeks. The authors found that psychological job demands and lower schedule autonomy were associated with postpartum depression.

Similarly, 436 women completed questionnaires five times during the first year postpartum (Gjerdingen and Chaloner, 1994). Employment had a significant impact on depression, especially longer work hours, and a maternity leave of less than 24 weeks. Other factors, such as maternal fatigue, loss of sleep, concern about appearance, and infant illness were also related to depression. Physical illness, previous mental illness, poor social support, fewer recreational activities, young age, and low income all contributed to depression as well.

Another study interviewed mothers three weeks before they started full-time out-of-home care for their babies, and followed them over the next six months. Employed mothers who were working, but wanted to be at home, were more depressed than mothers who were working and wanted to work. The children of mothers who wanted to be at home, but were working, were also more likely to experience unstable care. Early entry into care was related to higher income, less maternal depression, and the use of family home care (McKim, *et al.*, 1999).

A Canadian study of 447 mothers examined the relationship between employment status and depressive symptoms at six months postpartum (Des Rivières-Pigeon, *et al.*, 2001). The authors found that women on maternity leave, or women who were employed, had the lowest levels of depression. Women at home full-time were more likely to report a lack of social support, and to have an unwanted or mistimed pregnancy.

Women who have control over when (or if) they return to work have the lowest levels of depression. But other psychosocial variables, such as previous depression and lack of social support, continue to have an influence, in addition to maternity leave and employment. In the final section of this chapter, I describe the most influential of the social factors – social support.

## Social support

> This was the first grandchild on my side. I thought everyone would come to see me. My mom did, but only after I called and asked her to come. My dad came the next day, but only for the day. I was very isolated after the baby. I had no friends with babies. It was hard. I thought my family would come and everyone would hold the baby. Everyone

came to my house at Christmas and they spent six hours in the basement playing video games. I was really hurt by that. Nobody would help me. I've really never said anything. Maybe it would have been better if I had said something. [DeeDee]

Of the social factors considered, far and away the most influential factor is a woman's level of social support. As the research on non-postpartum depression has repeatedly demonstrated, lack of social support is related to depression. This is especially true when women are faced with stressful life events. Social support is also related to many of the factors described in the previous chapters. It increases self-esteem and self-efficacy, acts as a buffer when a woman is faced with a temperamentally difficult child, and can even alter a woman's attributional style. Any effort to prevent postpartum depression must include a strong component of social support. The social-support literature has included general support, partner support, and the impact of the social network. Social support even changes women's physiology. These studies are described below.

### General support

Social support helps prevent depression across the social strata. A study of 123 women at two weeks postpartum found that social support had a significant effect on depressive symptoms, functional status, and infant care, but did not moderate the effect of adverse birth events on these same outcomes (Hunker, *et al.*, 2009). In a study of 191 low-income women, Ritter, *et al.* (2000) found that women with good social support were less likely to become depressed. Moreover, women who had high levels of support were more likely to have high levels of self-esteem. Joanne describes a negative reaction from most of her friends, but notes that one friend continued to reach out to her.

> I was usually an outgoing person, but I didn't have the energy to relate to others. My friends didn't know what to do. They thought I had had a nervous breakdown. Many stayed away. Even now, many are surprised that I can still function. I had one friend who was very supportive and loving continually, even though she didn't understand. She brought meals, wrote little notes. She made no demands on my recovery. My mother-in-law and husband were helpful during that time too. [Joanne]

In a prospective hospital-based study, Webster and colleagues (2000a) found that low social support was strongly related to depression at 16 weeks postpartum. Several types of support were specifically related to depression including low support from friends, low family support, conflict with partner, and feeling unloved by partner. Fifty-one percent of the depressed women had a score of 25 or below on the Maternity Social Support Scale, while only 32% of the non-depressed women had a comparable score.

In another study, Webster and colleagues (2000b) found that social support was related to both depression and physical health. Women with low support during pregnancy were more likely to report poorer health during pregnancy and postpartum. They were more likely to delay seeking prenatal care, but to seek medical care more frequently once they did. And they were more likely to be depressed postpartum.

An Australian study (Haslam, *et al.*, 2006) found that women whose parents provided emotional support, and who had high self-efficacy, had lower levels of postpartum depression. This study included 247 pregnant and postpartum women. Mothers were assessed in their last trimester of pregnancy and at four weeks postpartum. Contrary to prediction, partner support did not influence levels of postpartum depression. The authors hypothesized that it was likely that support from the women's parents increased mothers' sense of competence and self-efficacy in caring for their new babies. In addition, support from parents may have been more specific than partner support to the needs of new mothers.

A qualitative study of 41 Canadian mothers found that social support was important for women's recovery from postpartum depression (Letourneau, *et al.*, 2007). In this study, mothers identified two types of support that were most helpful in their recovery: instrumental support (e.g. help with household chores), and informational support (e.g. information about postpartum depression). Affirmation support was more helpful when it came from other mothers who could empathize with their experiences, rather than from people who had never been depressed. Mothers also identified partners, friends, family, other mothers, and health-care providers as important sources of support. The mothers in this study indicated that they preferred one-on-one to group or telephone support, especially in the beginning. However, once mothers started to recover, they found that group support was helpful.

A study of 344 pregnant women found that 23 had screened positive for moderate-to-severe anxiety (Mann, *et al.*, 2008a). The researchers found that overall religiosity and social support were significantly associated with lower anxiety, whereas a history of psychiatric disorders was associated with a higher risk. Among the specific factors were self-rated religiosity, self-rated spirituality, and participation in religious activities. In another study with this same population, Mann, *et al.* (2008b) found that women who participated in organized religious activities were markedly less likely to report depressive symptoms (EPDS≥13). This finding was true even after controlling for the effects of social support and baseline depression scores. Religious attendance may have had a stress-buffering effect that specifically helps women as they make the transition to new motherhood.

### Partner support

Husbands or partners are key sources of social support. Several studies have found that when that partner support is not available, mothers are more likely to be depressed. A survey of 396 mothers in Canada found that partner support was significantly related to depressive symptoms (Dennis and Ross, 2006b). Women with depressive symptoms at eight weeks had significantly lower perceptions of relation-specific and postpartum-specific partner support than non-depressed women. In addition, women with depressive symptoms reported more conflict with their partners than did non-depressed women. The depressed women were more likely to indicate that their partners made them angry, tried to change them, and made them work hard to avoid conflict. Multivariate analysis revealed that three variables with regard to support were important: perceived social integration; partner encouragement to obtain help when needed, and partner agreement with how mother was handling infant care. The authors concluded that shared activities, problem-focused information and assistance, and positive feedback from the partner decreased a mother's likelihood of developing depression at eight weeks postpartum.

Another study attempted to determine the importance of social support with three samples of postpartum women: 105 middle-class white women, 37 middle-class mothers of premature babies, and 57 low-income African American mothers (Logsdon and Usui, 2001). Using structural equation modeling, the authors found that support received and closeness to partner were significant predictors of both self-esteem and depression. These predictors were the same for all three groups of mothers.

In comparing 193 mothers and fathers on levels of postpartum depression, Dudley and colleagues (2001) found that fathers may be even more influenced by the quality of the relationship than mothers. Mothers' depression was influenced primarily by their own personalities, and perinatal- and infant-related factors. In contrast, fathers were more influenced by the mothers' personality difficulties, unresolved past events, the mothers' current mental health, infant difficulties, and the state of their marriage/relationship. Depression in one partner was moderately correlated with depression in the other.

A study of 107 husbands and wives after the birth of their first child had similar findings. Lutz and Hock (2002) found that men who were less satisfied with their marriages were more likely to be depressed. For both men and women, fear of abandonment and fear of loneliness were significantly related to depressive symptoms. These relationships were stronger for men than for women in the sample.

In a qualitative study of nine mothers and five fathers, mothers all had a EPDS score greater than 13 at six to eight weeks postpartum (Tammentie, *et al.*, 2004). Support from partners, family members and friends was important during the postpartum period. The authors found that there was great discrepancy between what the mothers expected parenting to be like and what it was actually like for depressed mothers. More mothers than fathers strove for protection, perceived that the infant tied them down, and had high expectations of family life. Mothers and fathers felt overwhelmed by the amount of time and effort the baby took, and both felt exhausted by and inadequate for the task. Having a baby also changed their key relationships, and there was often no time for each other.

A related question is the impact of unmarried childbearing. Does marital status make any difference in maternal depression postpartum? Kiernan and Pickett (2006), using data from the U.K. Millennium Cohort Study (N=18,533), compared four sets of parents: married parents, cohabitating parents, solo mothers with a closely involved father, and solo mothers without an active partner. They were assessing whether partnership status was related to maternal smoking during pregnancy, breastfeeding, and maternal depression. The researchers found that all three aspects were inversely related to parental connectedness. The cohabitating mothers had worse health outcomes than the married mothers. Among mothers who were not married, smoking was more likely among the women without a regular partner. For breastfeeding, stronger parental bonds were associated with initiation of breastfeeding, with a significant difference between the cohabitating and the solo mothers. Maternal depression was associated with looser parental bonding. Among non-married mothers, this difference was most striking among cohabitating vs. solo mothers. The authors found the worse outcomes among the cohabitating mothers.

In a qualitative study of 535 first-time parents in Sweden, Ahlborg and Strandmark (2006) found that there were four factors affecting the quality of the relationships between couples: coping by adjustment to parental role (mutual support of each other as parents), the couple's intimacy (togetherness and love), coping by communication (verbal and non-verbal confirmation), and coping with external conditions (seeking support). The researchers suggested that these factors be discussed in parent groups as a way to ease stress between couples during the first postpartum year and prevent unnecessary separations and divorces. Similarly, Beach and colleagues (1994) noted that marital interventions not only have potential for increasing marital adjustment. Marital discord often precedes depression, and may be sufficiently difficult to provoke the onset of a first episode of depression. Marital interventions have considerable potential for both treating and preventing depression.

Partner support also proved helpful in the treatment of postpartum depression. From a sample of 29 women with postpartum depression, 13 were randomly assigned to receive psychoeducation for seven sessions. The second group had partners participate in four of the seven sessions. At the conclusion of the study, women whose partners were included in the intervention had significantly decreased depressive symptoms compared with the women whose partners were not included (Misri, *et al.*, 2000b).

When partner support is absent, support from friends can protect women from depression. A study of social support among women with critically ill children sought to determine whether friend support would buffer the negative effect of low spousal support (Rini, *et al.*, 2008). This study included 163 mothers of critically ill children. All were married and they were assessed at 3, 6, and 12 months after their children had received stem-cell transplants. The investigators found that women with low spousal and low friend/family support had the poorest function of all groups. The women with low spousal support but high friend/family support fared much better. In fact, their functioning was comparable to that of the women with high spousal support.

### The role of culture: social structures that protect new mothers

The above-cited studies focus on women's networks involving family or friends. Another type of research on social support has examined the role of the culture in which women live. Stern and Kruckman (1983), in their classic paper, found that depression, or even the postpartum blues, are virtually non-existent in many diverse cultures around the world. Although these cultures differed dramatically from one another, they had common elements. The characteristics of this type of cultural support are listed below.

#### A distinct postpartum period

In almost all the societies studied, the postpartum period was recognized as a time that is distinct from normal life. Postpartum is a time when mothers are supposed to recuperate, their activities are limited, and they are taken care of by female relatives. This was also common practice in colonial America, and was referred to as the "lying-in" period (Wertz and Wertz, 1989).

#### Protective measures reflecting the new mother's vulnerability

During the postpartum period, new mothers are recognized as being especially vulnerable. In some cultures, the postpartum period is considered a time of ritual uncleanness, while in others it is a time for mothers to rest, regain strength, and care for their babies. There were many rituals associated with vulnerability: certain foods mothers must either eat or avoid, wrapping of mothers' head or abdomen, and limitations on the amount of company they receive. All of these rituals protected the mother, and set aside the postpartum period as distinct from normal life.

#### Social seclusion and mandated rest

Related to the concept of vulnerability are the widespread practices of social seclusion for the new mother. During this time, she is supposed to rest and restrict normal activities. In the Punjab, women are secluded from everyone but female relatives and the midwife for five days. After the five days, there is a "stepping out" ceremony for the mother and baby. In other cultures, the time of seclusion can be for as long as three months. Seclusion and rest also allow mothers to recover, promotes breastfeeding, and limits their normal activities.

*Functional assistance*

In order to make sure that women get the rest they need, they must be relieved of their normal workload. Functional assistance involves care of older children, household help, and personal attendance during labor. As in the colonial period in the U.S., women often return to their families' homes to ensure that this type of assistance is available.

*Social recognition of her new role and status*

In cultures where there is a low incidence of the blues or depression, there is a great deal of personal attention given to the mother. This has been described as "mothering the mother." In these various cultures, the new status of the mother is recognized through social rituals and gifts. For example, in Punjabi culture, there is the ritual stepping-out ceremony, ritual bathing and hair washing performed by the midwife, and a ceremonial meal prepared by a Brahmin. When she returns to her husband's family, she returns with many gifts she has been given for herself and the baby. Ritual bathing, washing of hair, massage, binding of the abdomen, and other types of personal care are also prominent in the postpartum rituals of rural Guatemala, for Mayan women in the Yucatan, and for Latina women both in the U.S. and Mexico. Here is a description of one of these recognition rituals performed by the Chagga people of Uganda.

> Three months after the birth of her child, the Chagga woman's head is shaved and crowned with a bead tiara, she is robed in an ancient skin garment worked with beads, a staff such as the elders carry is put in her hand, and she emerges from her hut for her first public appearance with her baby. Proceeding slowly towards the market, they are greeted with songs such as are sung to warriors returning from battle. She and her baby have survived the weeks of danger. The child is no longer vulnerable, but a baby who has learned what love means, has smiled its first smiles, and is now ready to learn about the bright, loud world outside.
>
> (Dunham, 1992: 148)

Even in the absence of these types of ritual, mothers need physical nurturance. Professional postpartum doula Salle Webber describes what mothers need in the first few weeks after birth.

> In my work as a Doula, my focus is on the mother. I want to provide whatever it is that she needs to feel comfortable, nourished, relaxed, and appreciated: to facilitate a harmonious transition for both mother and child in those profound first days and weeks after birth. A mother needs someone who cares about how many times the baby woke to nurse in the night, how many diapers were changed, how her breasts are feeling. She may need her back massaged or her sheets changed, or she may need someone to provide an abundant supply of water or tea, salads ready-made in the refrigerator, a bowl of cut-up fruit. She needs to be able to complain about how little her mate understands what she's going through, and perhaps, some gentle reminders of all the contributions he has made. She needs someone to hold the baby so she can take a shower or even go to the bathroom; someone to answer the phone when she's napping; someone to water her plants or garden, to clean the kitchen and bathroom, to keep up on the family's laundry. She may have

many questions and concerns that only an experienced mother can understand. She needs patience and kind words and a clean and calm environment.

(Webber, 1992: 17)

### *What mothers usually face*

This is far cry from what mothers in the U.S. and other industrialized nations often receive postpartum. After a baby is born in mainstream U.S. culture, all the attention shifts from the mother to the baby. Many of the mothers interviewed for this book felt a profound sense of loss and abandonment by their medical caregivers and their families. In general, there was little acknowledgment of what these women had been through, both physically and emotionally, by giving birth.

> I really wanted someone to make me feel special. All the attention was on the baby. [Barbara]

> I feel a sense of anti-climax. I was used to being the center of attention. Then I had to go back to being a normal healthy person. I'm not begging for attention, but now everyone only pays attention to the baby. It would be nice to have some attention afterwards. While you're pregnant, you're feeling fat and slobby, and don't want it. After the baby, you want it. [Julie]

> I felt like I didn't matter. I felt like they weren't interested in me after I had my baby. My husband said "of course they are not interested. You've had your baby." The six-week visit seemed like an eternity away. I wrote [my midwife] a note to thank her. She didn't even mention it when I saw her at six weeks. When I felt great, they treated me nicely. Now when I feel so awful with this baby, no one seems to be available to me. [Karen]

> My doctor thought her job was done after my daughter was born. It's ridiculous to think the job is done just because you've delivered the baby. I called her a couple of times after, and she told me to see a social worker. I eventually left my OB. There were many reasons, but mainly because she left me high and dry after delivery. [Jan]

> After the birth, I had several people tell me that the most important thing was that I had a healthy baby. Yes, that is important. But what about me? No one pays attention to the fact that you've had major surgery. They would have paid more attention if you had had your appendix out. [Sally]

### *The health-enhancing effects of social support*

Support from other people is not simply a social nicety. It is essential for our very survival. Many of the studies on the health effects of social support have examined the health effects of marriage. But other studies have examined the impact of other types of social ties. These studies are described below.

In a review of the literature on marriage and health, Kiecolt-Glaser and Newton (2001) found that being married reduced premature mortality by 500% for men. For women, marriage reduced premature mortality by only 50% – probably because women have larger social networks outside marriage than men.

## Physiological effects of social support

Intimacy in couples had a stress-buffering effect and lowered the physiological reaction to job stress. Couples who spent time on intimacy had reduced daily cortisol levels, and this effect was present even when there was job stress (Ditzen, *et al.*, 2008). The authors concluded that their findings were in line with previous findings on the health effects of happy marital relationships.

There appears to be an immune system component of partner support. In a study of 61 nurses, women who reported insecure relationships with their partners had lower natural killer-cell cytotoxicity than their counterparts with secure attachments (Picardi, *et al.*, 2007). Perceived stress was also related to the lower natural killer-cell cytotoxicity. A secure attachment leads to feeling valued and worthy, and seeing their partners as trustworthy, reliable and available for support when needed. An insecure attachment is characterized by high-attachment-related anxiety, avoidance, or both.

## The physiological impact of marital strife

While the effects of marriage on health are generally good, ongoing marital strife is not. In fact, it increases the risk of heart disease, particularly for women. A 13-year longitudinal study of married women found that women with poor-quality marriages had higher rates of several markers for cardiovascular disease: low HDL cholesterol; high triglycerides; and higher body mass index, blood pressure, depression, and anger (Gallo, *et al.*, 2003).

In data from the Framingham Offspring Study, married men were half as likely to die during the follow-up period as unmarried men (Eaker, *et al.*, 2007). The Framingham Offspring Study is the second generation of data collection from the Framingham Heart Study, a major study of cardiovascular disease, now following the second and third generations of study participants. For women, marital status alone was not enough to prolong life; however, aspects of how women handled marital conflict were. Women who "self-silenced" in conflicts were four times more likely to die compared with those who did not. The findings were true even after adjusting for systolic blood pressure, age, body mass index, cigarette smoking, diabetes, and cholesterol.

Another way in which relationships may increase cardiovascular risk is by impacting sleep. Two recent studies have examined the relationship between security of adult attachments and sleep quality. Sleep is a physiologically vulnerable state. In order to sleep soundly, people must feel sufficiently secure so they can downregulate vigilance and alertness. And to do so, one must be secure in social relationships (Troxel, *et al.*, 2007).

In the first study, 78 married adults completed questionnaires about their sleep quality, quality of current partnership (secure vs. insecure attachment), and depression (Carmichael and Reis, 2005). The sleep questionnaire asked about seven aspects of sleep including perceived sleep quality, sleep latency (time to get to sleep), sleep duration, habitual sleep efficiency, sleep disturbances, and use of sleep medications. Married participants with anxious attachments reported poorer sleep quality, even after controlling for depression. Women with insecure attachments were concerned that their partners were emotionally unavailable and not trustworthy. The researchers indicated that one limitation to their study was that they used a self-report measure of sleep, rather than assessing sleep directly.

Troxel and colleagues (2007) addressed that limitation by using polysomnographic studies to assess sleep directly. In a study of 107 women with recurrent major depression, marital status and security of that relationship predicted quality and efficiency of sleep. If women had anxious attachments, particularly if they were separated or widowed, they had a significantly smaller percentage of stage 3–4 sleep than women who were currently partnered and who had secure attachments. The authors noted the importance of stage 3–4 sleep in protecting individuals from cardiovascular and metabolic diseases.

One intriguing question relevant to postpartum women is whether there are similar effects when women sleep near vs. away from their babies. What is the impact on sleep when women are separated from their babies at night? Do they also enter a state of hypervigilance? Do women who sleep near their babies have a higher percentage of stage 3–4 sleep? These are questions to explore in future studies, with important implications for how we counsel mothers. This is another reason that programs that seek to separate mothers and babies at night may prove ineffective. Mothers may be listening for their babies at night and not entering deep sleep as a result.

### When support is absent: social isolation and cardiac risk factors

Much of what we know about the health effects of social support comes from studying its absence – social isolation and an inability to trust others. This psychological state also triggers the inflammatory response. Individuals who expect the worst from people become hypervigilant to rejection in social relationships. And this world-view has discernable, physical sequelae.

A study of 6,814 healthy men and women found that participants with higher levels of cynical distrust, chronic stress, or depression had higher levels of inflammation (Ranjit, *et al.*, 2007). Inflammation included elevated C-reactive protein, IL-6, and fibrinogen. Chronic stress was associated with higher IL-6 and C-reactive protein, and depression was associated with higher IL-6. All are risk factors for heart disease.

Where you fall in the social hierarchy also has an impact on your cardiovascular health. If a woman perceives that she has low social status – because of education, ethnicity, vocation, or income level – it raises risk of cardiovascular disease via several physiological mechanisms. Low social status was associated with low-grade inflammation in a sample of 121 white and African American men and women (Hong, *et al.*, 2006). In this sample, researchers measured soluble intercellular adhesion molecule (sICAM) and endothelin-1 (ET-1). Both are measures of vascular inflammation. Men and women in the lowest social class had the highest levels of sICAM and ET-1. Low status was also reflected in the measure of C-reactive protein (CRP) in another study of middle-aged and older adults (McDade, *et al.*, 2006). In this sample, African Americans, women, and those with lower education had the highest levels of CRP. The authors concluded that psychosocial stress and health behaviors are both important determinants of systemic inflammation and increased cardiac risk.

While the research on cardiac risk factors may not seem immediately relevant to postpartum depression, it demonstrates that our social relationships either increase or decrease our vulnerability to stress. This vulnerability manifests through several physiological mechanisms, including inflammation. These findings indicate that humans are social animals and that social support, social integration, and perceived social status have measurable effects on health. Indeed, loved ones, and others in our social orbit, help regulate our internal states. What is particularly interesting about these findings is their continuity throughout the lifespan, from infancy to old age. With regard to new mothers, these findings tell us that social support is critical for new mothers – for both their physical and mental health. These findings also contradict commonly given advice that separates mothers and babies. This separation may trigger a stress response in mothers and be counterproductive to their recovery. Instead of separating them, an alternative is to support mother and baby together. This would down-regulate the stress response and allow mothers to gradually grow into their new role. Lewis and colleagues (2000) noted the importance of our relationships in maintaining our physical and mental health, and observed the following:

> Adults remain social animals; they continue to require a source of stabilization outside themselves. That open-loop design means that in some important ways, people cannot be stable on their own – not should or shouldn't be, but *can't* be.
>
> (Lewis, *et al.*, 2000: 86; emphasis added)

### *Summary*

Social factors have a significant role to play in the development of postpartum depression. Women who experience stressful life events during the childbearing years are at increased risk for depression, as are mothers at both ends of the age continuum. Low income can also make mothers vulnerable to depression, but not in all cases. Control over when to return to work can be protective, but lack of control increases risk. Social support can be an important buffer against life stress. Beyond a woman's immediate circle of family and friends, an entire culture can determine whether mothers are vulnerable to depression.

# Part III

# Treatment

# 10 Alternative and complementary therapies I

## Omega-3s, SAM-e, and exercise

Complementary and alternative treatment modalities are widely used for treating a variety of conditions, including psychiatric disorders (Freeman, 2009). Werneke and colleagues (2006) noted that up to 57% of psychiatric patients have used alternative treatments to treat depression and anxiety. With regard to perinatal depression, complementary treatments include Omega-3s, exercise, SAM-e, bright light therapy, and St. John's wort (Freeman, 2009). All show efficacy in treating depression. This chapter describes the efficacy of Omega-3s, SAM-e, and exercise. The other modalities are described in Chapter 11.

### Omega-3 fatty acids

> Overall, omega-3 EFA [essential fatty acids] are exciting therapeutic agents to explore in the context of psychiatric disorders. They hold the potential for primary prevention and contribute to other health benefits as well.
>
> (Freeman, *et al.*, 2006a)

Over the past 100 years, there has been a critical shift in the diets that Western populations consume: specifically, in the ratio of Omega-6:Omega-3 fatty acids. This shift has had a negative impact on our health. The amount of Omega-3s we consume has decreased dramatically while we have increased our consumption of Omega-6s. Omega-6s and Omega-3s are both polyunsaturated fatty acids (PUFAs) (see Figure 10.1). Omega-6s are proinflammatory and Omega-3s are anti-inflammatory. Omega-6 fatty acids are found in vegetable oils, such as corn and safflower oils, and are abundant in our diets. Omega-3s are found in fatty fish and some plant sources, and are much less so. While some Omega-6s are necessary for good nutrition, they become harmful when the ratio of Omega-6s to Omega-3s is too high – as it is in modern diets. Kiecolt-Glaser and colleagues (2007) noted that the hunter-gatherer diet had an estimated ratio of Omega-6s:Omega-3s of 2:1 or 3:1. The ratio in the typical North American diet today ranges from 15:1 to 17:1. Along these same lines, in Australia and New Zealand, the ratio is approximately 10:1 (Rees, *et al.*, 2005).

With regard to depression, the long-chain Omega-3s are of interest. These are eicosapentaenoic acid (EPA) and docosahexaenoic acid (DHA) (Bratman and Girman, 2003). Alpha-linolenic acid (ALA) is the parent Omega-3 fatty acid and is found in flax and other plant sources (see Figure 10.1). ALA is an essential fatty acid, and while important for good nutrition, it is too metabolically removed from the long-chain Omega-3s and has no efficacy in the prevention or treatment of depression (Freeman, *et al.*, 2006a).

Much of the research on the mental health effects of Omega-3s comes from studying populations who have high rates of fish consumption. These studies are described below.

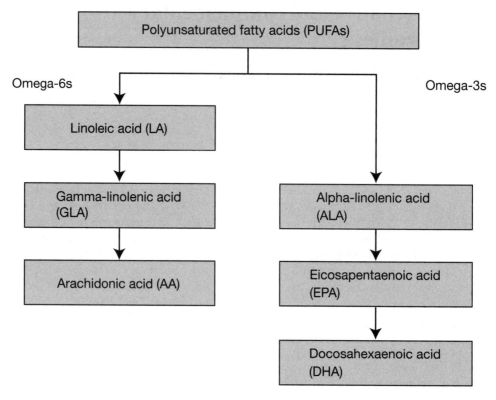

*Figure 10.1* Polyunsaturated fatty acids (PUFAs) (Wang, *et al.* Agency for Healthcare Research & Quality, 2004. Used with permission.).

### Omega-3s and depression in population studies

Populations who eat a lot of fish have lower rates of a variety of mental health problems, including postpartum depression. When comparing national rates of fish consumption with national rates of mental illness, researchers found that populations that ate less than 50 lb/23 kg of seafood a year (1 to 1.5 lb/500 g to 1.5 kg per person per week) had the highest rates of affective disorders (Noaghiul and Hibbeln, 2003). In a large population study, with more than 14,000 women from 22 countries, Hibbeln (2002) found that postpartum depression was up to 50 times more common in countries with low fish consumption. For example, the rate of postpartum depression in Singapore was 0.5%. In South Africa, it was 24.5%. Similarly, Rees and colleagues (2005) observed that the rates for postpartum depression in North America and Europe are ten times those in Taiwan, Japan, Hong Kong, and some regions of China.

Not all researchers have found a link between postpartum depression and fish consumption, however. In a study of 865 pregnant Japanese women, investigators failed to find lower rates of depression in women who ate more fish (Miyake, *et al.*, 2006). The researchers are likely to have encountered a ceiling effect as Japan has one of the highest fish-consumption rates in the world. In addition, Omega-3s were estimated from dietary questionnaires rather than measured directly in the plasma, which may have influenced the findings.

### Treatment with EPA and DHA

In addition to their efficacy in prevention, EPA and DHA can also be used as a treatment for depression and other psychiatric conditions. EPA, in particular, has an antidepressant effect for all patients, but also for specific populations, including pregnant and breastfeeding women (van der Watt, *et al.*, 2008).

In a review, EPA had efficacy in the treatment of depression in four of the six studies included (Peet and Stokes, 2005). The authors found that 1 g of EPA per day was the effective dose. Two grams had the same effects as one gram. Doses higher than two grams seemed to have the reverse effect. Similarly, in a meta-analysis of ten studies (N=329), Lin and Su (2007) found a significant antidepressant effect of EPA with DHA for patients with depression and with bipolar disorder. They did note some methodologic limitations of some of the studies they cited.

EPA and DHA were also used to treat major depression during pregnancy (Su, *et al.*, 2008). In this study, 36 pregnant women with major depression participated in a randomized clinical trial comparing a placebo to 3.4 g EPA/DHA (2.2 g DHA, 1.2 g EPA). Compared with those in the placebo group, subjects in the EPA/DHA group had significantly lower depression scores on the Hamilton Rating Scale for Depression at six and eight weeks postpartum, and had a higher (though non-significant) remission rate. EPA and DHA were well tolerated and there were no adverse effects for either mother or baby. The authors noted that this treatment was likely to have been effective because it halted the arachidonic-acid cascade. Arachidonic acid is a long-chain Omega-6 fatty acid and is proinflammatory (see Figure 10.1). People with mood disorders often have higher levels of arachidonic acid than the levels of those without mood disorders.

Not all studies have found that EPA/DHA are effective treatments, however. An open-label trial with mothers who had had previous episodes of postpartum depression found that fish-oil supplements did not prevent depression from occurring after a subsequent delivery. In this study, women were recruited between 34 to 36 weeks' gestation. The women were treated through to 12 weeks postpartum, with dosages of 1,730 mg EPA and 1,230 mg DHA per day. When four of the seven women recruited for the study became depressed, recruitment ceased. The authors hypothesized several possible explanations for their findings including an inadequate dose of EPA or DHA, administration that was too late in the pregnancy to prevent depression, and the wrong ratio of EPA to DHA. Even given their findings, however, the authors indicated that the results of other studies support continued investigation of EPA and DHA in the treatment of postpartum mood disorders (Marangell, *et al.*, 2004).

In a study of 59 women with perinatal major depressive disorder, women received either 1.9 g EPA and DHA per day or a corn-oil placebo (Freeman, *et al.*, 2008). Women in both groups also received supportive psychotherapy. The overall dietary intake of Omega-3s in both groups was low, with women eating less than half of a serving per month. At the end of the eight weeks of the study, both groups had significantly lower depression scores. There was no difference between the treatment and placebo groups. It is possible that the psychotherapy that both groups received may have made it impossible to determine the effects of the Omega-3s.

EPA is also useful for other conditions, including depression in bipolar disorder in a 12-week double-blind trial (Frangou, *et al.*, 2006). In this study, 75 patients were randomly assigned to one of three conditions for adjunctive therapy: placebo; 1 g ethyl-EPA, or 2 g ethyl-EPA. Both EPA groups showed substantial improvement over the placebo group after 12 weeks. A dose of 1 g was as effective as a dose of 2 g, and there was no advantage to 2 g over 1 g. Depression was measured by the Hamilton Rating Scale for Depression and the Clinical Global Impression scale. Summarizing their findings, the authors noted that EPA was well tolerated and safe, had an antidepressant effect, and may prove more acceptable to patients than pharmacologic interventions.

Hallahan and colleagues (2007) tested the efficacy of EPA/DHA supplementation in patients with recurrent self-harm. In this study, 49 patients with repeated acts of self-harm were randomized to receive a placebo, or 1.2 g EPA and 900 mg DHA per day. After 12 weeks, the patients receiving EPA and DHA had significantly improved depressive symptoms and lower daily stresses. The authors noted that these were significant markers for suicidality and that supplementation with EPA and DHA had lowered their risk.

A report by the American Psychiatric Association's Omega-3 Fatty Acids Subcommittee concluded that the preponderance of evidence points to a protective effect of EPA and DHA in mood disorders (Freeman, *et al.*, 2006a). EPA and DHA provided a significant benefit in unipolar and bipolar disorder, but the results are inconclusive for other psychiatric disorders. The researchers further noted that supplementation with Omega-3s could also help counter some of the metabolic and obesity effects of medications for psychiatric conditions.

Fish-oil capsules, the chief way to supplement with Omega-3s, were found to be tolerable for pregnant and postpartum women (Freeman and Sinha, 2007). In a study of 59 pregnant and postpartum women with major depression, participants received four capsules daily with either 1.84 g EPA and DHA, or corn oil. Thirteen women reported side effects; the most common were unpleasant breath or heartburn/reflux. Six women reported side effects in the Omega-3 group and seven in the placebo group. No participant dropped out of the study due to tolerability of side effects.

## Why it works: stress, inflammation, and EPA

EPA is a powerful anti-inflammatory that specifically lowers proinflammatory cytokines, and this probably explains its efficacy in treating depression. EPA mediates the inflammatory action of arachidonic acid by competing for the same metabolic pathways. In a large population study, high levels of Omega-3s (ALA, EPA, and DHA) in participants' plasma were related to lower levels of the proinflammatory cytokines IL-1$\alpha$, IL-1$\beta$, IL-6, and TNF-$\alpha$ and higher levels of anti-inflammatory cytokines, such as IL-10. For people with low levels of Omega-3s, the opposite was true: these people had high levels of proinflammatory cytokines and low levels of anti-inflammatory cytokines (Ferrucci, *et al.*, 2006).

In their review, Parker and colleagues (2006) noted that people with major depression had significantly higher ratios of arachidonic acid to EPA in both serum cholesteryl esters and phospholipids. High dietary proportions of Omega-6 fatty acids lead to high levels of arachidonic acid, rather than EPA, in the cell membranes of both tissues, leading in turn to a high proportion of inflammatory eicosanoids. An increase in arachidonic acid also affects production of EPA and DHA because it competes for the metabolizing enzymes.

Researchers have examined the impact of EPA and DHA on stress and stress-related inflammation. When college students were deficient in Omega-3s, they had a higher inflammatory response when exposed to a lab-induced stressor. In contrast, students with higher levels of EPA/DHA had a lower inflammatory response to stress (Maes, *et al.*, 2000). Similarly, Kiecolt-Glaser and colleagues (2007), in their study of 43 older adults, noted that previous stress and depression appear to "prime" the inflammatory response, making individuals more susceptible to subsequent stress. Even with modest supplementation with EPA and DHA, however, norepinephrine levels dropped.

A study from Japan had similar findings (Hamazaki, *et al.*, 2005). In a double-blind trial, participants took either a placebo or 762 mg of EPA/DHA per day for two months. The researchers noted that EPA concentrations increased in the red blood cell membranes in the supplemented group. The EPA/DHA group also had significantly decreased levels of plasma norepinephrine.

In summary, because of EPA and DHA's role in downregulating the stress response, they can help mothers become more stress resilient. This is especially valuable for women who are highly stressed or who have experienced trauma, as EPA and DHA increase resilience to stress and can decrease risk for postpartum depression (Kendall-Tackett, 2007, 2009).

### Additional effects of DHA in the perinatal period

During the perinatal period, DHA is also important to help prevent depression. In the Adelaide Mothers' and Babies' Iron Trail, a 1% increase in plasma DHA was related to a 59% decrease in risk of depressive symptoms postpartum (Rees, *et al.*, 2005). Pregnant women's diets are often deficient in DHA, which is unfortunate given babies' high need for it *in utero*. This deficiency may also put their mothers at risk for depression. As Rees and colleagues (2005) describe for mothers in Australia, during the last trimester of pregnancy, babies accumulate an average of 67 mg/day of DHA. The average intake for Australian mothers is 15 mg/day. In contrast, DHA consumption among Japanese, Koreans, and Norwegians is about 1,000 mg/day.

Because babies need DHA for brain and vision development, women's bodies will preferentially divert DHA to the baby, and the baby will take the DHA it needs from maternal stores. With each subsequent pregnancy, mothers are further depleted (Amir, *et al.*, 1996; Rees, *et al.*, 2005). Current recommended intake is 200 to 400 mg/day as a minimum dose. DHA appears to have a role in the prevention of depression, but according to two recent reviews, has no efficacy in *treatment* of depression when used alone (Peet and Stokes, 2005; Freeman, *et al.*, 2006b).

### Safety during pregnancy and lactation

EPA and DHA supplements are generally safe for peripartum women (Marangell, *et al.*, 2004; Shoji, *et al.*, 2006). A few studies have found very mild negative effects at high-dose levels. But in most studies, there were no adverse effects. These findings are summarized below.

### Studies during pregnancy

Most studies of pregnant women and EPA/DHA supplementation are population studies examining fish or fish-oil consumption. One study sampled 182 women from the Faroe Islands: a whaling, island community between the Shetland Islands and Iceland (Grandjean, *et al.*, 2001). The average fish consumption in this sample was 72 g of fish, 12 g of whale muscle, and 7 g of blubber per day. The researchers found that DHA level was the best predictor of gestational length, with a 1% increase in relative concentration related to a 1.5-day increase in gestation. However, an increase of 1% in relative EPA concentration was related to a 246 g decrease in birth weight. Even at these high levels of EPA and DHA consumption, however, the clinical effects were negligible.

Another study of 488 women in Iceland found increased risk for developing hypertension in pregnancy (OR=4.7) for women taking cod liver oil (Olafsdottir, *et al.*, 2006). There are some issues to consider, however, as we interpret the findings. First, cod liver oil contains not only

EPA and DHA, but three fat-soluble vitamins (A, D, and E) that can be toxic in large doses. Second, consumption of cod liver oil was estimated from questionnaire data – not directly measured in participant serum. Third, when data were divided into centiles, the authors noted a U-shaped curve, with the odds ratios of hypertension being the *lowest* for those with a modest supplementation, similar to findings of other studies. Their findings suggest that modest amounts of cod liver oil (0.1 g to 0.9 g) appear safe with no increased risk to the mother or baby. However, higher amounts of cod liver oil could be a problem.

Indeed, modest levels of cod liver oil supplementation appeared safe in another randomized trial of 341 women (803 mg EPA; 1,183 mg DHA per day). Mothers were supplemented from 18 weeks' gestation to three months postpartum (Helland, *et al.*, 2003). All the babies in this study breastfed for at least three months. There were no teratogenic effects noted. At 4 years of age, children whose mothers had taken cod liver oil during pregnancy and lactation had a higher Mental Processing Composite score. This score correlated with head circumference at birth, but not with birth weight or gestational age. Only pregnancy intake of DHA was significantly related to mental abilities at age 4.

Another line of research examined the effect of fish consumption during pregnancy and whether it protected offspring from allergic disease (Romieu, *et al.*, 2007). The rationale for the study was that the anti-inflammatory properties of Omega-3s modulate the immune system. The sample was a cohort of 462 pregnant women whose offspring were followed for six years after birth. The researchers found that 34% of infants had eczema at 1 year of age. At 6 years, 14% were atopic and 6% had atopic wheeze. After adjusting for potential confounds, the authors found that fish intake during pregnancy was protective against eczema at 1 year and against allergy/wheeze at 6 years. An increase in weekly fish intake from once to 2.5 times a week decreased the risk of eczema by 37%, and risk of positive skin prick test at age 6 by 35%. Risk was significantly lowered for non-breastfed children. There was no additive protective effect of mothers' fish consumption for breastfed infants.

In a meta-analysis, Szajewska and colleagues (2006) found that supplementation with EPA and DHA significantly increased the length of pregnancy. Supplementation did not influence percentage of preterm deliveries, rate of low-birth-weight infants, or rate of eclampsia/pre-eclampsia. The incidence of adverse effects from supplementation was low and most were mild (e.g. fish burps). One study included in the review reported an increase in blood loss at delivery among the fish-oil group. None of the other studies reported increased bleeding. Overall, neonates across studies did not differ in rates of adverse effects from non-supplemented neonates.

*Impact on breastfeeding*

EPA and DHA also appear to have no negative impact on breastfeeding babies, even at high dosages. Freeman and colleagues (2006b) conducted a small, randomized trial using three different dosages of EPA/DHA with 16 mothers with postpartum major depression (300 mg EPA/200 mg DHA per day; 840 mg EPA/560 mg DHA per day; or 1,680 mg EPA/1,120 mg DHA per day). Depression significantly decreased in all three groups. The study was limited by a small sample and no control group (therefore, not ruling out a placebo effect). But there were no adverse effects noted for mother or baby at any dosage level.

At very high dosages, EPA and DHA did create some small changes in breast milk fatty acid composition for 83 mothers who were supplemented from 20 weeks' gestation to delivery. These changes appeared to be beneficial, however, not harmful. Fish-oil supplementation significantly increased EPA and DHA concentrations in breast milk (Dunstan, *et al.*, 2004b) and in the erythrocytes of mothers and babies in the fish-oil group (Dunstan, *et al.*, 2004a). Higher levels of EPA/DHA were related to increased levels of IgA and sCD14 in the milk, potentially protective changes. The supplementation dosage used in this study was very high (2.2 g DHA/1.5 g EPA per day): *11 times* the recommended minimum of DHA. Dunstan and colleagues did express some concerns about what the alterations in fatty acid composition might mean. However, even at this high dosage, the cautions they raised were hypothetical rather than observed effects.

*Sources of EPA and DHA*

As the previously cited studies indicate, women are often deficient in long-chain Omega-3 fatty acids during the perinatal period. However, pregnant or breastfeeding women need to limit the amount of fish they eat, the prime source of EPA and DHA, because of contaminants in seafood. Fortunately, there are fish-oil supplements that are inexpensive, widely available, and tested for contaminants (see the U.S. Pharmacopeia website for a specific listing of brands that are tested for contaminants and that are USP verified: http://www.usp.org).

*Summary*

Increasing evidence suggests that DHA can help prevent depression in new mothers and that EPA is a useful treatment – alone, or in combination with medications and/or DHA (Freeman, *et al.*, 2006a). A review in the *British Journal of Psychiatry* summarized these findings as follows:

> There is good evidence that psychiatric illness is associated with the depletion of EFAs [essential fatty acids] and, crucially, that supplementation can result in clinical ameliora-tion. The clinical trial data may herald a simple, safe and effective adjunct to our standard treatments.
>
> (Hallahan and Garland, 2005: 276)

## S-Adenosyl-L-Methionine (SAM-e)

S-Adenosyl-L-Methionine (SAM-e) is another supplement that is effective in treating depres-sion. SAM-e is a substance that naturally occurs in the body and is crucial to cell metabolism in all animals. It is derived from the amino acids methionine and adenosine triphosphate. Our bodies manufacture methionine from protein. SAM-e contributes to a process known as methylation that regulates serotonin, melatonin, dopamine, and adrenaline. It also regu-lates neurotransmitter metabolism, membrane fluidity, and receptor activity (Bratman and Girman, 2003). If people have low levels of B6, B12, or folic acid, SAM-e breaks down into homocysteine. High homocysteine levels are harmful to cardiovascular health and have been related to depression (Folstein, *et al.*, 2007). Moreover, high levels of homocysteine during pregnancy raise the risk of spina bifida and other birth defects (Health Quest Radio News & Science, 2000). Folate should not be used as a monotreatment for depression, but can be combined with SAM-e. Supplementation with 400 to 1,000 mg of folate daily would be likely to prove a useful adjunct to treatment (Freeman, 2009).

A meta-analysis of 28 studies indicated that SAM-e decreased depression significantly more than a placebo and that it was comparable to antidepressant medications in its effective-ness (Agency for Healthcare Research and Quality (AHRQ), 2002). The authors of this report noted that, in placebo trials, SAM-e was providing an active treatment. Clinically, patients improved, but SAM-e did not completely eradicate depression.

SAM-e has also been used to treat postpartum depression (Cerutti, *et al.*, 1993). In this study, women were randomly assigned to receive 1,600 mg of SAM-e, a placebo, or usual care. By the tenth day, women receiving SAM-e had significantly lower depression scores than women in the placebo group. By day 30, however, the difference between the SAM-e and placebo group was no longer significant. The difference was still significant, however, between the women receiving SAM-e and the usual-care group.

To date, there have been no studies that treat pregnant women for depression with SAM-e (Freeman, 2009). However, the recent AHRQ report summarized five studies on SAM-e used antenatally for cholestasis in pregnancy with no adverse effects for either mother or baby. SAM-e is generally very well tolerated. The standard dose is 200 mg twice a day, with rapid titration up over the next one to two weeks. It may take as much as 1,600 mg/day to achieve an initial response in depression, but a maintenance dose can be as low as 200 mg twice a day (Bratman and Girman, 2003).

There are two downsides to this supplement. First, it is expensive. Even at discount stores, SAM-e can cost as much as $1.00/pill. This cost can be prohibitive for many. Second, SAM-e degrades easily. Consumers have no way of knowing whether the SAM-e that they purchased was handled correctly. Consequently, consumers may pay top dollar for an inert substance.

At this time, the impact of SAM-e on breastfeeding is also unknown. Since it naturally occurs in the body, it is most likely safe, but there is no research to confirm this. However, no adverse effects have been reported via breastfeeding (Freeman, 2009). In summary, SAM-e shows promise for treating postpartum depression. It also appears to be safe for pregnancy and lactation, but there are still some unknowns, so mothers should be aware of these.

## Exercise

Exercise is another effective treatment for depression in general, and postpartum depression in particular (Daley, *et al.*, 2007). Traditionally, exercise has been recommended for people with mild-to-moderate depression. But as two clinical trials have found, exercise can also alleviate major depression as effectively as medications. Exercise can also be safely combined with other modalities.

### *Exercise for depressed people*

A number of studies have demonstrated the effectiveness of exercise in boosting mood. In a study from Finland (N=3,403), exercise two to three times a week lowered depression, and helped with feelings of anger, distrust, and stress (Hassmen, *et al.*, 2000). Men and women who exercised perceived their health and fitness as better than non-exercisers, and this has been associated with lower levels of depression. Exercise also increased feelings of social integration.

The efficacy of exercise was also demonstrated in a randomized trial of patients with major depressive disorder. In this study, 156 patients (>50 years old) with major depression were randomized into one of three treatment groups: aerobic exercise alone, sertraline alone, and a combination of exercise and sertraline. After four months, exercise was as effective as sertraline in alleviating depression. The more striking findings, however, occurred at ten months. At that time, the exercise-only group had a significantly lower rate of relapse than either the medication alone or medication/exercise groups. The authors speculated that this was because, by learning to exercise, those in the exercise-only group had a coping tool that they could use when faced with life stressors (Babyak, *et al.*, 2000). This study is particularly noteworthy because it was the first to try exercise as a treatment for major depression.

In 2007, this same group of researchers replicated their findings (Blumenthal, *et al.*, 2007). In this study, 202 adults with major depression were randomized to one of four conditions: sertraline, exercise at home, supervised exercise, or a placebo control. After four months of treatment, 41% of the patients were in remission and no longer met the criteria for major depression. Efficacy rates by treatment were as follows: medication=47%, supervised exercise=45%, home-based exercise=40%, and placebo=31%. The exercise condition was 45 minutes of walking on a treadmill at 70% to 85% maximum heart rate capacity, three times a week, for 16 weeks. The home-exercise group received the same instructions, but was not supervised and had minimal contact with the research staff. The authors concluded that the efficacy of exercise was comparable to medications. The supervised program was especially effective, but the home program was also comparable to medications. All treatments were more effective than the placebo.

A study of 230 pregnant women examined the relationships between depressive symptoms, body-image satisfaction, and exercise in the first, second, and third trimester of pregnancy and at six weeks postpartum (Downs, *et al.*, 2008). Depressive symptoms and body image in early pregnancy predicted depression later in pregnancy. Exercise moderated these effects. In a sample of 80 women with postpartum depression at six weeks, women were assigned to exercise three times a week or to receive standard care (Heh, *et al.*, 2008). Women who exercised were significantly less depressed at five months than the standard-care group.

The mood-altering effects of exercise appear fairly quickly. In a study of 26 women, Lane and colleagues (2002) found that women's moods significantly improved after each exercise session. Depressed mood was especially sensitive to exercise and decreased significantly after each session.

### Exercise is also anti-inflammatory

One reason why exercise works as a treatment for depression is because it lowers inflammation. Chronic inflammation affects the body's composition and metabolism in several ways, including the loss of body protein and the accretion of fat (Roubenoff, 2003). For example, cachexia, or loss of lean muscle mass, is at least partially mediated by the proinflammatory cytokines IL-1$\beta$, IL-6, and TNF-$\alpha$. Exercise can reverse these inflammatory-mediated changes.

Initially, exercise acts as an acute physical stressor and raises IL-6 and TNF-$\alpha$. Over a longer period of time, however, exercise lowers inflammation. Older adults, for example, are one group with higher levels of proinflammatory cytokines since levels naturally increase as we age. Indeed, researchers hypothesize that this age-related rise in inflammation creates vulnerability to diseases, such as heart disease, cancer and Alzheimer's (Kiecolt-Glaser, *et al.*, 2007). Because of this increased vulnerability of older adults, they are frequently the population of choice for studies on exercise, depression, and inflammation. The results of these studies are helpful for understanding the mechanism for exercise's impact on depression.

A study of adults aged 60 to 90, tested the effects of physical activity on perceived stress, mood, and quality of life. The researchers also assessed serum IL-6 and cortisol. The patients (N=10) assigned to the exercise group were instructed to walk for 30 minutes, five times a week for the ten-week study. The control group was ten older adults who were not engaging in physical activity. After the ten-week exercise intervention, the subjects had significantly lower stress on the Perceived Stress Scale, and improved mood and quality of life on the SF-36 Health Questionnaire. They reported better physical functioning, more vitality, better mental health, and less bodily pain. They also had a significant decrease in serum IL-6 (Starkweather, 2007).

Exercise also had a positive effect on wound healing, and this is an indirect measure of systemic inflammation (Emery, *et al.*, 2005). In this study, participants were randomized into exercise and control conditions, and were then given a punch biopsy so that researchers could monitor participants' rate of wound healing. For the exercise group, wounds healed in 29 days. In the control group, it took 38 days. Exercise for one hour a day, three days a week lowered perceived stress and improved wound healing. This study is of interest because we know from these researchers' other studies that wound healing is impaired when stress or hostility levels are high (e.g. Kiecolt-Glaser, *et al.*, 2005). Stress and hostility both increase systemic inflammation. When systemic inflammation is high, wound healing is impaired because proinflammatory cytokines are in the blood stream and not at the wound site where they belong. The study by Emery and colleagues (2006) indicates that exercise improves wound healing by lowering levels of circulating systemic cytokines and diverting them to the wound site.

Overall level of fitness is also related to inflammation (Hamer and Steptoe, 2007). The sample in this study was 207 men and women from London. Participants who responded with higher systolic blood pressure to a lab-induced stress also had a higher IL-6 and TNF-$\alpha$ response. The TNF-$\alpha$ response to stress was five times greater in the low-fitness group compared with that in the high-fitness group. Participants who were physically fit had a lower inflammation response when under stress, which is likely to have protected them from both depression and chronic disease.

### Exercise and breastfeeding

As the above-cited studies indicate, exercise is helpful in lowering systemic inflammation and treating depression. Yet mothers may be concerned that it will negatively impact breastfeeding. Research studies have generally found that exercise had no negative effects on breastfeeding (Amorin, *et al.*, 2007). An Australian study of 587 new mothers (Su, *et al.*, 2007) examined the relationship between mothers' exercise, the initiation and duration of breastfeeding, and the effect of exercise on infant growth. Mothers were interviewed seven times over the first year. At six to twelve months, exercise had not decreased breastfeeding duration. At twelve months, exercise had no significant impact on infants' growth. Researchers concluded that exercise while breastfeeding is safe and important for maintaining health.

A more specific question regarding exercise and breastfeeding is whether exercise causes lactic acid to build up in mothers' milk. In a study of 12 women, milk and blood samples were taken after a non-exercise session, after maximal exercise, and after a session that was 20% below the maximal range (Quinn and Carey, 1999). The researchers found that in women with an adequate caloric intake, moderate exercise neither increased lactic acid in breast milk nor caused babies to reject it. When women exercised in the "hard" range (using the perceived-exertion scale), lactic acid increased. The authors recommended exercise in a moderate range because it neither increases lactic acid accumulation in the breast milk nor alters babies' willingness to breastfeed.

In summary, exercise is a highly effective treatment for depression – alone or in combination with other treatments, and it has no negative effect on breastfeeding. Exercise can be a viable alternative treatment if mothers refuse medications. The one challenge with exercise is getting depressed mothers to do it because it is often the last thing depressed people feel like doing. But they may be motivated to try when they realize it's an effective alternative to medications. The study by Blumenthal and colleagues (2007) found a slightly higher remission in the supervised vs. at-home exercise groups. This is probably due to compliance rates being higher because participants knew people expected them to show up to exercise. It's easier to skip exercise in an unsupervised home program. The supervised program also provided at least some social support. A similar approach, perhaps involving a mothers' exercise group, may be useful for mothers who want to give this modality a try.

## Summary

Omega-3s, SAM-e, and exercise are all effective treatments for depression – even major depression. All of these modalities can be safely combined with other treatments and have no negative impact on breastfeeding.

In the next chapter, other complementary and alternative treatments for depression are described, including bright light therapy, St. John's wort, kava, and combined modalities.

# 11 Alternative and complementary therapies II

## Bright light therapy, herbs, and combined modalities

As described in the previous chapter, there is a range of effective, evidence-based, complementary and alternative treatments for depression in new mothers. In this chapter, bright light therapy, St. John's wort, kava, acupuncture and combination therapies are described. Most of these treatment modalities are effective for even major depression.

### Bright light therapy

Some people dread the change of seasons. Shorter, darker days mean fatigue, oversleeping, overeating, and having a general sense of malaise: a pattern known as seasonal affective disorder (SAD) (Sullivan and Payne, 2007). In the northern hemisphere, seasonal affective disorder is depression that occurs during late fall and winter months, as darkness occurs earlier in the day. Symptoms include depression, lethargy, difficulty waking, impaired concentration, lack of interest in social activities, and craving carbohydrates, which can lead to winter weight gain (National Alliance on Mental Illness (NAMI), 2007). Seasonal depression is quite common – much more so than major depression. In a study of 93 Midwestern undergraduates, 28% had seasonal affective disorder vs. 9% who had major depression (Sullivan and Payne, 2007).

For more than 20 years, bright light therapy has been used to successfully treat seasonal affective disorder. Response is often within days (NAMI, 2007). Light therapy can also be helpful for other affective disorders, including non-seasonal depression, antenatal and postpartum depression, bipolar disorder, some eating disorders, and certain sleep disorders (Oren, et al., 2002; Terman and Terman, 2005). An expert panel for the American Psychiatric Association concluded that bright light therapy was an effective treatment for both seasonal and non-seasonal depression, with results comparable to those of antidepressants (Golden, et al., 2005).

In a recent clinical trial, patients were randomized to receive light therapy at 10,000 lux, for 30 minutes a day and a placebo medication; or 100 lux (placebo light) with 20 mg fluoxetine (Lam, et al., 2006). A total of 96 patients with seasonal major depression participated for eight weeks. The researchers found that light therapy was as effective as fluoxetine in relieving symptoms, with an identical clinical response rate for even severe depression. By one week, patients in the light-therapy group had a greater response to treatment, but this difference disappeared at subsequent assessment points. There were more side effects with fluoxetine, but both treatments were generally well-tolerated, with no overall difference in adverse effects.

### Light therapy in pregnant and postpartum women

To date, only a few studies of bright light therapy have included pregnant and postpartum women, with mixed findings in terms of effectiveness. The larger literature on light therapy in general, however, suggests that this modality is worth investigating further. For example, bright light alleviated depression in two case studies of new mothers who suddenly became depressed after the birth of their babies (Corral, *et al.*, 2000). These mothers refused antidepressants, but agreed to a trial of bright light therapy. Both of these women responded to bright light therapy, and had significantly lower rates of depressive symptoms after treatment.

In a study of fifteen women with postpartum depression, ten were assigned to receive light at 10,000 lux for six weeks, and five were assigned to dim red light (600 lux). After six weeks, both groups improved and there was no significant difference between the groups (Corral, *et al.*, 2007). An open-label trial with 16 pregnant women with major depression found that there was a 49% improvement in depressive symptoms after three weeks of treatment with bright light (10,000 lux). Based on these results, the authors recommended a randomized trial to further test the efficacy of this intervention with depressed pregnant women (Oren, *et al.*, 2002).

### Light intensity, duration, and timing of light exposure

There are several characteristics of light related to its effectiveness as a treatment. These characteristics include light intensity, duration, and timing of light exposure. Researchers have investigated a wide range of light intensities and several appear effective. Light intensity is measured in lux, which is brightness by proximity. Lights at closer distances have a higher lux than the same lights that are further away.

Lights with intensities of 10,000 lux appear to be most effective. At this level of intensity, 30 to 40 minutes of exposure is sufficient. Two studies with light exposures of 30 to 40 minutes at 10,000 lux achieved a 75% remission rate in depression. It took two hours to achieve similar remission rates at 2,500 lux. And in some cases, even with longer exposure, lower-intensity lights were not as effective (Terman and Terman, 2005). Another potential problem with longer exposure times is that patients are less likely to comply. This may particularly be true for mothers of young children, who probably won't find it practical to sit in front of a light box for two or three hours.

Another study used a Litebook™ LED (1,350 lux) for 30 minutes, and found that that amount of light significantly lowered depression scores compared with a placebo light (Desan, *et al.*, 2007). This was a small trial (N=23), and patients were assessed after one, two, three, and four weeks of treatment. By four weeks, 57% of patients in the LED condition were in remission compared with 11% of patients in the control condition. The authors speculated that this lower intensity light worked because it was in the 450–480 nm range, and that melatonin rhythms were best shifted by those wavelengths. Because of this concentration in short wavelengths, even lower-intensity light might prove as effective as brighter light, while using smaller, more convenient devices.

### Timing

Timing of light exposure also makes a difference. Morning exposure to bright light is generally more successful than light exposure later in the day. In their review of 25 studies, Terman and Terman (2005) found significantly higher remission rates with morning exposure (53%), compared with mid-day (32%) and evening (38%) exposure.

One exception to the use of morning light is in patients with bipolar disorder. Morning light exposure can increase risk of a manic episode. This problem can be addressed by timing light exposure to later in the day and having patients continue on their medications during light treatment (NAMI, 2007; Terman and Terman, 2005).

### Dawn simulation

Because of the effectiveness of morning light exposure, a variant to standard light therapy has recently been added to the repertoire of possible treatments: dawn simulation. As the name implies, dawn simulation refers to a light that comes on before a patient is awake, and gradually increases in intensity over a period of 15 to 90 minutes (the length can be tailored to individual preference). The advantage to this treatment is that it does not require sitting in front of a light box for an extended time, making it a more practical alternative for new mothers or mothers of young children. Although a relatively new technique, it is showing promise as a treatment for seasonal depression (Golden, *et al.*, 2005). Some newer lighting devices are both light boxes and dawn simulators.

One theory about why dawn simulation is effective is that its impact occurs during the early dawn interval, when melatonin levels wane and core body temperature rises. The early dawn interval is when circadian rhythms are most susceptible to light-elicited phase advances. According to this theory, depression is more likely to be triggered when it is still dark outdoors in the early dawn interval. To test this theory, Terman and Terman (2006) randomly assigned 99 adults with seasonal major depression to one of five treatment conditions. These included dawn simulation, dawn light pulse, post-awakening bright light therapy (30 minutes at 10,000 lux), negative air ionization at high flow rate, and ionization at low flow rate. After three weeks of treatment, patients who received bright light therapy (57%) and dawn simulation (50%) had the greatest improvement in symptoms. The researchers concluded that bright light therapy still appeared to be the most effective. However, if there are problems with non-compliance or non-response, dawn simulation or dawn pulse are viable alternatives.

### Why light is effective

Researchers have proposed a number of possible mechanisms to explain why bright light alleviates depression. Most explanations have to do with modifying the internal circadian clock. Our circadian rhythms, or daily patterns of sleep and arousal, are regulated by the pineal gland, which secretes melatonin. The suprachiasmatic nucleus of the hypothalamus regulates synthesis of melatonin. The pineal gland responds to light via light receptors in the retina. The superiority of morning-light exposure is likely to be due to the diurnal variations in retinal photoreceptor sensitivity, with greater sensitivity to morning light. Indeed, exposure to evening light can lead to insomnia and hyperactivation in some people (NAMI, 2007; Terman and Terman, 2005).

Preliminary evidence indicates that there is an inflammatory component to seasonal depression as well. Lam and colleagues (2004) hypothesized that during winter, proinflammatory cytokines increase for patients with seasonal depression. In a study of 15 patients, and a matched group of normal controls, those with SAD had significantly higher levels of IL-6. After two weeks of bright light therapy, symptoms improved, and 64% of patients had at least a 50% reduction in depressive symptoms. However, light therapy did not lower inflammation after two weeks. The authors concluded that seasonal depression involves activation of the immune-inflammatory system, which is not immediately altered by light therapy (Leu, et al., 2001).

### Safety issues

Because light boxes can be relatively expensive (about $100 U.S.), and appear to be simple, patients often consider assembling a unit themselves. However, just because they can, doesn't mean they should. Clinicians generally recommend that patients don't use homemade devices for several reasons. First, it is difficult for consumers to find lights that are of sufficient brightness to generate a therapeutic effect. Second, some patients have experienced excessive irradiation, and corneal or eyelid burns with homemade devices. Finally, homemade devices often use incandescent lights, which are not recommended because 90% of light output from incandescent bulbs is on the infrared, or heat, end of the spectrum. Not only can infrared exposure at high intensity burn the lens, cornea, and retina, but it is on the wrong end of the color spectrum for a therapeutic effect (Terman and Terman, 2005). The National Alliance on Mental Illness (2007) recommends bulbs with a color temperature between 3,000 and 6,500 degrees Kelvin, and are in the white-to-blue range of the color spectrum. These do not harm patients' eyes.

Light boxes with high levels of exposure to UV can also cause eye damage. The National Alliance on Mental Illness recommends lights that are encased in a box with a diffusing lens that filters out UV radiation (NAMI, 2007). Patients wanting to try light therapy should use a lighting apparatus from a reputable dealer. Since price may be an issue, many hospitals, and some manufacturers, have loaner programs that allow patients to try the lighting device in their homes before buying them.

### Summary

Bright light therapy is a generally safe, well-tolerated treatment option for seasonal depression, and it's useful for non-seasonal depression as well. Bright light therapy is also breastfeeding friendly and can be used during pregnancy. Although the initial cost of therapeutic light boxes can be high, a single purchase will last for years. For patients who dread the change of seasons, this investment is often well worth the price, especially if they want to avoid medications during pregnancy or breastfeeding.

## Herbal antidepressants

Herbal medications have a long history of use around the world. Despite their increasing popularity in the U.S., many healthcare providers are uncomfortable with patients medicating themselves for something as serious as depression. To make matters worse, patients often do not tell their doctors that they are taking herbs for fear of censure. This can be dangerous because of the potential for herb–drug interactions. It is important for healthcare providers to know if patients are taking herbs. To facilitate communication, it's helpful to know some of the possible reasons that patients turn to herbal medications.

### Why patients take herbs

From the patient's perspective, herbs offer a number of advantages. If you understand why women might prefer these modalities, you can talk more comfortably with them about their choices, and women are more likely to be forthcoming about using herbs.

- *Control*. One reason patients prefer herbs is that they can control their own health care. Instead of having to wait for a doctor's appointment, they can address their depression right away. They also have control over when they start treatment and when they stop.
- *Privacy*. Patients may be ashamed to admit that they are depressed and are frightened by the possibility that their employers or others will find out that they are taking antidepressants. Unfortunately, on occasion, medication information *does* get released to employers via insurance forms or just plain gossip – even with confidentiality regulations in place. Further, antidepressant use can influence hiring and promotion decisions in some types of job. Even if that's not the case, patients may still not want others to know.
- *Costs*. Newer and name-brand antidepressants can be expensive, especially if not covered by insurance. In contrast, herbs are generally reasonably priced, and can be purchased at discount and warehouse stores. The savings each month can be substantial compared with name-brand non-generic prescription drugs. This is becoming less of an issue as many frequently used antidepressants are available in generic form. Nevertheless, cost can still be a concern for some mothers.
- *Side effects and safety*. The side-effect and safety profiles of herbs are significantly better than those associated with medications (Klier, *et al.*, 2006; Schultz, 2006). For some, side effects of antidepressants prove intolerable and are a common reason why patients stop taking them. Most herbs have very low incidence of adverse effects. For example, according to one recent review, risk of adverse effects associated with St. John's wort was 10 times lower than that associated with standard antidepressants (Schultz, 2006). Along these same lines, although antidepressant use during pregnancy is probably safe, many women fear teratogenic effects of medications taken during pregnancy and therefore may be reluctant to take antidepressants at that time (Dennis and Allen, 2008).
- *Patient compliance*. Patient compliance is an often important issue. Just because women are prescribed antidepressants, doesn't mean they will take them. In one study of depressed men and women in New York City (N=829), only 28% were still taking their antidepressants three months later (Olfson, *et al.*, 2006). Patients were more likely to stop taking them if they were Hispanic, had less than 12 years of education, or had a low income. They were more likely to continue taking their medications if they had more than 12 years of education, had participated in psychotherapy at some point, and had private health insurance.

The two most common herbs used for depression are St. John's wort and kava. These are described below.

### St. John's wort

St. John's wort (*Hypericum perforatum*) is the most widely used herbal antidepressant in the world (Dugoua, *et al.*, 2006). Herbalists have used St. John's wort since the Middle Ages. At that time, it was used to treat insanity resulting from "attacks of the devil." It derives its name from St. John's Day (June 24) because it blooms near this day on the medieval church calendar. "Wort" is the old English word for a medicinal plant. It is native to Great Britain, Wales, and northern Europe. And since settlers brought it to North America in the eighteenth century (Balch, 2002; Humphrey, 2003), it is now a common wildflower in the northeastern and north-central U.S.

*Efficacy of St. John's wort*

A large body of evidence indicates that St. John's wort effectively treats depression (Sarris, 2007; Werneke, *et al.*, 2006). A number of clinical trials have compared the efficacy of various St. John's wort extracts to either a placebo or an antidepressant. In one trial, 375 patients were randomized to receive either St. John's wort (*Hypericum perforatum* Extract WS 5570) or a placebo for six weeks to treat mild-to-moderate depression (Lecrubier, *et al.*, 2002). At the end of six weeks, patients receiving St. John's wort had significantly lower scores on the Hamilton Depression Rating Scale, and significantly more patients were in remission than among patients receiving the placebo. Both groups had similar rates of adverse effects. Fifty-three percent of the patients in the St. John's wort group responded to treatment, compared with 42% of the placebo group.

Two randomized trials compared St. John's wort to the tricyclic antidepressant imipramine. The first randomized trial compared St. John's wort (*Hypericum* extract ZE 117) to imipramine for 324 outpatients with mild-to-moderate depression (Woelk, 2000). After six weeks of treatment, it was found that St. John's wort was as effective as imipramine in lowering depressive symptoms. Adverse effects were significantly more likely in the imipramine group, with 63% reporting adverse effects compared with 39% reporting adverse effects in the St. John's wort group. In addition, only 3% in the St. John's wort group dropped out of the study due to adverse effects vs. 16% of the imipramine group. The author concluded that St. John's wort is therapeutically equivalent to imipramine, but better tolerated by patients.

The second trial compared St. John's wort (*Hypericum* extract STEI 300) with a placebo and imipramine. The subjects were 263 primary-care patients with moderate depression. The authors found that St. John's wort was as effective as imipramine for moderately depressed patients after four, six, and eight weeks of treatment (Philipp, *et al.*, 1999). Patients in this trial also tolerated St. John's wort better.

Two clinical trials compared St. John's wort with sertraline for major depression. In the first study, 340 adults with major depression were randomly assigned to receive either *H Perforatum*, a placebo, or sertraline for eight weeks (Hypericum Depression Trial Study Group, 2002). Subjects responding to the medication could opt to receive still-blinded treatment for another 18 weeks. Depression was assessed at baseline, and again at eight weeks. The rate of full response was low and almost identical for both the St. John's wort and sertraline groups (24% vs. 25%). The low response rates for both medications suggest limitations to the study. Eight weeks may not have been sufficient time for patients with severe depression to recover. Alternatively, the dosages may have been too low. The authors noted that their findings were not unusual in that approximately 35% of studies of standard antidepressants show no greater efficacy than the placebo.

Another study that same year had opposite findings. This study (van Gurp, *et al.*, 2002) included 87 patients with major depression recruited from Canadian family practice physicians. Patients were randomly assigned to receive either St. John's wort or sertraline. At the end of the 12-week trial, both groups improved, and there was no difference between the two groups. However, there were significantly more side effects in the sertraline group at two and four weeks. The authors concluded that St. John's wort, because of its effectiveness and benign side effects, was a good *first choice* for a primary-care population.

St. John's wort was also compared with paroxetine in a study of 251 patients with moderate-to-severe major depression (Szegedi, *et al.*, 2005). In this study, patients were randomly assigned to receive 20 mg paroxetine or 900 mg St. John's wort (*Hypericum* extract WS 5570) per day. After two weeks, dosages for non-responders were doubled: 1,800 mg St. John's wort or 40 mg paroxetine. After six weeks of treatment, the response rates for St. John's wort were 70%, and 60% for paroxetine. The remission rates for St. John's wort were 50% vs. 35% for paroxetine. The authors concluded that St. John's wort was as effective as paroxetine, and better tolerated.

Anghelescu and colleagues (2006) also compared the efficacy and safety of *Hypericum* extract WS 5570 to paroxetine for patients with moderate-to-severe depression. The acute phase of treatment lasted for six weeks, with another four months of follow-up to prevent relapse. The patients improved on both treatments with no significant difference in efficacy between paroxetine and St. John's wort. The authors noted that St. John's wort was an important alternative to standard antidepressants for depressed patients.

*Mechanism for efficacy*

Researchers still do not understand the exact mechanism for St. John's wort's antidepressant effect. Linde, *et al.* (1996) noted that hypericum extracts have at least ten constituents that probably cause its pharmacological effects. St. John's wort is standardized by percentage of hypericin, one of the active constituents. Hypericin was once considered the primary antidepressant component. Researchers no longer believe that this is true (Bratman and Girman, 2003). More recently, researchers have recognized hyperforin as the possible antidepressant constituent (Lawvere and Mahoney, 2005; Muller, 2003; Wurglies and Schubert-Zsilavecz, 2006; Zanoli, 2004). Hyperforin appears to inhibit the reuptake of the monoamines and GABAergic activity (Kuhn and Winston, 2000; Werneke, *et al.*, 2006). It may relieve depression by preventing the reuptake of serotonin, using the same mechanism as the selective serotonin reuptake inhibitors (SSRIs) (e.g. fluoxetine, sertraline). Indeed, Muller (2003) noted that only hyperforin (and its structural analogue, adhyperforin) inhibit neurotransmitter reuptake.

St. John's wort, and particularly hyperforin, also appears to be anti-inflammatory (Balch, 2002; Dell'Aica, *et al.*, 2007; Kuhn and Winston, 2000; Wurglies and Schubert-Zsilavecz, 2006) and it modulates cytokine production (Werneke, *et al.*, 2006). Hyperforin has had anti-nociceptive (anti-pain) and anti-inflammatory effects in animal studies (Abdel-Salam, 2005). It inhibits the expression of another inflammatory marker – intercellular adhesion molecule (Zhou, *et al.*, 2004). In vitro effects show that St. John's wort is anti-oxidant, anti-cyclooxygenase-1, and anti-carcinogenic (Zanoli, 2004).

Only recently has St. John's wort been shown to specifically lower levels of the proinflammatory cytokines involved in depression (Hu, *et al.*, 2006). The study used an animal model to test whether St. John's wort could counter the toxic side effects of chemotherapy. The investigators specifically explored whether St. John's wort had an impact on the levels of proinflammatory cytokines, including IL-1$\beta$, IL-2, IL-6, IFN-$\gamma$, and TNF-$\alpha$. They found that St. John's wort did inhibit proinflammatory cytokines and intestinal epithelium apoptosis. Although this was not a study of depression, it was the first to demonstrate that St. John's wort inhibits the cytokines that are high in depression.

*Dosage*

The dosage of St. John's wort is 900 mg per day (300 mg three times per day), standardized to 0.3% hypericin and/or 2% to 4% hyperforin (Lawvere and Mahoney, 2005). It generally takes four to six weeks to take effect (Bratman and Girman, 2003; Ernst, 2002; Kuhn and Winston, 2000). St. John's wort reaches peak level in the plasma in five hours, with a half-life of 24 to

48 hours. Herbalists often combine it with other herbs to address the range of symptoms that depressed people have. Some of these herbs include lemon balm, kava, schisandra, rosemary, black cohosh, and lavender (Humphrey, 2007; Kuhn and Winston, 2000).

Unfortunately, it can be challenging for women to know if a brand of herbs they purchase is of good quality. As of this writing, the U.S. Pharmacopeia does not verify brands of St. John's wort. However, ConsumerLabs.com does rate brands of herbs. For a small subscription fee, women can access this resource, and read the ratings of specific brands of herbal products.

## Safety concerns

Taken by itself, St. John's wort has an excellent safety record, with a very low frequency of adverse reactions (Ernst, 2002; Humphrey, 2003; Muller, 2003). Approximately 2.4% of patients who take St. John's wort develop side effects. The most common are mild stomach discomfort, allergic reactions, skin rashes, tiredness, and restlessness. Like other antidepressants, St. John's wort can trigger an episode of mania in vulnerable patients or patients with bipolar disorder (Bratman and Girman, 2003). St. John's wort can also cause photosensitivity. A review of 38 controlled clinical trials and two meta-analyses on St. John's wort found its safety and side-effect profile to be better than that of standard antidepressants. The incidence of adverse effects ranged from 0% to 6%, which is ten times less than adverse effects associated with antidepressants (Schulz, 2006). There is also a significantly lower rate of drop-out from studies due to side effects in St. John's wort trials than there is from studies of standard antidepressants.

Some have expressed concern that St. John's wort functions as a monamine oxidase (MAO) inhibitor. It has been shown to be function in this way in mice, but not in rats or humans (Bladt and Wagner, 1994; Bratman and Girman, 2003). As I describe in Chapter 13, patients who take MAO inhibitors cannot eat or drink anything with tyramine, a substance found in aged foods. Yet, St. John's wort is widely used in countries such as France without dietary restrictions, and people in these countries regularly consume cheese and red wine (both of which contain large amounts of tyramine).

More concerning is St. John's wort's interactions with several classes of medications. Studies suggest that the mechanism is likely to involve the drug-metabolizing enzyme CYP3A4 and the transport protein P-glycoprotein (Schulz, 2006). This enzyme accelerates the metabolism of anticoagulants, anticonvulsants, cyclosporins, birth-control pills, protease and reverse transcriptase inhibitors used in anti-HIV treatments, and others, leading to lower serum levels of the medication than prescribed (Dugoua, et al., 2006; Ernst, 2002; Hale, 2008; Schulz, 2006). It can also interact with prescription antidepressants, causing a potentially fatal episode of serotonin syndrome (Bratman and Girman, 2003; Looper, 2007; Schulz, 2006; Werneke, et al., 2006). Prescription antidepressants should not be taken while taking St. John's wort (Harkness and Bratman, 2003), and any mothers who are taking St. John's wort need to tell their healthcare providers that they are taking it.

## St. John's wort and breastfeeding

St. John's wort is generally safe to take while breastfeeding (Dugoua, et al., 2006; Hale, 2008; Humphrey, 2007). In a case study, Klier and colleagues (2002) examined the pharmacokinetics of St. John's wort in four breast-milk samples (including both fore and hind milk) from a mother taking the standard dose of St. John's wort (300 mg three times per day). They tested the samples for both hypericin and hyperforin, and found that only hyperforin was excreted into breast milk at a low level. Both hyperforin and hypericin were below the level of quantification in the infant's plasma.

More recently, Klier and colleagues (2006) tested 36 breast-milk samples from five mothers taking 300 mg of St. John's wort three times a day. The researchers also tested the plasma of the five mothers and of two infants. As in their earlier case study, they found that only hyperforin was excreted into breast milk, at low levels. The relative infant dose of hyperforin was 0.9% to 2.5% of the mother's dose, a level of infant exposure comparable with that of antidepressants. No side effects were noted in either mothers or babies.

A recent review found that there is good evidence to support use of St. John's wort while breastfeeding (Dugoua, *et al.*, 2006). The authors found that St. John's wort affects neither milk supply nor infant weight. They noted that it could cause infant colic, drowsiness or lethargy, although only a few cases have been reported. The authors concluded that common and traditional use of St. John's wort caused minimal risk for breastfeeding women and their babies. They did express some concern about use of St. John's wort during pregnancy, however.

### Summary of St. John's wort

St. John's wort is another effective alternative to antidepressants that may be more acceptable for some women. Its standard use is for mild-to-moderate depression, but it has also been used for major depression. However, some caution is in order. Even though St. John's wort is a "natural" alternative to medications, it, too, is a medication and should be treated as such. It should never be used with antidepressants. Mothers need to tell their healthcare providers that they are taking it as it can interact with a number of different medications. If used with safety concerns in mind, normal use of this medication does not appear to be harmful for mothers or babies. Although hyperforin is excreted into breast milk, it appears in very low levels in infant plasma, and in some cases was undetectable (Hale, 2008; Humphrey, 2007).

### Kava

Kava (*Piper methysticum*) is another botanical that may be prescribed for depression. It has a long history of use in the Polynesian islands. Kava produces relaxation, and is also believed to be antiseptic and anti-inflammatory. Its more common psychotropic use is for anxiety (Ernst, 2002) and it operates on the same receptors as the benzodiazepines (e.g. Xanax). Kavalactones (the active ingredient) also promotes relaxation of the skeletal muscles, and has been used for chronic pain conditions and sleep disorders (Kuhn and Winston, 2000). It is often mixed in preparations with St. John's wort to treat anxiety and depression, although some recommend that people with depression avoid kava (Kuhn and Winston, 2000). In a recent systematic review on herbal preparations for use with anxiety disorders, Ernst (2006) concluded that only kava had anti-anxiety effects in humans.

However, even though it has a long history of use in other cultures, there have been some serious concerns about this herb. Although side effects are relatively rare, occurring in approximately 2% of patients, they are serious (Ernst, 2002, 2006). Kava interacts with other medications including antidepressants, benzodiazepines, alcohol, and sleeping pills, and has potentially dangerous side effects including liver damage (usually with a high dose; van der Watt, *et al.*, 2008). The U.S. Food and Drug Administration has issued a consumer advisory. It is currently contraindicated for breastfeeding mothers (Balch 2002; Hale 2008; Kuhn and Winston, 2000).

*Summary*

At this time, kava is an herb most mothers should avoid because of safety concerns. If non-breastfeeding mothers want to take this herb, they should not self-medicate with it but should take it only under the guidance of a licensed herbalist, naturopath, or other healthcare professional who is knowledgeable about herbs.

## Combined modalities and other techniques

At this point, there is not a large empirical base on the efficacy of other alternative treatments for postpartum depression. However, some of these approaches are promising, and could be considered as possibilities for treating depressed mothers. These modalities include acupuncture, Ayurvedic medicine, homeopathy, aromatherapy, massage, and traditional Chinese Medicine (Mantle, 2002).

A randomized clinical trial compared acupuncture with sham acupuncture and massage, and found that acupuncture was helpful in alleviating major depression in pregnant women (Manber, *et al.*, 2004). The response rate over ten weeks was 69% for acupuncture, 47% for sham acupuncture, and 32% for massage. With pregnant women, however, acupuncture should be used with caution as some acupuncture points may cause uterine stimulation and could potentially trigger premature labor and delivery (Freeman, 2009).

There is also a synergistic effect of combining multiple modalities. In a study of 112 women (aged 19 to 78 years) with mild-to-moderate depression, walking outside in the sun 20 minutes a day, plus taking a vitamin supplement decreased depression and improved overall mood, self-esteem, and general sense of well-being (Brown, *et al.*, 2001). In a Finnish study of healthy adults (aged 26 to 63 years), patients were randomly assigned to three conditions: aerobics class with bright light, aerobics class with normal illumination, and relaxation/stretching sessions in bright light. The study period was eight weeks. The authors found that bright light and exercise relieved depression. For atypical depression, bright light was more effective than exercise. The authors concluded that twice-weekly administration of bright light, alone or with physical exercise, can alleviate seasonal depression (Leppaemaeki, *et al.*, 2002).

A recent Cochrane review (Dennis and Allen, 2008) examined evidence related to massage therapy and depression-specific acupuncture for treating antenatal depression. The authors concluded that the sample was too small and too non-generalizable for them to make a specific recommendation. Nevertheless, they identified little risk associated with these treatments and mothers may find them helpful.

## Conclusion

Bright light therapy, St. John's wort, and combined modalities are all effective treatments for depression. These modalities are also generally low-cost, not harmful, and mothers can initiate them themselves. These modalities also have the advantage of having a minimal impact on breastfeeding. They can be offered as an alternative to mothers who refuse to take medications. At present, pregnant or breastfeeding women should avoid kava. Mothers who are not breastfeeding should use kava only when under the care of an experienced provider. As with other treatments for depression, mothers should be monitored to determine whether these techniques are reducing their depression. If not, other options should be added, or used instead.

# 12 Community interventions and psychotherapy

In a wide variety of cultures, mothers with depression often indicate that they prefer having someone to talk with rather than being treated with medications (Dennis and Chung-Lee, 2006). In this chapter, I describe the efficacy of community support and psychotherapy. These modalities have been effective in both preventing and treating depression.

## Community interventions

Community-based care and peer support is an important way for mothers to interpret, negotiate, and experience social norms of motherhood (Dennis and Chung-Lee, 2006). This support can be administered in a wide range of ways. One review found that proactive telephone support, where providers initiated the contact, was helpful in at least four areas related to maternal/child health: preventing smoking relapse, preventing low birth weight, increasing breastfeeding duration and exclusivity, and decreasing the risk of postpartum depression (Dennis and Kingston, 2008). The authors indicated that telephone support, delivered by professionals or lay people, is a flexible, efficient, cost-effective and accessible form of health care. Telephone support can be the primary intervention or it can be a component of a multi-modal form of intervention.

Peer support was also helpful in preventing postpartum depression in a Canadian study (Dennis, et al., 2009). In this study, 701 women were identified as being at high risk for depression via an online screening system. They were randomized to receiving either standard care or to receiving telephone support from a mother who had previously experienced and recovered from postpartum depression. The peer volunteers were matched to the mothers based on ethnicity and area where they lived. The volunteers initiated contact 48 to 72 hours after randomization and were asked to make a minimum of four contacts with mothers, and then as many as they deemed necessary. Women received on average eight contacts. The retention rate among the volunteers was also high, suggesting that it was a rewarding activity for them as well. At 12 and 24 weeks postpartum, a research nurse blinded to treatment conditions followed up by telephone. The incidence of depression was 14% in the intervention group and 25% in the control group at 12 weeks. More than 80% of women in the intervention group were satisfied with intervention and would recommend it to a friend. The authors concluded that this was an accessible intervention and effective for mothers from diverse cultures. They also noted that lay people who have experienced similar problems could have a positive effect on maternal psychological well-being.

Healthcare providers can also provide support to new mothers. In a study of 2,064 women, half were assigned to an intervention of flexible care provided by midwives, and the other half were assigned to standard care. At four months postpartum, women in the flexible-care group had significantly better mental health than women in the standard-care group. The authors concluded that midwife-led, flexible, tailored-to-individual-needs care significantly improved new mothers' mental health and reduced the risk of postpartum depression (MacArthur, *et al.*, 2002).

A study of 623 women from England had different results. This study sought to determine whether additional support in the first month postpartum increased maternal health and breastfeeding rates, and decreased the risk of postpartum depression (Morrell, *et al.*, 2000). Half of the women were assigned to receive home visits, and the other half were assigned to receive standard care. At six weeks postpartum, there were no significant differences in health status, use of social services, depression or breastfeeding rates. The mothers were very satisfied with the health visits, however.

A study from South Africa found that home visiting improved mother–infant interaction, but did not decrease depression (Cooper, *et al.*, 2002). In this study, 32 women were randomly assigned to receive home visits by trained community volunteers, or to receive usual care. The home visitors provided emotional support, and taught mothers to be more responsive to their babies using items from the Neonatal Behavioral Assessment Scale. This intervention had no significant impact on maternal mood (although depression scores were lower for mothers in the intervention group). However, it was significantly associated with mothers being more positive with their babies.

Community-based care even helps in the general population. Simon, *et al.* (2000) found that telephone follow-up by a care manager significantly improved patient compliance with antidepressant treatment. The telephone follow-up consisted of a five-minute introductory telephone call, and two 10- to 15-minute calls at eight and sixteen weeks after the initial prescription. The case managers communicated with doctors about whether there were side effects, or whether the patient might be under-medicated (i.e. still showing moderate levels of depression). The case managers also assisted with arrangements for follow-up visits, but did not provide psychotherapy. This intervention resulted in a 50% improvement in depression scores, and a lower probability of major depression at the six-month follow-up than was found for those in the standard-care condition.

In contrast, a review of 22 randomized trials found that universal postpartum supportive care for low-risk women was not effective for any outcome variable (Shaw, *et al.*, 2006). The studies reviewed covered a wide range of interventions (home visitation, peer support, telephone counseling, case management), and a wide range of maternal outcomes (e.g. depression, home environment, child abuse and neglect, parent knowledge). These programs were helpful for high-risk women, however. Home visitation and peer support produced reductions in EPDS scores.

*Education*

Education is a key component of many community-based programs that aim to reduce the risk of depression and help mothers have more positive interactions with their babies. The results in respect of the effectiveness of these programs, however, have been mixed. In one education program (Elliot, *et al.*, 2000), women identified during pregnancy as being vulnerable to depression were randomly assigned to either a preventive intervention or a control group. At three months postpartum, 19% of the women in the "Preparation for Parenthood" group had scores in the depressed or borderline depressed ranges compared with 39% of the mothers who received standard care. These findings were only for first-time mothers.

Dennis (2005) found no preventive effect of antenatal and postnatal classes, lay home visits, or early postpartum follow-up in another review. She did find a beneficial effect of home visiting by a professional and a positive trend towards significance with debriefing. She concluded that there was no clear evidence to recommend antenatal and postnatal classes, early postpartum follow-up, continuity of care models, psychological debriefing in the hospital, or interpersonal psychotherapy. Interventions that target at-risk women, which are individually based, or which are initiated in the postpartum period are more likely to be beneficial.

Another study found that education during pregnancy was not helpful in reducing postpartum depression (Hayes, *et al.*, 2001). In this study, women were randomly assigned to either an education condition or to normal care. Depression was assessed during pregnancy and at two points postpartum. There were no differences between the control and intervention groups. Further, there was no relevant influence of social support or demographic variables. There was an improvement in depressive symptoms for both groups over time: mothers were more likely to be depressed during pregnancy than at either point postpartum. The authors concluded that their findings challenge two strongly held beliefs by professionals in the perinatal health field. First, that depression can be reduced through education. And second, that interventions done during pregnancy can endure into the postpartum period.

A study on depression in general compared problem-solving treatment and eight sessions on prevention of depression, with a control comparison group in a European community sample (Dowrick, *et al.*, 2000). There were 452 participants aged 18 to 65 who were identified through a community survey as having depressive disorders. The level of depression was 17% less than in the control group, and six months after the intervention, the depression-prevention group had a rate of depression that was 14% lower than the control group. The authors concluded that problem-solving and psychoeducation reduced severity and duration of depressive disorders and improved mental and social functioning. The problem-solving course was more acceptable than the prevention-of-depression course, but both were effective in reducing depression among participants.

In summary, community-based programs show promise in helping women make a smooth transition to motherhood. However, education programs appear to have only limited effectiveness, but can be effective for high-risk women. To be most effective, community-based programs must take place alongside more traditional, individually focused interventions for depression. Moreover, we need research that demonstrates the effectiveness of these programs in preventing or ameliorating postpartum depression.

## Psychotherapy

Another way in which mothers can experience support is through psychotherapy. In clinical trials, psychotherapy has proven as effective as medications in treating depression, with lower rates of relapse (Rupke, *et al.*, 2006). Researchers have found two types of psychotherapy to be highly effective in treating for depression in new mothers: cognitive-behavioral therapy and interpersonal psychotherapy. These studies are described below.

### Cognitive-behavioral therapy (CBT)

In numerous clinical trials, CBT has proven to be as powerful as medications for treating depression and a whole range of co-occurring conditions, such as anxiety, chronic pain, and obsessive-compulsive disorder (Rupke, *et al.* 2006). Moreover, patients who received cognitive therapy were less likely to relapse and drop out of treatment than those who received medications alone (Antonuccio, *et al.*, 1995; Rupke, *et al.*, 2006).

Cognitive therapy is based on the premise that distortions in thinking cause depression. It teaches patients to recognize and counter these thoughts (Rupke, *et al.*, 2006). The goal is to help patients identify distorted beliefs and replace them with more rational ones. Cognitive therapy is *not* simply learning to think "happy" thoughts. It is powerful enough to change the brain. Two studies compared cognitive therapy with medications for patients with obsessive-compulsive disorder (Baxter, *et al.* 1992) and panic disorder (Prasko, *et al.*, 2004). In both studies, the outcome variable was change in positron emission tomography (PET) scans of the brain before and after treatment. Before therapy, groups in both studies showed abnormalities in brain metabolism. After treatment, both groups had improved PET scans, but there was no difference *between* the groups. In other words, cognitive therapy caused the same changes in the brain that medications had.

Cognitive therapy has also been used to treat postpartum depression. In a study from England, 87 women with postpartum depression were randomized to one of four conditions: fluoxetine or placebo, plus one or six sessions of CBT (Appleby, *et al.*, 1997). Health visitors who attended a brief training program provided the therapy. The sessions were designed to offer reassurance and advice on topics of specific concern to new mothers. The initial session was one hour, and subsequent sessions were 30 minutes each. Four weeks after treatment, all four groups had improved. Not surprisingly, women receiving fluoxetine improved significantly more than women receiving the placebo, and women receiving six sessions of counseling improved significantly more than women who only received one session. There was no advantage to women receiving both medication and counseling beyond the first session. CBT was as effective as medication.

A study from Australia compared standard care, group cognitive therapy, or individual counseling for women with postpartum depression. After 12 weeks, both types of psychological treatment were superior to standard care, and the researchers concluded that individual counseling was as effective as group cognitive therapy (Milgrom, *et al.*, 2005).

Researchers added cognitive therapy to medications to treat moderate-to-severe postpartum depression (Misri, *et al.*, 2004). In this study, depressed, anxious mothers were assigned to receive paroxetine alone or paroxetine with group cognitive therapy. Mothers in both groups improved after treatment and there was no significant difference between the groups. From these results, there appeared to be no additional benefit of adding cognitive therapy to medications.

A small trial of 23 mothers with postpartum depression tested whether reducing depressive symptoms would also lower parenting stress (Misri, *et al.*, 2006). In this study, mothers were randomized to receive either medication or CBT. All of the mothers in the study were experiencing clinically significant levels of parenting stress before treatment. At the end of the study, both cognitive therapy and medication monotherapy decreased maternal stress. Rather than targeting stress directly, the treatments lowered postpartum depression, which led to a corresponding drop in parenting stress.

A study from Korea randomly assigned 27 pregnant women with depression to either a CBT intervention or a control condition (Cho, *et al.*, 2008). The CBT intervention consisted of nine bi-weekly, one-on-one, one-hour sessions that took place antenatally. The components included educating patients about depression, scheduling pleasant events, and changing negative thoughts to positive ones. Regarding marital relationships, the intervention consisted of promoting understanding of their spouses. In the control group, patients were educated about depression in one prenatal session. The authors found that CBT administered prenatally was an effective preventive measure for postpartum depression and that it also improved marital satisfaction. The intervention used standard CBT techniques, but focused on behavioral techniques to improve marital relationships.

Cognitive therapy was not effective in preventing depression in mothers of very preterm babies, however (Hagan, *et al.*, 2004). In this study, 101 mothers of very preterm babies received six sessions of cognitive therapy. They were compared with 98 mothers who received standard care. There were no differences in onset or duration of depression between the two groups, and 37% of mothers were depressed. The authors indicated that mothers of very preterm infants had high rates of stress and depression, and that a six-week intervention did not alter the prevalence of depression in this group.

A study from Glasgow, with a non-postpartum sample, combined cognitive therapy with mindfulness meditation in an eight-week course for people with relapsing, recurring depression (Finucane and Mercer, 2006). With a sample of 13 patients, the mean pre-course depression score was 35.7. After the course, it was 17.8. Anxiety had a similar decline. Mindfulness was added to treatment to address the ruminative thinking style that increases vulnerability to relapsing depression. Ruminative thinking involves rehashing personal short-comings and problematic situations. This style of thinking perpetuates, rather than relieves, stress. Mindfulness teaches patients to let go of negative thinking and to be open to what is there without aversion or attachment. Patients in this trial found the addition of mindfulness helpful in preventing subsequent episodes of depression.

In summary, what we think, and how we frame the world, has a substantial impact on our mental health. Cognitive therapy is a powerful way to treat even major depression. Not only does it treat depression, but it can also produce measurable changes in the brain that are comparable to those produced by antidepressants. It also has no impact on breastfeeding, and is a viable, effective alternative to medications for the treatment of depression.

### Interpersonal psychotherapy

Interpersonal psychotherapy is another type of psychotherapy that has also proven effective in the treatment of postpartum depression. For example, an NIMH-collaborative research study, interpersonal psychotherapy was as effective as tricyclic antidepressants and cognitive therapy, and was effective for almost 70% of the patients (Tolman, 2001).

Interpersonal psychotherapy is based on attachment theory, and the interpersonal theories of Harry Stack Sullivan. It is time-limited and focuses on the client's interpersonal relationships. Disturbances in the key relationships are hypothesized as being responsible for depression (Stuart and O'Hara, 1995). Interpersonal psychotherapy addresses four problem areas: role transitions, interpersonal disputes, grief, and interpersonal deficits. On a client's first visit, a specific problem is identified, and the client and therapist begin work on that issue. Mothers complete an interpersonal inventory and review information about key relationships, the nature of current communications, and how having a baby has changed those relationships (Grigoriadis and Ravitz, 2007). In the case of postpartum women, the goal of interpersonal psychotherapy is to help them with role transitions and changes in roles they have already established. A related goal is to assist women in building, or making better use of, existing support (Grigoriadis and Ravitz, 2007).

In a study of 120 women with postpartum major depression (O'Hara, *et al.*, 2000), women were assigned to either interpersonal psychotherapy or wait-list conditions for 12 weeks. The therapists were trained in interpersonal psychotherapy, and they followed a standardized treatment manual. O'Hara and colleagues (2000) found that women in the therapy group had significantly lower depression scores than women in the wait-list group at four, eight, and twelve weeks after treatment. The rate of recovery from depression was also significantly higher for women in the therapy group, and they scored better on postpartum adjustment and social support. The authors noted that interpersonal therapy was effective for women with postpartum depression. It reduced depressive symptoms and improved social adjustment. The authors felt that interpersonal psychotherapy represents a viable alternative to pharmacotherapy, especially for women who are breastfeeding.

Klier and colleagues (2001) also found interpersonal psychotherapy effective for 17 women with postpartum depression. In this study, interpersonal psychotherapy was used in a group setting. Women had significantly decreased depression after attending the group, and this was still true at the six-month follow-up. The authors noted some limitations in their study, such as small sample size, lack of a control group, and possible bias in the therapist's assessment of the women. Reay and colleagues (2006) had similar findings in their preliminary study of 18 mothers with postpartum depression. In this study, mothers participated in a program of interpersonal psychotherapy with two individual sessions and eight group sessions. Mothers' depression decreased significantly after treatment. However, 67% of the mothers were also on antidepressants and there was no control group.

Another study compared interpersonal psychotherapy with parenting education for 50 low-income, pregnant women with major depression (Spinelli and Endicott, 2003). Both interpersonal psychotherapy and the education condition were administered over 16 weeks. Women in their sample had a number of severe risk factors for depression: 47% had a history of childhood abuse (28% sexual abuse, 25% physical abuse, 6% both), and 73% had a history of major depression. In addition, many had chaotic home environments, unstable relationships, or partners involved in criminal activity. At the end of 16 weeks, significantly more women in the treatment group had a reduction in depressive symptoms of 50% or more on the Hamilton Depression Scale and the Beck Depression Inventory. The authors concluded that interpersonal psychotherapy was an effective first-line treatment for depression during pregnancy.

Another study also found interpersonal psychotherapy helpful in preventing postpartum depression in high-risk women (Zlotnick, *et al.*, 2006). In this study, 99 low-income pregnant women were randomly assigned to receive standard antenatal care, or standard care plus an intervention based on interpersonal therapy. The goals of the intervention were to improve women's close, personal relationships; change their expectations about these relationships; build their social networks; and help them master their transition to motherhood. The intervention was four 60-minute group sessions during pregnancy, with one "booster" session after delivery. At three months postpartum, 4% of the intervention group became depressed compared with 20% of the control group.

Interpersonal psychotherapy was used to treat low-income, depressed adolescents in five school-based mental health clinics in New York City (Mufson, *et al.*, 2004). In this study, 63 teens with depression or dysthymia were randomly assigned to receive 16 weeks of interpersonal psychotherapy or 16 weeks of treatment as usual. "Treatment as usual" included whatever individual psychotherapy the teens would have received if the program were not in place. The sample was 84% female, and 71% Hispanic. By the end of the intervention, teens receiving interpersonal therapy had significantly fewer depressive symptoms, had better social functioning, greater clinical improvement, and a greater decrease in clinical severity on the Clinical Global Impressions Scale. The authors noted that the largest treatment effects occurred for the older and more severely depressed adolescents. They also noted that although medications are often seen as frontline treatment for depressed teens, these were difficult to access through school clinics. Moreover, minority families were reluctant to accept antidepressants. Of the four teens in the study who were prescribed antidepressants, all had poor compliance with taking medications. The authors concluded that this school-based program was a viable alternative to medications for depressed, low-income adolescents.

In addition to data from clinical trials, two recent literature reviews indicated that interpersonal psychotherapy is effective and well-suited to the treatment of postpartum depression. In a review of four clinical trials, Weissman (2007) found that women who received 12 to 16 weeks of interpersonal psychotherapy showed a significant reduction of symptoms compared with women who received standard care. Weissman also indicated that interpersonal psychotherapy can be provided by mental health professionals, healthcare providers, or trained laypeople. Grigoriadis and Ravitz (2007) also concluded that interpersonal psychotherapy is an effective treatment for postpartum depression. They indicated that this approach can be easily integrated into primary-care settings, and that it is short-term, highly effective, and ideally suited to the needs of postpartum women.

### Anti-inflammatory effects of psychotherapy

Although evidence is quite preliminary, both cognitive therapy and interpersonal psychotherapy probably have an anti-inflammatory effect. Interpersonal psychotherapy's effect is due to an increasing amount and quality of support, which has been described in Chapter 9.

With regards to the effects of cognitive therapy, it is instructive to examine the literature on the health effects of hostility. Hostility is of interest because it is a particular way of looking at the world. People high in hostility tend to attribute negative motives to others, have difficulty trusting others and establishing close relationships. Hostility also specifically raises inflammation. In one study, hostility was associated with higher levels of circulating proinflammatory cytokines (IL-1$\alpha$, IL-1$\beta$, and IL-8) in 44 healthy, non-smoking, premenopausal women. The combination of depression and hostility led to the highest levels of IL-1$\beta$, IL-8, and TNF-$\alpha$ (Suarez, *et al.*, 2004). There was a dose-response effect: the more severe the depression and hostility, the greater the production of cytokines.

More recently, Suarez (2006) studied 135 healthy patients (75 men, 60 women), with no symptoms of diabetes. He found that women with higher levels of depression and hostility had higher levels of fasting insulin, glucose, and insulin resistance. These findings were not true for men, and they were independent of other risk factors for metabolic syndrome including body mass index, age, fasting triglycerides, exercise regularity, or ethnicity. These findings were significant since pre-study glucose levels were in the non-diabetic range. The author noted that inflammation, particularly elevated IL-6 and C-reactive protein, may mediate the relationship between depression and hostility, and the risk of type 2 diabetes and cardiovascular disease, possibly because they increase insulin resistance.

In another recent study, Kiecolt-Glaser, *et al.* (2005) found that couples who were high in hostility had higher levels of circulating proinflammatory cytokines. As a result, the rate of wound healing for the high-hostility couples was 60% slower than that of low-hostility couples. High-hostility couples had high levels of cytokines circulating systemically, where the cytokines were more likely to impair health and increase the risk of age-related diseases.

Cognitive therapy specifically addresses beliefs like hostility. Since negative cognitions increase inflammation, we could predict that reducing their occurrence would lower inflammation. That is indeed what Doering and colleagues (2007) found in their study of women after coronary bypass surgery: clinically depressed women had a higher incidence of in-hospital fevers and infections in the six months after surgery, due, in part, to decreases in natural killer-cell cytotoxicity. An eight-week program of CBT reduced depression, improved natural killer-cell cytotoxicity, and decreased IL-6 and C-reaction protein. Because the immune system was functioning more effectively, this intervention decreased post-operative infectious diseases. Another study by these same authors found that depressed women were more susceptible to systemic infections after coronary bypass surgery due to depression's impact on natural killer-cell cytotoxicity (Doering, *et al.*, 2008). Major depression increased their risk of infections, such as pneumonia and upper respiratory infections.

### *Summary of psychotherapy*

Cognitive therapy and interpersonal therapy are both effective treatments for postpartum depression. At this time, there is more empirical support for cognitive therapy. In addition, mothers may have an easier time locating a practitioner who can provide it. But interpersonal psychotherapy shows a lot of promise for both preventing and treating postpartum depression. Indeed, at some point, interpersonal psychotherapy may supplant cognitive therapy as the frontline psychotherapy for postpartum depression.

## Trauma-focused treatment

As described in Chapters 6, 7, and 8, women may come into the postpartum period with significant histories of psychological trauma. Trauma may be due to current events, such as their birth experiences, or to events that took place in the past, or both. Trauma treatment involves a combination of patient education, peer counseling, and psychotherapy. Medications can also be used and are described in Chapter 13. The combination of all these modalities provides the best overall care.

### *Patient education*

Women who have been traumatized by birth events, past abuse or other events, are often frightened by posttraumatic reactions. Education is the first component of a treatment plan. It can reassure women that they are not going "crazy," which many actually fear, and lets them know that they are not alone in their reactions. Patient education contains four key elements: normalization, removing self-blame and doubt, correcting misunderstandings, and establishing clinician credibility (Friedman, 2001). Patient education is always used as an adjunct to other treatment modalities (Friedman, 2001). However, most clinicians agree that it is an important component of any type of therapeutic approach. The components of patient education are as follows.

### *Normalization*

Normalization lets women know that their symptoms are similar to those experienced by millions of people who have been through traumatic events. This can create a profound sense of relief. Women learn that there is no stigma attached to their reactions, nor is it a result of their "weakness." Rather, normalization communicates that symptoms of PTSD are a common human response to trauma.

### *Removing self-blame and self-doubt*

Many survivors of traumatic events blame themselves for being in harm's way, and are ashamed that they did not take some kind of heroic steps to avoid the trauma or get out of the dangerous circumstance. Education can help patients realize that they did the best they could under the circumstances. Patient education can also help women evaluate how realistic their heroic fantasies are. It can communicate that their "failure" to act was due to the overwhelming nature of the event itself, and that the overwhelming nature of the event is part of the definition of trauma.

### Correcting misunderstandings

Patient education, and education of family members and friends, can help people understand the woman's behaviors in terms of trauma symptoms. Behaviors that seem strange or upsetting can be explained when seen through the lens of the woman's experiences. This can help those in a woman's support network work with, rather than against, treatment goals.

### Clinician credibility

Finally, patient education can help establish clinicians as knowledgeable about psychological trauma, and reassure them that the clinicians understand what patients are experiencing. This enlists patients' cooperation in treatment and can facilitate the development of trust.

## Peer counseling

Peer counseling uses an approach similar to that of Alcoholics Anonymous®, in that everyone involved in the group has had personal experience of trauma. Examples of postpartum peer counseling includes groups for women who had cesarean or other difficult births, mothers of premature or ill infants, mothers who have experienced previous childbearing loss, and mothers who are abuse survivors. The relationships in the peer group are equalitarian, and there is no authority figure or professional who leads the group. These groups can also "meet" online. Peer counselors often serve as role models for new clients, and demonstrate that it is possible to move beyond traumatic experiences (Friedman, 2001).

## Trauma-focused psychotherapy

When people are traumatized, they develop a conditioned response that pairs the traumatic event with certain environment cues (e.g. sights, sounds, smells) and bodily sensations (e.g. pain), a process known as fear conditioning. In trauma-focused psychotherapy, there are two specific goals. The first is for people to unlearn the conditioned response that triggers PTSD symptoms. The second is to address PTSD-related cognitions about themselves and others.

Psychotherapy is generally the treatment of choice for people with PTSD. Two of the most effective individual treatments are CBT and Eye Movement Desensitization and Reprocessing (EMDR). These techniques are described below.

### Cognitive-behavioral therapy (CBT)

CBT in trauma treatment is designed to counteract conditioned fear responses, and to normalize abnormal thoughts, behaviors and feelings of patients with PTSD. Three common forms of CBT are exposure therapy, cognitive therapy, and stress-inoculation training.

## EXPOSURE THERAPY

Exposure therapy is specifically designed to alleviate the conditioned emotional response to traumatic stimuli that has been engendered by the traumatic event. After a traumatic event, patients naturally tend to avoid any memories of it, or any stimuli that remind them of their trauma. When patients avoid processing their trauma, however, it inhibits their recovery. Exposure therapy helps patients master their fears, and counters the belief that they are weak or incompetent (Foa and Cahill, 2002).

Exposure therapy begins when patients are asked to imagine the traumatic event. In a single session, patients are asked to repeatedly describe what happened, and their thoughts and feelings that occurred during the trauma (Foa and Cahill, 2002). During their narratives, patients are asked to report their level of distress every ten minutes. If treatment has been successful, then patients can confront their traumatic pasts without triggering PTSD symptoms, especially intrusive thoughts or hyperarousal. This form of treatment is highly effective (Foa and Cahill, 2002; Friedman, 2001). However, van der Kolk (2002) cautions that too much exposure to traumatic memories can backfire, and actually precipitate PTSD symptoms, such as hyperarousal and sensitization.

## COGNITIVE THERAPY

As described earlier, cognitive therapy addresses distortions in thinking. Women who have been traumatized often see the world as a dangerous place and see themselves as helpless (Foa and Cahill, 2002; Friedman, 2001). The goal of cognitive therapy is to help patients identify these automatic thoughts, and to replace them with more accurate ones (Foa and Cahill, 2002). This form of therapy is also highly effective in reducing symptoms of PTSD (Friedman, 2001).

## STRESS-INOCULATION TRAINING (SIT)

SIT uses a combination of methods to help survivors cope with anxiety, trauma-related stimuli, and threatening situations. SIT is based on social-learning theory, which states that traumatic events create behavioral, social, and cognitive fear responses. SIT includes relaxation techniques, biofeedback, cognitive restructuring, and assertiveness training to help patients deal more effectively in social relationships. Stress-inoculation training is as effective as exposure therapy for reducing PTSD symptoms, and these improvements last over time (Friedman, 2001).

### Eye Movement Desensitization and Reprocessing (EMDR)

EMDR is another treatment that has proven effective for many people who have experienced traumatic events. It is based on the hypothesis that saccadic eye movements can reprogram the brain, and therefore can be used to help alleviate the emotional impact of trauma. (Saccadic eye movements are the quick eye movements that jump from one fixation point to another.)

During EMDR, women imagine a traumatic memory, or any negative emotions associated with that memory. Then women are asked to articulate a belief that is incompatible with their previous memory (e.g. on their personal worth). While women are remembering this event, they are asked to use their eyes to follow the clinician's fingers that are making rapid movements. During treatment, women are asked to rate the strength of both the traumatic memory and the counteracting positive beliefs (Friedman, 2001).

Studies have demonstrated that this method of treatment is effective: 50% to 70% of patients no longer met criteria for PTSD after receiving EMDR treatment. In contrast, only 20% to 50% of women who received supportive therapy no longer met PTSD criteria (Friedman, 2001).

### The efficacy of psychotherapy for trauma treatment

Overall, it appears that CBT is the most effective treatment for PTSD. Of the forms of CBT, exposure therapy has the best empirical support (Foa and Cahill, 2002). In one study that directly compared CBT with EMDR, patients assigned to the CBT group had significantly fewer symptoms post-treatment than patients assigned to EMDR. Those who received CBT were almost three times as likely to have recovered from PTSD at the three-month follow-up (Devilly and Spence, 1999). However, EMDR is also effective in treating all three clusters of symptoms and can be a useful addition to treatment regimens (Friedman, 2001). Stress-inoculation training has also proven effective for the treatment of rape-related PTSD. Exposure therapy appears to be most effective for those with low levels of functioning before beginning treatment, whereas stress-inoculation training is helpful for patients with high levels of anxiety (Foa and Cahill, 2002). However, van der Kolk (2002) cautions that, particularly in the case of complex PTSD, there are still many questions about what is the optimal treatment. He states that what appears to be most important is to give patients a sense of mastery that will allow them to live in the present rather than the past, and to be no longer held captive by their memories.

## Conclusions

Research on treatment is a newer part of the literature on postpartum depression. It confirms that postpartum depression can be successfully treated with psychotherapy. When mothers can talk with others about their postpartum experiences, it alleviates their symptoms and eases their transition to motherhood. This research demonstrates that social relationships are vital to mothers' mental health and that supportive care – through either community support or psychotherapy – is a vital part of the treatment arsenal.

In the next chapter, I summarize the final treatment option: use of antidepressant medications.

# 13 Antidepressants in pregnant and breastfeeding women

Antidepressants are often the first line of treatment offered to depressed patients in healthcare settings. Antidepressants are often necessary for more serious depressions, but may be used for mild and moderate depression as well (Geddes, *et al.*, 2007). While not all women are willing to take them, they do have their place in the repertoire of treatments for depression.

## Helping mothers weigh their options

When helping mothers weigh their options about whether to take medications, one factor to consider is the severity of their depression. A mother who is severely impaired will probably benefit from medications (Chaudron, 2007). It's also important to consider the type of symptoms they have. Medications are especially helpful in treating the following symptoms: sleep disturbance (including early-morning awakening, decreased sleep efficiency, frequent awakenings through the night and possibly hypersomnia), appetite disturbance (eating too much or too little), fatigue, decreased sex drive, diurnal variations in mood (e.g. feeling worse in the morning), restlessness or agitation, impaired concentration, and "pronounced anhedonia" (the inability to experience pleasure) (Preston and Johnson, 2009).

Another factor is her feelings about being on medications. Some mothers may resist being on antidepressants. In a review of 40 studies, Dennis and Chung-Lee (2006) found that women were often reluctant to take antidepressants, even after education about their relative safety. Among the concerns they mentioned were fear of addiction, side effects or possible harm to their infants, and the stigma associated with taking antidepressants. In a study from France (Chabrol, *et al.*, 2004), 405 new mothers were asked about the acceptability of treatments for depression including psychotherapy by consultation, psychotherapy by home visit, and antidepressants. The researchers found that psychotherapy in both forms was more acceptable than antidepressants – even after information was provided to the mothers about the effects of antidepressants on breast milk. However, the information the researchers provided on antidepressants may have influenced this response. Below is a partial account of what they told mothers with regard to antidepressants. Given what they said to mothers, the mothers' refusal to take medications was hardly surprising.

> However, the effects of the antidepressants on the developing brain of the child and the long-term consequences are unknown. In the case of breastfeeding it is therefore recommended not to prescribe antidepressants except in the cases where the advantages can clearly be shown to outweigh the potential risks.
>
> (Chabrol, *et al.*, 2004: 7)

Wisner, *et al.* (1996) recommended that mothers be actively involved in the decision about whether to use medications. If mothers feel they are being forced to wean and/or forced to take medications against their will, they are more likely to be non-compliant with treatment and risk an exacerbation of symptoms. If a mother wants to continue breastfeeding, there are many good reasons to support her in that. Wisner and colleagues (1996) recommended that mothers and fathers be included in the discussion of risk and benefits associated with breastfeeding with medications, not breastfeeding, and being raised by a chronically depressed mother.

## Factors to consider in medication use

Making a decision about which antidepressant to use can be complex (Chaudron, 2007). In selecting an antidepressant, Remick (2002) recommended the following considerations. First, has the patient been on a particular antidepressant before and did she have a positive response to it? Second, if a patient is possibly suicidal, a tricyclic or monoamine oxidase (MAO) inhibitor would not be a good choice since these medications are potentially lethal in overdose or in combination with certain foods. Third, the side-effect profile of the medications should also be considered. These side effects include sedation, weight gain, orthostatic hypotension, and sexual dysfunction, and can be more or less troubling for individual patients. Fourth, another consideration is other medications a patient is currently taking; possible drug–drug interactions should also guide the choice. Finally, costs of a medication need to be considered. The newer medications are considerably more expensive than the older antidepressants that are available in generic form. For patients without prescription coverage this can be a deciding factor.

## Types of antidepressant

There are four major types of antidepressant. All work to increase the amount of neurotransmitters serotonin, norepinephrine, or dopamine available in the brain. These categories are described below.

### *Tricyclics*

Tricyclic antidepressants (TCAs) are the oldest, and least expensive, of the antidepressants. They have a solid track record of effectiveness and include medications such as Pamelor (nortriptyline), and Elavil (amitriptyline). They are effective, but tend to have side effects that people do not like, so patient compliance is often a problem with TCAs. Once patients start to feel better, they may chose to discontinue the medications, and this can negatively affect their treatment.

TCAs have another serious drawback: the risk of suicide. Tricyclics can be lethal in too large a dose. If these medications are used, patients must be closely monitored, and not given sufficient medication in each prescription period to provide the means for patients to kill themselves. MAO inhibitors should also be avoided if there is a suicide risk. Preston and Johnson (2009) recommend the following medications as alternatives to TCAs for suicidal patients, or for those at high-risk for suicide: fluoxetine (Prozac), sertraline (Zoloft), paroxetine (Paxil), or bupropion (Wellbutrin).

### Selective serotonin reuptake inhibitors (SSRIs)

SSRIs include such commonly used medications as fluoxetine (Prozac), sertraline (Zoloft), paroxetine (Paxil), citalopram (Celexa), and escitalopram (Lexapro). As their name implies, they work specifically on serotonin receptors. While these medications have side effects, there are fewer than in the case of the other antidepressants, and their dosing schedule is less complex. SSRIs are effective for approximately 80% of patients (Institute for Clinical Systems Improvement, 2000; Preston and Johnson, 2009).

One of the major complaints of patients using SSRIs are their sexual side effects, in the general population and in postpartum women (di Scalea, *et al.*, 2009). A study of 70 postpartum women examined these effects and compared two antidepressants: nortriptyline (a tricyclic) or sertraline (an SSRI). The women were randomly assigned to receive one of these medications for major depression in an eight-week clinical trial. At the beginning of the trial, 73% complained of three or more sexual concerns. By eight weeks, only 37% mentioned sexual concerns. Those whose depression remitted were significantly less likely to report sexual concerns than women whose depression did not remit. This finding was independent of the medication type that they were on. The authors concluded that sexual concerns are more a function of depression rather than a side effect of a particular medication. What this might mean is that mothers who continue to report sexual side effects may still be depressed, and this bears further scrutiny.

Because SSRIs have the potential for interacting with other medications, a careful history of other medications (prescription, other-the-counter, and herbal) should always be taken. SSRIs can be dangerous if taken with MAO inhibitors, non-sedating antihistamines (e.g. Hismanal), tricyclic antidepressants, and lithium because they may increase levels of each. There can also be problems if they are taken with carbamazepine and St. John's wort (Preston and Johnson, 2009). If switching from an SSRI to St. John's wort, the wash-out period is five days.

### Mixed-function antidepressants

Some of the newer types of antidepressant are venlafaxine (Effexor) and mirtazapine (Remeron). Venlafaxine is a selective norepinephrine reuptake inhibitor (SNRI) and is a frontline treatment for depression and PTSD. Mirtazapine is a tetracyclic antidepressant, and is classified as a noradrenergic and specific serotonergic antidepressant. It is most useful as an add-on medication to enhance the effectiveness of other antidepressants, such as buproprion and venlafaxine, in cases of severe or treatment-resistant depression. Both are rated as L3 in *Medications and Mothers' Milk*, ("moderately safe"), and should be prescribed only if the benefit outweighs the potential risk to the infant (Hale, 2008).

### Monoamine oxidase (MAO) inhibitors

MAO inhibitors are also very effective antidepressants, but they have fallen out of favor because of the strict dietary restrictions associated with their use. MAO inhibitors include phenelzine (Nardil), isocarboxazid (Marplan), and tranylcypromine (Parnate). When taking these medications, patients cannot eat or drink anything with tyramine, a byproduct of bacterial fermentation, which is common in foods such as red wine and cheese. When these foods are consumed with an MAO inhibitor, hypertensive crisis or even death can occur. MAO inhibitors are not widely used in the U.S., but may be prescribed for refractory depressions. They are also effective in the treatment of atypical depression (Institute for Clinical Systems

Improvement, 2000). These medications are enjoying a renaissance of use, however, because if the dietary restrictions are observed, some feel they are safer than tricyclics and have fewer side effects (Preston and Johnson, 2009).

These medications are the only antidepressants that are contraindicated for breastfeeding mothers. There is some concern that the medications may cause permanent changes in the baby, and the risk does not outweigh the benefits.

## Dilemmas in treating pregnant women

The dilemmas involved in treating pregnant women for depression are not new, but the array of treatment choices and spectrum of mood and anxiety disorders are. This often leaves clinicians in a "gray zone" of whether to treat or not (Chaudron, 2007). The benefits probably outweigh the risks, but we should not be glib because there *are* some risks associated with using medications during pregnancy (Freeman, 2007; Yonkers, 2007). These are described below.

### In utero *effects of antidepressants*

> When a clinician is faced with the dilemma of managing mentally ill pregnant women, no decision is risk free.
>
> (Misri, *et al.*, 2006: 1031)

In treating depression, the toughest choices involve using a medication during pregnancy. Prenatal exposure carries risk of fetal complications – although these are statistically rare – that need to be thoroughly discussed with the mother. In short, providers need to be able to decide which medication best fits with a particular patient, and to help the patient accept it without stigma or guilt (Chaudron, 2007). These complications must be balanced with the impact of untreated depression, which also increases the risk of complications (see Chapter 2).

### *Antidepressants and preterm birth*

One possible risk of antidepressants use in pregnancy is the increased risk of preterm birth. In a recent study of pregnant women with depression, more than 20% of infants with continuous exposure to SSRIs during pregnancy were delivered preterm (Wisner, *et al.*, 2009). This study included 238 women who were assessed at 20, 30 and 36 weeks' gestation. The patients were divided into three groups: depression with no SSRI exposure, SSRIs with either continuous or partial exposure, and untreated major depression with either continuous or partial depression exposure. Women were on the following medications: 34% sertraline, 25% fluoxetine, 23% citalopram or escitalopram, and 18% other medications. At study end, 20% of the infants with continuous SSRI exposure were preterm. However, the rate of preterm birth among the mothers with continuous *untreated depression* was also 20%. The rate of preterm birth among the non-exposed or partially exposed groups ranged from 4% to 9%. All other outcomes did not differ between the groups.

Suri, *et al.* (2007) also examined the impact of prenatal antidepressant exposure on 90 women, 49 of whom had major depression and were treated with antidepressants while pregnant. There were 22 women with major depression who were not treated with antidepressants, and 19 healthy comparison women. The primary outcomes were infants' gestational age at birth, birth weight, one- and five-minute Apgar scores, and admission to special care nursery. The rates of preterm birth were 14.3% for women taking antidepressants, 0% for women who were depressed but not on medications, and 5.3% for the healthy controls. The rates of admission into special care were 21%, 9%, and 0% for the three groups, respectively. Dose of medication was also significantly related to preterm birth, with higher doses leading to shorter gestational ages; preterm was 20% in the high-dose group, 9% in the low-dose group, and 0% in the no-antidepressant group. Birth weight and Apgar scores did not differ significantly. The authors concluded that medication status, not depression, was related to gestational age at birth.

In a large population study in British Columbia, Canada (N=119,547), infants exposed to SSRIs *in utero* were compared with the infants of mothers who were depressed and not treated, and with those of non-depressed mothers. The percentage of SSRI exposure ranged from 2.3% to 5% over the 39-month recruitment period. Birth weight and gestational age were significantly less for the SSRI-exposed infants than for the infants of depressed mothers who were not treated. The most commonly used medications were paroxetine (44.7%), fluoxetine (27.2%), sertraline (25.6%), fluvoxamine (4.6%), and citalopram (3.3%) (Oberlander, *et al.*, 2006).

Timing of medication exposure influences the complications associated with their use. First- and third-trimester exposure are the times of greatest concern.

### First-trimester exposure

A prospective study collected data from women whose babies were born between 1995 and 2003. There were 200 neonates exposed to antidepressants *in utero* and 1,200 controls (Maschi, *et al.*, 2008). The purpose of this study was to assess the impact of antidepressants on newborns exposed during pregnancy. There were three groups that differed in the timing of when they took antidepressants: before conception and during first trimester, during the second and third trimesters, and before conception and during the entire pregnancy. The most commonly used medications were paroxetine (58 cases), fluoxetine (32 cases), and amitriptyline (26 cases). As in previous studies, there was a finding of significantly increased risk of preterm birth for exposed- vs. non-exposed infants. This was particularly true for the chronically exposed group.

Of 200 exposed infants, 14 experienced adverse events and 3 required NICU/SCN admission. No statistically significant difference was found after adjusting for prematurity, birth weight and sex of the neonate. There were no significant effects found by medication type. Three cases (5%) of neonatal complications were reported with paroxetine exposure, one of which required admission to the NICU. In contrast, in a sub-group of the non-exposed group, there were 17 complications (5%), six of which required NICU admission. One case of cardiac malformation was reported following paroxetine exposure in the first trimester, and a total of 2% of the control group had malformations, none of which were cardiac malformations. A major limitation of these findings is that data were collected via maternal interview, and therefore may have underreported especially the minor effects (Maschi, *et al.*, 2008).

Similarly, the results of the Sloane Epidemiology Center Birth Defects Study recently confirmed that SSRIs do not significantly increase the risk of birth defects overall. The researchers included three birth defects in their study: craniosynostosis, omphalocele, and heart defects (Louik, *et al.*, 2007). Sertraline increased the risk of omphalocele (OR=5.7) and septal defects (OR=2.0), and paroxetine increased the risk of the heart defect right ventricular outflow tract obstruction (OR=3.3). It should be noted that even with these odds ratios, only 1.7% to 4.7% of infants with these defects were exposed to SSRIs in the first trimester. The authors concluded that the overall risk of having a child affected by SSRI use was only 0.2%.

First-trimester exposure may also increase the risk of miscarriage. In a sample of 937 pregnant women exposed to antidepressants prior to and during early pregnancy, there were 122 spontaneous abortions, including three ectopic pregnancies (Einarson, *et al.*, 2009). In their comparison group of 937 non-exposed pregnant women, there were 75 spontaneous abortions and no ectopic pregnancies. Logistic regression analysis indicated that antidepressant exposure and prior spontaneous abortion were the risk factors for current spontaneous abortion. The authors concluded that antidepressant exposure in the first trimester is associated with a small, but statistically significant, risk of miscarriage. It also increased the risk of mothers' decision to terminate the pregnancy. They urged caution in interpreting these results because one must also consider the effect of underlying depression.

### *Third-trimester exposure and discontinuation syndrome*

In neonates, third-trimester exposure is related to SSRI withdrawal or "discontinuation" syndrome (Cipriani, *et al.*, 2007; Looper, 2007). Discontinuation syndrome includes acrocyanosis, tachypnea, temperature instability, and irritability (Oberlander, *et al.*, 2004). When comparing exposed and non-exposed infants, the rates of complications were 13.9% for neonatal respiratory distress (vs. 7.8%), 9.4% for jaundice (vs. 7.5%), and 3.9% for feeding problems (vs. 2.4%). The length of hospital stay was significantly longer for exposed infants, suggesting that SSRI exposure created an independent effect. The authors concluded that exposure to prenatal SSRIs increased risk of low birth weight and respiratory distress, even when maternal illness severity was accounted for (Oberlander, *et al.*, 2006). These findings were contrary to what the researchers expected in that they predicted that reducing depression would lessen adverse neonatal complications associated with maternal depression. The effects were compounded for children who had been exposed to SSRIs *in utero* and whose mothers were currently depressed.

A large study (N=997 infants, 987 mothers) sought to prospectively investigate the neonatal effects of exposure to tricyclic and SSRI antidepressants during the third trimester (Kallen, 2004). The medications used included tricylic antidepressants, such as clomipramine and amitriptyline, and SSRIs including citalopram, paroxetine, fluoxetine, and sertraline. Following exposure, there was an increased risk for preterm birth (OR=1.96) and low birth weight (OR=1.98). After exposure to antidepressants, especially tricyclic drugs, there was an increased risk for low Apgar scores (OR=2.33), respiratory distress (OR=2.21), neonatal convulsions (OR=1.90), and hypoglycemia (OR=1.62). Infant outcomes after exposure to paroxetine were not worse than those associated with exposure to other SSRIs. The author concluded by noting that there were neonatal effects of antidepressants used in late pregnancy, and that the SSRIs may be the drugs of choice during pregnancy.

In a prospective study of neonates, newborn behavior was compared between babies exposed to medication in the second and third trimester of pregnancy (N=46), and non-exposed babies (N=23). Among babies exposed to medications, some were exposed to SSRIs alone. The SSRIs used in the study included fluoxetine, sertraline, and paroxetine. The second group was exposed to an SSRI and clonazepam (Oberlander, *et al.*, 2004). Maternal drug levels were assessed during pregnancy and at delivery. Infant drug levels were assessed via cord blood and at Day 2 postpartum. All but one of the babies was born healthy and at full term. Thirty percent of the exposed infants showed symptoms of discontinuation syndrome. These symptoms were more common in the SSRI/clonazepam group (39%) than in the SSRI-only group (25%). The most common symptoms were mild respiratory distress, and in some rare cases, hypotonia. Indeed, all the infants with symptoms had respiratory distress. The symptoms were self-limiting, and when these infants were assessed at two and eight months on the Bayley Scales of Infant Development, there were no significant differences between the exposed and non-exposed groups. Discontinuation symptoms were especially likely when paroxetine was combined with clonazepam as clonazepam appeared to change the metabolism of paroxetine (Oberlander, *et al.*, 2004).

In a study of two-month olds, Oberlander and colleagues (2005) compared three groups of infants: those who had had prenatal SSRI exposure; those with both pre- and postnatal SSRI exposure, and infants with no exposure. They found 30% of the breastfeeding infants had detectable drug levels. When they were present, the infant medication levels were substantially lower than milk and maternal levels. The developmental effects of postnatal SSRI exposure have not yet been found and the effects of exposure to SSRIs via breast milk seem to be minimal (Oberlander, *et al.*, 2005).

In a review of 13 published articles, Moses-Kolko and colleagues (2005) noted that exposure to SSRIs late in pregnancy increased overall risk of neonatal behavior syndrome (OR=3.0) compared with early or no exposure, suggesting medication withdrawal. Tapering these medications in the third trimester may be advisable. Most of the studies they reviewed reported on the effects of fluoxetine and paroxetine. Neonates exposed to SSRIs primarily displayed central nervous system, motor, respiratory, and gastrointestinal symptoms. These symptoms are generally mild and self-limiting, and can be managed with supportive care. Severe symptoms are rare, and no reported neonatal deaths have occurred that are attributable to SSRI exposure.

### *Childhood effects of pre- and postnatal SSRI exposure*

Two studies examined longer-term effects of pre- and postnatal exposure to SSRIs. Both studies included the same cohort of patients and were designed to assess "behavioral teratogenecity" that may have occurred in the wake of SSRI exposure *in utero* and breast-milk SSRI exposure. Behavioral teratogenecity included internalizing and externalizing behaviors as indicated on the Child Behavior Checklist. Internalizing behaviors include emotional reactivity, depression, anxiety, irritability, and withdrawal (Misri, *et al.*, 2006). Externalizing behaviors include levels of activity, impulsiveness, non-compliance, verbal and physical aggression, task persistence, problem solving, disruptive acts, and emotional outbursts (Oberlander, *et al.*, 2007).

In these studies, 22 mother-infant dyads who were exposed prenatally to SSRIs were compared with 14 non-exposed mother-infant dyads. Of the 22 depressed mothers, 5 were taking fluoxetine, 14 paroxetine, and 3 sertraline. Nine of these women were also taking olanzapine. The exposure to the medication was substantial, averaging 181 days of prenatal exposure and 60 days postnatal for SSRIs and 41 days postnatal for olanzapine (Misri, *et al.*, 2006; Oberlander, *et al.*, 2007). Amazingly, mothers in this study remained symptomatic even after treatment for depression: 64% still had anxiety symptoms, 73% had symptoms of depression. At the four-year visit, 59% had anxiety symptoms and 50% had depressive symptoms (Misri, *et al.*, 2006).

With regard to medication exposure, there were no significant differences in either parent or caregiver ratings of internalizing behaviors. Independent raters also rated the child's behavior in a laboratory setting where they were blind to the child's medication status, and there were no differences between exposed and non-exposed groups. When the entire cohort was measured, mothers were more likely to report symptoms in their children when they were anxious or depressed. This was not true for teacher ratings and the relationship remained even after prenatal exposure was added to the model. Maternal mood was more predictive of mother-reported internalizing behaviors than of prenatal medication exposure (Misri, *et al.*, 2006).

Similarly, there was no difference at age 4 between the exposed and non-exposed groups in externalizing behaviors (Oberlander, *et al.*, 2007). Current maternal depression and anxiety were more predictive of externalizing at age four than prenatal medication exposure. Umbilical cord blood levels were associated with externalizing behaviors at 4 years, but once current maternal depression was added to the model, it only accounted for 11% of the behavioral outcome. Exposure was related to the child's lower persistence in the laboratory observation, and poor neonatal adaptation predicted increased aggressiveness at age 4. The authors concluded that current maternal stress and mood were better predictors of externalizing behaviors, regardless of prenatal depressed mood or medication exposure. This study was the first to consider the dual role of prenatal SSRI exposure and current maternal mood.

## Breastfeeding and medications

Breastfeeding is another route by which babies can be exposed to medications. With regard to breastfeeding, some have argued that we don't know the clinical significance of medications transferred via breast milk, nor do we know the long-term effects (Cipriani, *et al.*, 2007; Field, 2008; Melzer-Brody, *et al.*, 2008; Payne, 2007). Commonly cited adverse effects of medication exposure via breast milk include infant irritability, poor-quality or uneasy sleep, and poor feeding. Most of these effects have been documented in case studies, however, where there may have also been prenatal exposure. In contrast, studies with larger samples generally find no adverse effects. Any risk/benefit analysis must also weigh up the risks of infant exposure to mothers' medications against the risks of *not breastfeeding*, which is associated with considerable morbidity. In most cases, the risks associated with breastfeeding on medication are still less than the risk of not breastfeeding (Hale, 2008; Payne, 2007). And, as documented in Chapter 2, not treating depression with either medications, or with non-pharmacologic approaches, is never an appropriate option.

### *Does medication cross into breast milk?*

A study of 14 breastfeeding mother–infant dyads assessed maternal and infant platelet levels of 5-HT as an indication of medication transfer before and after 6 to 16 weeks of treatment for postpartum major depression (Epperson, *et al.*, 2001). The infants' plasma showed little to no change in platelet 5-HT levels after breastfeeding. Sertraline, and its major metabolite, desmethylsertraline, were at or below the lower limit of quantification. When sertraline is administered in typical clinical doses, it usually has a negligible effect on platelet 5-HT transport even in young, exclusively breastfed infants.

Paroxetine has also been studied with regard to breastfeeding in a study of 25 mother-infant pairs. The researchers found detectable levels of paroxetine in all maternal serum samples and in 24 of 25 breast-milk samples. However, in the infant serum samples, paroxetine was below the lower limit of detection. The mean infant dose of paroxetine was 1.1% of the maternal dose (Misri, *et al.*, 2000a). There were no adverse effects in any infants.

A recent meta-analysis of 67 studies of antidepressant levels in breastfeeding infants pooled data from 337 research cases, including 238 infants (Weissman, *et al.*, 2004). The researchers analyzed data on 15 different antidepressants and their major metabolites, and found that antidepressants were detectable in breast milk for all the antidepressants they studied. Fluoxetine produced the highest proportion of elevated infant levels and the highest mean infant level. Citalopram was also relatively high. Only one infant across studies had an elevated paroxetine level, and that infant had also been exposed prenatally. All other infant paroxetine levels were zero, and this included three infants with prenatal exposure.

Weissman and colleagues (2004) indicated that there are many factors that influence transfer of medication to infants via breast milk. They noted that some potentially serious short-term effects have been noted in case reports of infants exposed to antidepressants via breastfeeding, but that the infants' symptoms could be due to withdrawal and re-exposure via breast milk. Compared with other antidepressants, fluoxetine was more likely to accumulate in breastfeeding infants. There was also a case report of an infant with no prenatal exposure having symptoms following exposure to citalopram via breastfeeding. This infant's level was 13% of the average maternal dose (Weissman, *et al.*, 2004).

With regard to long-term effects, the researchers noted that low or undetectable infant plasma concentrations alone cannot reassure us that the antidepressant will have no effect on the rapidly developing brain, or indicate whether chronic, low-dose exposure poses a risk. However, studies with asymptomatic infants are reassuring. Moreover, although antenatal exposure differs from exposure via breastfeeding, prenatal exposure provides a "loading dose" that far exceeds any exposure from breast milk and can thus distort findings regarding exposure via breast milk. In addition, studies often fail to account for other confounds, such as maternal smoking or alcohol use, both of which can affect infant metabolism (Weissman, *et al.*, 2004).

In summary, breastfeeding infants' exposure to paroxetine, sertraline, and nortriptyline is unlikely to lead to detectable or elevated plasma drug levels. In contrast, infants exposed to fluoxetine had higher levels of exposure, especially if they had been exposed prenatally. Citalopram exposure may lead to elevated levels in some infants, but more data are needed. Although these appear safe for the majority of babies, some adverse effects have been identified through case studies. Therefore, breastfeeding mothers should be advised to watch for any possible signs of adverse reactions including irritability, poor feeding, or uneasy sleep. Premature babies or others with impaired metabolite efficiency should especially be monitored for adverse effects (Weissman, *et al.*, 2004).

Escitalopram, as a newer antidepressant, was not included in the review by Weissman and colleagues (2004). However, it too has a favorable profile for breastfeeding mothers. A recent study examined the transfer of escitalopram and its metabolite into breast milk from eight women who were taking escitalopram for postpartum depression (Rampono, *et al.*, 2006). The mothers had been taking the medication for an average of 55 days. The total relative infant dose for the combination of escitalopram and its metabolite was 5.3% of the maternal weight-adjusted dose (3.9% for escitalopram; 1.7% for demethylescitalopram). The levels were undetectable in four infants and at very low levels in two others (two infants did not have their blood tested). Based on the infant dose calculations, the authors concluded that escitalopram is preferred to citalopram for treatment of depression during breastfeeding, and is safe for breastfeeding women.

With regard to medications and breastfeeding, Yonkers (2007: 1458) makes the following observation.

> The take-home messages are that breastfeeding has many benefits, the amount of medication in breast milk varies according to when the drug is taken and what part of breast milk is assayed, but usually maternal use does not lead to substantial levels in the neonate. However, it is best that neonates be monitored for difficulty feeding, weight

gain, sleep or state changes, etc. … if the mother is undergoing antidepressant treatment while breastfeeding.

## The anti-inflammatory effects of antidepressants

Until recently, researchers believed that antidepressants' efficacy was due to their effects on the monoamine neurotransmitters, such as serotonin and norepinephrine. That conceptualization is accurate but probably incomplete. In a review of the literature, Maes (2001) noted that most major classes of antidepressants – including tricyclics, SSRIs, SNRIs, heterocyclics (e.g. trazodone) and MAO inhibitors – downregulate proinflammatory cytokines, including IL-1β and TNF-α, and increase glucocorticoid receptor functioning. Long-term therapy normalizes the inflammatory response system, including downregulating IL-6 and acute-phase proteins (such as C-reactive protein). Maes (2001) concluded that antidepressants may have their effect because of their immunoregulatory effects, an effect since noted by several others (Kubera, *et al.*, 2004; Pace, *et al.*, 2007; Roumestan, *et al.*, 2007; Szelnyi and Vizi, 2007; Vollmar, *et al.*, 2007). In addition, anti-inflammatory COX-2 inhibitors, such as Celebrex, boost the effects of the antidepressant reboxetine (Pace, *et al.*, 2007). COX-2 is a signaling molecule that can contribute to glucocorticoid resistance. Blocking it decreases glucocorticoid resistance.

Antidepressants also decrease levels of acute-phase proteins, such as C-reactive protein. A study compared C-reactive protein levels in cardiac patients with major depression before and after treatment with one of the SSRIs: sertraline, fluoxetine, or paroxetine. In these patients, C-reactive protein dropped significantly after treatment, independent of whether depression resolved (O'Brien, *et al.*, 2006).

Another study tested the anti-inflammatory effects of the antidepressants, fluoxetine and desipramine, in two animal models of human disease (Roumestan, *et al.*, 2007). In the model of septic shock used in this study, both antidepressants decreased TNF-α levels. In the model of allergic asthma, fluoxetine and the steroid prednisolone reduced several types of leukocytes, including macrophages, lymphocytes, neutrophils, and eosinophils. The authors concluded that antidepressants had a direct peripheral anti-inflammatory effect. They noted that antidepressants can be useful in treating inflammatory conditions – especially those with co-morbid depression – noting that antidepressants may allow patients to cut down on steroid use.

An in vitro study of inflammation was designed to test whether the antidepressant venlafaxine would modulate the inflammatory response (Vollmar, *et al.*, 2008). Venlafaxine is a norepinephrine-serotonin reuptake inhibitor. In a astroglia-microglia co-culture, the researchers demonstrated that venlafaxine was anti-inflammatory and decreased IL-6 and IL-8.

Another study compared the antidepressants venlafaxine, fluoxetine, and imipramine in three groups: older adults with treatment-resistant depression; age-matched adults without depression, and young, healthy control volunteers (Kubera, *et al.*, 2004). The researchers found that imipramine, venlafaxine and a combination of fluoxetine and 5-HTP lowered IL-6. None of the medications lowered TNF-α. They speculated that the therapeutic activity of antidepressants is at least partly due to their impact on IL-6. They also found that tricyclic antidepressants, SSRIs, serotonin norepinephrine reuptake inhibitors, and 5-HTP, all downregulated the immunoregulatory system by suppressing the IFN-γ/IL-10 production ratio (Kubera, *et al.*, 2001).

In a review of the literature, O'Brien and colleagues (2004) noted that antidepressants have immunoregulatory effects, particularly by increasing production of IL-10, an anti-inflammatory cytokine. They proposed that future antidepressants target immunoparameters by either blocking the actions of pro-inflammatory cytokines or increasing the production of anti-inflammatory cytokines.

In summary, several recent studies have demonstrated that antidepressants have action beyond their impact on the monoamine neurotransmitters. They downregulate inflammation and at least part of their efficacy is likely to be due to their immunoregulatory effects.

## Phases of depression management with medication

In this final section, the phases of depression management with medication are described. Management of depression with medication has three main phases: acute, continuation, and maintenance (Lesperance and Frasure-Smith, 2000; Preston and Johnson, 2009). Knowing about the phases of management can help you communicate a treatment plan more effectively with mothers on medications.

Before medication starts, mothers and their doctors should observe the infant for alertness, activity, sleep, and feeding patterns. Wisner, *et al.* (1996) also advise that serum levels of infants younger than ten weeks be measured once mothers have settled on their minimum effective dose. In infants older than ten weeks, the serum levels should be measured only if there are behavior changes from baseline. Wisner and colleagues (1996) recommended charting any discussion of medications with mothers, as well as discussions about weaning, attempting non-drug treatments, and the mother's competence to consent to treatment.

### *Acute phase*

The acute phase occurs during the first six to twelve weeks of the depressive episode. It begins with the first dose and lasts until the patient is asymptomatic (Preston and Johnson, 2009). The objectives during this stage are to rapidly reduce symptoms of depression, and to monitor patients for the risk of suicide. It is important to evaluate whether the antidepressant you prescribed is effective. If it is not, there are two possible explanations that may account for the effect: the dose is inadequate, or treatment has not been sufficiently lengthy for an adequate response (Institute for Clinical Systems Improvement, 2000; Preston and Johnson, 2009). Assessments should include an evaluation of symptoms, work or school productivity, and whether interpersonal relationships have improved.

In this phase, it is also important to talk to patients about what they should expect from medications. Patients who are adequately educated are more likely to comply with treatments when they understand side effects, and have realistic expectations about what medications will do. Preston and Johnson (2009) recommend that the following information be given as part of educating patients about medication use.

1   Medications may take 10 to 21 days before patients notice a difference in symptoms.
2   When symptoms do improve, it is likely that they will be the ones with a biological basis, such as sleep disturbance. Medication may not help with more psychologically based symptoms, such as self-esteem.
3   Treatment is working when patients are sleeping better, have less daytime fatigue, and have some improvement in emotional control.
4   There may be side effects, but these can be managed.
5   The total length of time to be on antidepressants varies for each individual.
6   Antidepressants are not addictive.

### Continuation phase

The continuation phase lasts from four to nine months. The objective during this phase is to prevent a relapse of symptoms, which can occur if treatment is terminated during this time (Lesperance and Frasure-Smith, 2000). If symptoms have not improved, or if the patient has relapsed, it is appropriate to re-evaluate both the diagnosis and patient compliance. Are there co-morbid conditions (especially substance abuse) that are keeping treatments from being effective? Is the medication effective for the patient or should another be tried? Is the patient complying with treatment and taking the medications at the appropriate intervals?

A larger dose may be needed in some cases, or the patient may need to be on the medication for a longer period of time. Preston and Johnson (2009) noted that the most common mistake that family physicians make is to under-medicate their depressed patients. This is also true for patients with anxiety, who often require substantially higher dose for symptoms to remit. Generally, the length of an adequate trial is four to six weeks. If the medication is not effective after that time, another medication should be considered, or an additional medication could be added to the regimen (Institute for Clinical Systems Improvement, 2000).

### Maintenance phase

This phase should be initiated for patients who have had multiple episodes of depression or who have particularly severe or difficult-to-treat episodes and are therefore at high risk of recurrence. This phase may be for life in some patients, particularly those who have had three or more episodes of major depression.

## Conclusions

Conventional antidepressants are an important part of the treatment arsenal for women with postpartum depression and related conditions. These medications can treat even severe depression, and all but one type are compatible with breastfeeding. They can be combined with other modalities (except for St. John's wort) described in the previous chapters to give mothers additional tools to reduce inflammation, improve their sleep, cope with future life stresses, and increase their sense of competence and self-efficacy.

# 14 Postpartum depression and psychosis

## One woman's story

When I was working on the first edition of this book, a young woman named Jenny contacted me. She told me that she had suffered from postpartum depression and psychosis in the recent past, and was anxious to share her story for the benefit of other mothers. What made Jenny's story unique was that she had kept a diary before and during her experience, and as she recovered.

She has shared her diary with me, as well as the medical records from the state hospital. They provide a fascinating glimpse inside postpartum mental illness. This story was so compelling, I wanted to include it in this edition as well.

When preparing to write *Depression in New Mothers*, I contacted Jenny again. Eleven years had elapsed since our first contact. During that time, she has had four more children with no recurrence of postpartum psychosis or depression. She has also published her own full-length account of her experiences. In preparation for this volume, Jenny provided a brief update of her life today.

## Background

Jenny relates her illness to a number of different factors. She feels she was vulnerable to postpartum illness because of her health history and her life-long struggle with severe allergies. In addition to her health history, she experienced a series of stressors in both the pre- and postpartum periods, which are described below. In the years that have elapsed since our first contact, she has also recovered memories of two previous sexual assaults: one during childhood, the second during her hospitalization. She has added this information to her account.

Jenny was 20 years old when she had her first child. Her marriage and the birth of her daughter within less than a year constituted two major life changes within a relatively short span of time. Nevertheless, she was happy with her new life and joyfully celebrated the birth of her first child. She was also buffered from the potential negative effects of these stressors by a large and supportive family, a close relationship with her parents, and strong religious faith.

> Michelle H. was born exactly 76 hours ago. December 1, 1988 at 10:44 p.m. This will be a landmark day in my life. I was so overjoyed and emotionally ready for her to be here, and now she's here. [My husband], Mom, Dad, and my sister and her husband were all there. It was an awesome moment.

As thrilled as she was with the birth of her daughter, her birth experience was stressful. Jenny does not feel that it was the sole or even main cause of her illness. Rather, it was the first link in a chain of events that led to her illness.

## The birth experience

Jenny was very involved in the care she received during her pregnancy. Before the baby was born, she carefully prepared herself for labor and delivery, read extensively, exercised, and did yoga. Three weeks before her due date, she read two books on the Bradley method of natural childbirth. While she had always wanted to have natural childbirth, these were the first books she had read that articulated what she wanted. Unfortunately, the hospital where she was to deliver specialized in high-risk patients and tended to intervene frequently, even in routine births – the hospital's rate of cesarean births was an alarming 50%. Since it was so close to her due date, she had no choice but to proceed with her doctor and the hospital. Even after making the decision to proceed, she knew it would be difficult to have a natural delivery in that setting.

> My alarm grew as the week progressed. [My husband] and I went on a tour of [the hospital] and I freaked out. I had done everything backwards. I chose my doctor then the hospital, then three weeks before giving birth, I discovered the method I wanted to use. Not exactly ideal. According to Bradley, you choose the facility, then the doctor and you know the method before you get pregnant. Anyway, the past four weeks have been hell as I've tried to convince [my husband], my doctor, my mom, and mostly myself that this was the method I wanted to use. At one point, I seriously considered changing doctor/hospital but we recognized that most doctors won't take on a patient this late in the game.
>
> Knowing I'd have a fight on my hands, I read the Bradley Method three times to fully acquaint myself with the techniques (all relaxation, deep breathing, concentration) and all the arguments for not having "procedures" done at the hospital, to me or the baby.

During her lengthy labor (more than 24 hours), one of the more negative aspects was the way she describes being treated by the hospital staff. At one point, she was alone in a hospital room on a table. She had only a sheet over her, and she was very cold. An intern, who was apparently inexperienced, came in and gave her a rough and lengthy examination. Another doctor examined her, then the intern and the other doctor discussed Jenny's progress with each other in front of her.

> Then I began having a hard contraction. She [the second doctor] put her hands on my abdomen and instructed the intern to do likewise. They both were pushing and poking. I about lost control. I realized that he was the teachee and she was the teacher and I was the guinea pig. When my contraction was over I said "don't ever touch me while I'm having a contraction again."

At this point, Jenny asked to see her husband who had been outside the room talking to her doctor on the telephone.

> When I saw him [her husband] I almost started to cry. I had asked three nurses for a blanket because I was frozen. I was cold, hurting and those dumb doctors had been using my laboring body to teach each other what a contraction should feel like.

At this point, Jenny and her husband were given the option of going home, walking, or being admitted to a labor room. She could not be admitted to the birthing room, as she requested, because she was only 2 to 3 cm dilated. They decided to go home. The Bradley method states that solitude, quiet, physical comfort, and physical relaxation are essential for the laboring woman. During the hours at the hospital, none of these were available. She labored at home for the next few hours and started to make progress. She arrived at the hospital again, hoping to go directly to the birthing room after being checked at her doctor's office.

> When we arrived at the hospital, I was cold, tense, and nervous that I would get a lot of crap from the hospital staff. I sat in a wheelchair during nine contractions. As usual, they had miscommunicated the doctor's request for me. One nurse said I had to go to triage to "get checked." Another said I couldn't drink anything when she saw me take a sip of Vernors pop. Another said the birthing room wasn't prepped. (We had called half an hour before from the clinic to tell them we were on our way.) No time to prep? Bull! I sat in that wheelchair getting madder and madder. Finally, I asked the admitting nurse if I could go labor in a labor bed until I was ready because I was having a hard time controlling my contractions. She called the birthing room to ask. They said "No, we're just about done." I had two more contractions while they finished. I was almost crying by now. I kept thinking of how wonderful I had felt at home, the contractions didn't even hurt while I was in the shower with the hot air [sic] beating on my back.

She sat in the lobby of the hospital in a wheelchair for 30 minutes while in active labor. Once she got into the birthing room, she continued to have trouble with the hospital staff over the issue of continuous fetal monitoring. Prior to coming back to the hospital, her doctor had agreed to intermittent fetal monitoring (ten minutes every hour), but the nurses kept insisting that she have continuous fetal monitoring. At one point, they even threatened to make her leave if she did not comply. When she was five centimeters dilated, her doctor ruptured her membranes. Three hours later her daughter was born. In spite of the difficulties, it was a joyous occasion.

## The postpartum period

Approximately eight weeks after her daughter was born, Jenny and her husband moved to another state. This pulled Jenny away from her support network, including her close-knit family. During this time, her husband's back went out, adding to the stress of their move, as he was unable to help with either childcare or the move. Nevertheless, Jenny was happy in her new role and enjoyed their new home.

> It's so wonderful to be a mother. I've dreamed and planned to be one all my life. She [her daughter] is everything to me, besides [her husband], and I would die for her. She's pretty and personable and I'm flattered that she wants to be with me most. It makes me feel good to see that satisfied look on her little face when she's done eating and I love to think that her little body is receiving nourishment and growth from my body.

Within approximately six weeks of their move to another state, Jenny developed postpartum psychosis. During the weeks prior to her psychosis, she had read a book about allergies that listed a number of food and environmental allergens. This book recommended a five-day fast as a way of locating allergy-producing substances. Having suffered from allergies all her life, she took this very seriously. She started to fast, even though she was breastfeeding, in an attempt to locate the foods and substances that caused allergic reactions. She was also getting fewer and fewer hours of sleep each night, insisting she could handle everything. As the days went by, she became increasingly manic. In this state, she took everything to its extreme, including trying to purify her body and her household environment by getting rid of all plastic and turning off her heat because there was a natural gas leak in her home. Here is her retrospective description of what happened to her. She wrote this account shortly after she was released from the psychiatric hospital.

> It started slowly, then built to a peak. I became paranoid about being clean, purity, being perfect. I wanted to be a savior: save the town, the ward, the state, everyone. I wanted the millennium to start. I wanted to go to the temple to see Christ face to face. I wanted to live the word of wisdom perfectly. I cut out sugar, chocolate, meat and ate only whole organic foods. I fasted. [My baby] looked hungry when my mom arrived. I kept freaking out, thinking [my husband] was going to die, someone was going to kill me, steal [my baby], etc. It was hell!
>
> I sang hymns all the time to ward off evil thoughts and spirits. I ran to Main street, staying in the light, cast Satan out of [town], took my clothes off to my garments, sat down in the Lotus position looking at the sun, and waited. A police woman came up and tried to talk to me. She called [my husband]. He came and tried to get me to come home. They threw me in the ambulance and I came to. I put on my clothes, declared I was fine, and did my banking. [My husband] flipped out. He called the bishop, and my parents. I asked my mom to come down.

Her parents and husband took her to the hospital where she had delivered, but she refused to check herself in. From there, she went to the state hospital for nine days in her parents' state, then a private hospital for nine days, then back to the state hospital for six days, and finally back to the private hospital for two weeks. After her release, she convalesced at her parents' home for one month before returning home with her husband.

## The hospital diary

The next section of Jenny's story is taken from the diary she kept while in the state and private mental hospitals (the first time at each one). She wrote this account while she was hospitalized for postpartum psychosis. Much of the journal is dedicated to trying to make sense of what had happened to her. The following are excerpts from her diary.

> *March 29, 1989* This is going to be the most important journal I've ever kept. I'm in a mental hospital. [name of state hospital] On Friday, I'm moving to a new hospital. [name of private hospital]. I'm confused though. Talking helps. I'm hoping this journal will help. I asked mom to bring it to me. Everyone here is very nice. They are all trying to help me get better.

> *March 30, 1989, 7:19 a.m.* I woke up this morning and my breasts were aching (forced weaning). I asked the nurse for some Tylenol. She brought me some and I feel better. I exercised, prayed, watched the news, ate a banana that Mom gave me yesterday (day before yesterday), and I feel good. I cried this morning because I miss [my baby]. I want to nurse her so bad but I've accepted that I won't be able to ever again – that hurts. I loved to think that it was my body that helped to make her grow. What a lift! But I can deal with it. I miss her smilin' face.

*7:43 a.m.* I've been thinking of an analogy to what has happened. It goes like this. Imagine yourself getting kicked in the head. But there is no tissue damage, no blood, no bruise, only your brain has been hurt. The hurt is very bad and you try to make it better but don't know what to do. You scream and cry and try to hurt yourself. You act totally irrational. As time goes by, the hurt starts to heal, somehow. The cells repair themselves (analogy), the tissue rebuilds, all that is really needed is some time, rest, good food, a listening ear and a notebook with a pen. The memory comes back and with it dark images, so evil, and bad that you cry, but also light, God, hope, love and peace. These images fight each other for space in your conscious [sic]. As time goes by, the light is the one that prevails and sanity or at least peace is restored. The dark images return sometimes to scare and frighten but eventually the light prevails and everything is OK. Now, I just need time to understand why and sort things out. It hurts to think I went through so much. Sometimes I'm embarrassed by my behavior. I want to crawl under a rock. But I'm also relieved because so much that was unexplainable is now understood.

I'm still not myself. I have so many questions. And every time I ask one of the patients, they either look at me crazy or they give me their philosophy on life. The nurses try to answer my questions, but they are very busy and the doctors are great but they have even less time and many demands. It's OK, Mom said [private hospital] will be much better and they'll answer my questions and clear up any confusions. I can't wait to go. I just know it's got to be better than this place. I don't hate it here, but I can see that it's holding me back from getting better.

*8:55 a.m.* I can't help having the feeling that the nurses and everyone keep lying to me and there is some major plot against me. They tell me one thing, then do another. They told me the gynecologist would be here at 8:30. Well, it's long past. They don't understand that to me a minute is like an hour and a day is like a month. Even five minutes seems like a year. Time is relative I know, but I wish they would tell the truth. I'm so confused as it is.

I wish they'd come soon. I don't want them to take any blood. I hope they don't. I really am afraid to go see these doctors. I don't know them and they are going to touch the most private parts of my body. I usually don't have a problem with this, but now I'm scared. It's weird how you can change so quickly. I still am confused. I want answers NOW!!

*12:10 p.m.* I finally saw the doctors at 9:30 a.m. It's so hard to wait! They were cool. Wanted to take some blood but I said "no." Wanted to do a pelvic, I said "no way." I'm feeling too vulnerable right now. I need some time before they do these things again. I still think I'm going to refuse drugs at any cost. I'm having a hard enough time getting control and I really think what I need is some sleep.

I would say 95% of this problem is physical. The doctors and everyone keep talking about "chemical" but I think sleep deprivation is a real disease and I haven't had "good" sleep in so long. And the food changes that I imposed upon myself were a large part of this too so I understand why – at least some of the whys, but I still have quite a few to figure out. I have a lot of questions, but each second something new comes to me. The greatest thing is the way [my husband] and the family are supporting me. They are the greatest in the world. They have been visiting, bringing me food, talking on the phone and in person. They don't realize how much that helps. For four days, I was in isolation. I didn't know where I was, what was going on or where any of my family were, and I was scared to death. So scared, hurt, afraid, lonely, I wanted to die, that was all that I wanted.

About 10 times during the isolation, I thought OK, this is it, here I go, and then something would happen and I would be released for another few minutes, hours, seconds until the next death wish came. It peaked on Saturday night when I wanted to die for the last time. My tongue was lolling around in my head, I was dazed and confused. I hurt all over, my body was convulsing but all I wanted to do was die. The doctor was truly hurting my arm with the I.V. and instead of dying, I fell asleep. It was so depressing. When I woke up on Easter Sunday, I couldn't understand why I was alive. I didn't know what Christ wanted me to do. I had done everything I could to purify my life and body and he still didn't want to see me face to face.

[After receiving a blessing that night from her father, the death wishes stopped.] Then I became suspicious of everyone. I thought they were trying to poison me with the food. I thought they were draculas taking my blood. I pulled out the I.V. and the catheter because I *knew* God wanted me to do it.

*March 31, 1989 8:00 a.m.* Today has finally arrived! I get to leave this pit of despair. Everyone is so pathetic here. I was *so* angry last night. I kept imagining doing terrible things. The thing is I'm a good person. I want to do what's right. I have a daughter who needs me, a husband who needs me, and I don't need to be in this shit-hole prison. So why the hell am I here?????? I didn't commit any crime and I practically have to ask permission to pee. They try to poison me with this shit they call food and surround me with so much smoke it's like a bar. I hate it here. I keep seeing myself in [town name], singing hymns, and casting out Satan. The policewoman came up to me and asked me to get dressed. Poor lady. As I was sitting there in the full Lotus position with my hands in the symbol of knowledge pose, all I can remember is this guy walking by and saying to her, "This isn't exactly Mr. Rodger's neighborhood, is it?" And me, wanting to laugh but knowing I couldn't because it was too solemn a moment, and Satan would get my soul if I moved before [my husband] got there. Then he arrived and said, "Jenn, you've gotta come home," and I did, but I was very sick.

At this point, she was transferred to the private mental hospital. The following are excerpts taken from her diary written at that time.

*March 31, 5:00 p.m.* I'm finally here. It's nice. I'm exhausted. The orientation helped. I have so many questions but mostly I want to rest. I feel nervous, tense, overwhelmed. I had an in-tense [sic] evaluation, a medical check-up, an evaluation with a shrink (he was nice, not Dr. S., but a good guy).

*April "Fools" Day, 1989.* Just met with Dr. S. He's an ass. Really. Wants me to take drugs. I just kept saying "nope." He can't force me unless I have another psychotic episode. I'm going to do everything I can to avoid that. But I *refuse* to fall into their mode of medicate, medicate, medicate. All I need is some sleep, some good food, and a chance to get my wits about me. He kept tryin' to say I needed drugs. He doesn't know a damn thing about me except that I did some outrageous things out of the norm.

I'm not just going to roll with it folks. I'm going to fight them every step of the way and I'm going to question everything. Sorry if that's in-con-VIEN-ient, but it's the way it goes. I'm going to get along with everyone and get the hell out of here.

*Later.* This place is awful. What I was just thinking is if it is such a great place and does so much good, why the hell has my roommate been here *six* times? ... She is *so* doped up and screwed in the head by all the probing, searching to find out why, that I think she's on the verge of suicide. Well, she told me she was. Everyone here seems doped up, suicidal and depressed.

I think this *all* could have been avoided *if* Mom and Dad had taken me home, put me to bed and let me sleep it off. But I was in a psychotic state when they showed up and I know they were scared by my behavior. So, like everyone else, take her to DRS. GOD. *They* will make everything better. Bullshit! All they did was scare the shit out of me and isolate me from my family.

This place is the same. They have buckets of pills, lots of analysis and isolation. *Most* of the people here need these things because they are suicidal. I am *not* suicidal. I'm just a tired Mom who was put in a situation [new home town] that was hard to handle and freaked out. I had too too too much pressure. No sleep (for a month) and I changed my eating habits. Those things plus all the pressure of the move, my callings, [my husband's] calling, Bradley Method of childbirth classes, fear of Satanism in [new town], pressure to be the best wife, best mother, best friend, best ward member, best sister, best daughter, best actress, best children's theater director, best temple-goer, cleanest house, cleanest healthiest body, cleanest healthiest well-behaved baby, best body, best reader, best student, best sister-in-law, best daughter-in-law, best gardener, best reader, most intelligent church-goer, best talker, best listener, best EVERYTHING, was *too* much. I need a vacation. That's what [hospital] is to me. I'm going to sleep, read, eat, and write – journal, letters, and I'm not going to listen to my doctor too much.

I'm very suspicious of a doctor who doesn't even know me coming in and telling me I "need" drugs to make me "feel good." Sorry, that just doesn't cut it. If he said "you have an infection, I want you to help it get better," I'd take them. But I *don't* believe in "feel good" drugs and dammit *nobody* is going to make me take them. I'm not going to become one of "these" zombies who walk around pretending everything is fine. I know that I have a problem. I want to know what caused it, what I can do to avoid it in the future, and how I can get better.

*April 1st, 7:40 p.m.* Well it's been a helluva day. I've been harassed by just about every-body to take the drugs (yes, including [my husband] and Mom). [After a discussion with her doctor] he began pushing the drugs earnestly. He even tried to "bargain" with me. "I'll let you see your baby if you take the medicine." Nope. Those types of statements make me so curious to know *why* he feels the drugs are so important. I am *convinced* that the psychosis I experienced in [state name] was worst when I had no sleep, was eating little or fasting and when I was really tired. Nobody else seems to be ... I admit I have a problem. I want to get better and I want to know why but I *have* to do it *my* way. This is just like the birth. Hopefully, they'll understand.

## The psychiatric evaluation

During the time that this diary was written, the doctors at the mental hospitals were keeping their own records. The following are excerpts from these records that describe Jenny's illness from the medical perspective. The first entries were made at the time Jenny was discharged from the state hospital to the private hospital. Below are excerpts from the "combined psychiatric examination and summary note."

## Mental status

This is a 21-year-old, white female who appears to be her stated age. She is of moderate build. The patient is very agitated and disoriented. Her affect is blunted. Her mood went from hostile to tearful and scared. The patient denied being depressed but stated that she was very tired. The patient denied any suicidal or homicidal thoughts. She was preoccupied with religious grandiose delusions, stating "I was chosen by Jesus to fill a mission on this earth. I don't need a doctor. Jesus will heal me. I will fast until he comes to heal me." The patient is oriented to person and time. The patient seems to be confused regarding the events of the last four or five days. The patient's long-term memory appears to be intact. Her judgment and insight are poor.

## Clinical course and treatment in the hospital

The patient was admitted on 3/23/89 from [other hospital] on a Medical Certificate. The patient was admitted with four-point restraints due to her being uncooperative to admission procedures. She was nonverbal and her behavior was unpredictable. The patient was put into seclusion. She was refusing meals and drank five, eight-ounce glasses of water. On 3/24/89 the patient remained in seclusion. She was very agitated and delusional. She received 2.5 mg of Haldol and refused to talk to the doctor and refused to take a shower or use the bathroom. On 3/25/89, the patient continued to be hostile, refused to put clothes on, or to eat or drink. The patient voided on the floor, refusing to use the bathroom. Haldol was given to the patient. She received Benadryl 25 mg due to a dystonic reaction from Haldol. The patient continued to refuse fluids and was transferred to [other facility] to monitor input and output and dehydration. The patient had IV and Foley catheter. She was placed in four-point restraints due to her kicking the staff and not keeping her clothes on. On 3/26/89, the patient continued to refuse fluids or food. On 3/27/89, she was up and responding to verbal questioning. The patient cleaned herself up. While in the bathroom, the patient pulled out the IV and Foley. The patient began drinking fluids and her mother brought food from home. She began to eat the food brought from home well. The patient was transferred back to Receiving C. The patient became oriented and began to remember what had been happening in the last week. From 3/28/89 to 3/30/89, the patient continued to be cooperative, discussed stressors, and discussed mental illness. Arrangements were made to transfer the patient to [private hospital]. On 3/31/89, the patient was transferred to [private hospital] for continued hospitalization.

This next section is taken from the "psychosocial history." The informants were Jenny's husband and her parents. Jenny was not interviewed herself "due to her extreme psychosis."

According to the informants, the patient found her natural childbirth experience frustrating due to her unrealistic expectations. The method that the patient chose conflicted with the standard hospital fetal monitoring techniques. This created numerous conflicts for the patient throughout the labor and delivery. Consequently, the patient left the hospital twelve hours after the birth, with the baby. The family indicated that the patient and her child were released appropriately, even though the physician recommended that they stay an additional one or two more days. The patient and the child were released under the care of the patient's mother, who provided the patient with rest and helped in caring for the newborn.

This is the patient's first psychiatric hospitalization. The onset was sudden, with a direct connection to the recent birth of her daughter. According to the informants, throughout the delivery of the child, the patient was hostile and suspicious of physicians. The patient had opted for a particular type of natural childbirth, three weeks prior to the birth of the baby. She discussed this with her obstetrician, who did not prepare her for certain discrepancies between hospital policy and the method of natural childbirth. The informants report that, even after the birth, the patient sustained her hostile and angry feelings.

The informants report that the symptoms escalated when the patient and her husband moved to [new state] in February of 1989. The husband hurt his back and could not help with the move and/or childcare. Therefore, the patient was left to cope with a new living situation in a new city, care of a newborn infant, and her first experience in moving away from her family. The family reported that the patient made statements to the effect that she could do it all, and did not need to eat or sleep, and that she was a very strong person. Resultant to this situation, the patient began to distort and exaggerate her religious philosophies and books that she was reading, interpreting these as "special messages from God." The patient began to make statements that she had heard the voice of God and began exhibiting confused behaviors. She would stare at the sun, believing that she was getting certain communications from God.

She read a book about allergies, and based upon certain chapters of this book, she threw out all of the plastic in the home, including the baby's bassinet, cleaning supplies, and turned off the heat. Because the baby had no place of its own to sleep, the child then slept with the patient and her husband, significantly interrupting the patient's sleep pattern to the extent that she did not sleep for several days. Also, based upon her reading, she refused to eat or drink anything but spring water. She has lost 20 pounds in three weeks. The patient sang religious hymns repetitively and was found on a public street in her underwear, staring at the sun. At this time, three days prior to her admission, the husband returned to [home state] with the patient and his daughter in order to seek the support of the patient's parents and assistance in obtaining mental health services.

After going to the private hospital, Jenny was sent back to the state hospital for her "uncooperative attitude" regarding the administration of medications. These next excerpts are from the discharge summary from her second stay at the state hospital. It is during these six days that she went to court to try to avoid having to take anti-psychotic medications.

## Reason for admission

This 21-year-old, white female was admitted on a Medical Certificate. She was transferred from [private hospital] because of her uncooperative behavior with the treatment. She was refusing to have any lab work done or comply with any medication. Before she was at [private hospital] she was at [state hospital]. Although she did go for a hearing and agreed to treatment, she did not cooperate when she went to [private hospital]. She has been for treatment. She has been having delusions.

## Clinical course

The patient stayed on the Fourth Level until 4/18/89. She remained very uncooperative and guarded and paranoid. She was very much suspicious. She was very negative and was not responding to any questions. She was observed to be singing in the hallways and humming. She did not understand the need for treatment. She was approached for the physical examination and for the psychiatric evaluation almost every day. She did not cooperate very much except for the last few days. She was much more cooperative and did give some information. She provided that she had been acting very manic and hyperactive in the past. She agreed that she was doing some bizarre things. She has been scared and afraid and paranoid. Through the counseling she was willing to go to the private hospital and get treatment.

The next section is from the psychosocial history. The informants for this report are Jenny's parents. There is a great deal of overlap with the history reported at the time of first discharge. There are also some differences, which provide additional information about her illness.

The patient is described as tending to be enthusiastic, generally does well at most things she attempts but tends to be "hard on herself if she finds herself falling short of her own expectations." She's considered to be very bright and creative, theatrically inclined and artistic. She enjoys being involved but tends to be very strong willed "not shy about expressing her opinions."

Although the family sees her emotional problems as starting on the day of daughter's delivery, the patient's obstetrician indicated that he thought he noticed manic symptoms approximately three weeks previously [Note: he did not note these symptoms in her medical records, however]. The patient had planned on natural childbirth at [hospital name], in the birthing room, but at the time of the delivery became very angry when her doctor broke her waters and insisted on exercising certain hospital procedures which she objected to. She also was angry with her parents and husband for not backing her up, at the time of the birth there were five family members in the birthing room. The parents indicate that the patient was somewhat obsessed with having natural childbirth and that some of her expectations were unrealistic. The mother feels that she was not psychotic at the time of the birth, but did become so following her move to [another state]. The patient became even more inclined to believe what she read in various books, particularly being obsessed with a book on allergy, to the point she ran up considerable phone bills telling people to read the book then went on a three-day fast, while nursing her baby. She started perceiving her husband as being evil and unclean because he works with computers and was not sympathetic to her expectations. It appears that her husband expressed some regrets at the idea of "never having a Big Mac or chocolate chip cookies again." She allegedly would not let her husband in the house on their anniversary because "God told me not to let you in." In several phone calls to her mother she said, "Satan is causing it."

## Analysis

The author of the psychosocial report apparently recognized that Jenny's illness had multiple causes. The report specifically mentions fatigue that was aggravated by and related to her mania, problems with social support brought on by her move to another state, and high expectations for herself as a wife and mother (wanting to be the best at everything). Fasting may have resulted in a metabolic imbalance that in combination with other factors, triggered the psychosis. The lack of social support in the new town may have also allowed her illness to progress as far as it did.

What is particularly interesting is the apparent lack of understanding about the role of

Jenny's birth experience in her illness by both her family and the people treating her. They viewed her expectations as "unrealistic." According to Jenny, clinicians at the state hospital tended to focus on her birth experience in some cases to the exclusion of all the other underlying factors. They focused on it while dismissing her feelings about it, as if naming her expectations as "unrealistic" would make her sense of disappointment and anger disappear. These issues and her perceptions of these events were important to her, however. Ironically, had her feelings been validated and had she been allowed to express them, her feelings of anger and disappointment could have dissipated. As it was, they continued to exert an influence.

## 2003 update: Information on past sexual abuse

In 2001, four days after the death of Jenny's older brother, she started to have memories of being sexually abused as a baby. These memories were accompanied by a variety of sensations and feelings. She was re-hospitalized in the summer of 2001 for a weekend of care for suicidal and homicidal feelings towards her perpetrator. During this time, she also had memories of being raped while in the state mental hospital on the first night of her arrival. She remembers being orally and vaginally assaulted by four orderlies while in four-point restraints, then taken to a seclusion room where she was thrown naked onto a mat. She has no evidence for these experiences except her memories, and the fact that she developed oral herpes simplex II a few months after being released from the hospital. These assaults in the state hospital could explain her additional paranoia and fear while she was being treated. It also helps to explain her desire for death as well as periods of blackout/amnesia during certain points of her hospitalization.

## The road to recovery

Jenny's recovery from her postpartum illness was a lengthy process. After her first stay in the private mental hospital, she was transferred back to the state hospital for six days. During this time, she went to court in order to avoid taking anti-psychotic medication. The account of her continuing recovery is taken from an interview conducted for the first edition of this book.

> During the six days back in the state mental hospital, I was literally a prisoner until I went to court. I had no friends, except for the other patients. Everyone was pressuring me. I called TV stations and reporters. One reporter was very supportive and wrote an article on postpartum depression. While I was there, I was crazy. I'd sing patriotic songs and talk about my rights. During that time I was totally confused. I demanded a jury trial, which was my right. But they treated it like a joke. I wasn't a zombie.
>
> My sentence was 90 days, forced medications if necessary. When I heard that, my heart literally broke. I couldn't fight it anymore. Back at the hospital, my mom yelled at me for three hours. She said that I had to take the drugs and come home and take care of my baby. I finally couldn't fight anymore.
>
> I went back to the private hospital and started on Lithium and Stelazine. I started to self-destruct and overeat. They told me it would "fix" the chemical imbalance in my brain. I didn't know it [Stelazine] was a tranquilizer. When I started on the drugs, I was confused, couldn't finish a thought, tired (I slept 16–20 hours a day), and depressed. The drugs worked though. They stopped the mania and racing thoughts. I'm not against drugs, only the improper use of drugs. Once I complied, I could do what I wanted. I was totally cooperative and even warm to my doctor, doing everything he said.

After two weeks in the private hospital, she was released and stayed for five weeks at her parents' home. She then went home to her husband.

> A big part of my recovery was going home to [new state] and facing my demons. I was worried about having no friends, about isolation. It was important to face what I was frightened of and being forced to be a mom again.

In order to help her recover, she took her medications faithfully. She also began to put on weight and gained 50 pounds during that time. She started having severe PMS after coming home from the hospital. One psychiatrist told her she'd be on Lithium for the rest of her life. That news was devastating. She called Depression After Delivery (DAD) and got a referral for a new psychiatrist. She went on progesterone, which helped with her PMS, and stopped Lithium, but she was still on Stelazine. She started on Prozac and got really depressed. She was hospitalized again, and was suicidal. Another doctor took her off Stelazine, which helped, and doubled her dosage of Prozac.

She identified several activities as helping her to recover. She started a support group for postpartum depression, was a DAD phone volunteer, and became a Bradley childbirth educator. "That was really important. Being around these happy couples who accepted me as a normal person." She had one 20-minute flashback about a year after her release from the hospital. "That was scary. I thought I had beaten it. I didn't go on Lithium or back in the hospital. It helped not to emphasize it." A pivotal moment came when she read an article in *Newsweek* about Prozac. It was then that she decided to try to wean herself away from the medications.

> During that time, I was having highs and lows; really manic. I started looking for alternatives. During this time, I was obsessed with getting pregnant again to show I could do it right. I prayed. I discovered homeopathic [sic], which cleanses the body. I discovered Chinese herbs. I feel this was from the Lord. Otherwise, I'd be on antidepressants again. It really helped. Going off of the drugs was like detox. I cried for a whole week. I think all the suppressed emotions of the last year came out.
>
> I went through all the stages of grief, especially grief itself. It was so healing to have this time. I gained an additional 50 pounds. I didn't understand. I couldn't figure out what was happening until I read a book on detox – this is part of it. I still had severe PMS. I became a hermit. I was still obsessed with becoming pregnant, and I was somewhat depressed. Spiritually, I was completely depressed – I didn't want to talk to God. But it was a healing time, a happy time. I started to feel again. I could sing, feel joy, enjoy [my baby], my husband.
>
> In January, I began a weight loss program with Chinese herbs and lost 30 pounds. I've paid lots of attention to nutrition. I have a semi-vegetarian lifestyle. I eat organic foods and drink distilled water. I've had no drugs for over a year. I use homeopathics, do yoga, and exercise faithfully.

Jenny has identified six factors that helped her heal. These included time to heal, the support of her husband, adequate nutrition (including fruits, vegetables, and dietary supplements), grieving over her lost time with her daughter, prayer of friends and family, and having another baby (thus moving on with her life).

Overall, Jenny is philosophical about her experience and feels that good has come of it. She summarized her feelings this way.

I don't regret that this happened. I don't feel bitter. I feel grateful to have had this experience. I didn't a year ago, but I do now. I feel empowered. Now I can empathize with other women, and I have placed myself in a key position to help other women. I don't know if I would have done this if I hadn't had this experience. I'd rather have had this experience than a normal easy birth. It uncluttered my life. It was the ultimate growth experience. I don't feel like I'm 23, I feel like I'm 50. I also feel that it was necessary. God allows things to happen to allow us to grow. Mental illness was not part of my plan, but it empowered me like nothing else could have to do what I needed to do.

## 2003 update

Jenny is now 35. In the past 12 years, she has given birth to four additional children. Recognizing postpartum as a vulnerable time, she and her husband have taken extreme measures to be sure that she gets her rest and is not unduly stressed after childbirth. She has not experienced a relapse of her psychosis, and has found alternatives to allopathic care.

## 2009 update

Jenny is now 41. As a loud blogging voice on the Internet, she feels passionate about mothers being given alternative options to allopathic drugs and hospitalizations when suffering from postpartum emotional distress. As a promoter of gentle home birth, she believes non-traumatic birth is the first step in preventing depression and psychosis. She successfully used the Ayurvedic Mother Baby postpartum program to help her heal after her fifth birth, and believes all women would be well served to research and use this healing modality to prevent postpartum mood disorders. Her books, columns, and insights can be found on the web at http://naturalfamilyco.com and http://naturalfamilyblog.com

# Epilog
## Some final thoughts

As you can see, there is much you can do to help mothers suffering from postpartum depression. In surveying the whole of working with new mothers, I have a few final suggestions to help you on your way.

### Listen to mothers

I always put this suggestion in for people like me. I'm a teacher, and I like to teach and tell people what I know. I have to remind myself to listen first. Just letting a mother tell her story can be therapeutic in and of itself. It will also allow you time to figure out what the mother's real concerns might be. Sometimes mothers know and can articulate what is bothering them. They just need someone to hear them, and validate what they are saying. Other mothers may not fully understand why they feel so bad. They just need to tell their story. I always know that I need to listen more when I start getting "Yeah, but …" in response to a suggestion. If we listen, and the mother feels we've truly heard her, she'll be more likely to follow our suggestions.

### Let mothers know about factors that might be influencing their emotional state

After listening carefully, then it is time to share what you know. Sometimes mothers really do not know why they feel bad. This can be true even years later. Dozens of times, I've been teaching a seminar and had participants come up and say that they never realized that a crying baby (or some other factor they identified with) could have caused their emotional distress. And these women are generally healthcare professionals with grown children. Having someone simply name the factors involved can be validating to mothers, and it lets them know that they are not the only ones who have experienced what they are going through.

### Offer specific suggestions that can help

Once you have narrowed down the cause (or causes) of a mother's distress, offer her some strategies to alleviate the problem. For example, if she is in pain, teach her some ways to alleviate it. If she is having breast pain, make an immediate referral to a lactation specialist to address the problem. If a mother is highly fatigued, brainstorm with her about how she can get more rest. Also be sure to rule out physical problems. If she has a baby with a difficult temperament, put her in contact with other mothers you know who have babies with this type of temperament.

## Help her mobilize her own support system, including offering referrals to people or organizations that can offer long-term support

Your role is pivotal in terms of helping mothers identify depression and referring them to the sources of help they need. But you cannot be a mother's long-term source of support. It's not practical, and in the long run, is not in the best interest of the mother. What you can do is help mothers find support among their own network, and in their communities.

One of the most helpful things you can do is give mothers "permission" to get help and support. So often, mothers labor under the belief that they must tough things out themselves. Over the years, I've had many mothers relate to me the apocryphal tale of the mother in the field who gives birth, and gets right back to work. Yes, unfortunately, this does happen – especially in impoverished communities. But it is far from ideal and, as I described in Chapter 9, does not happen in many of the non-Western cultures with low rates of depression. In fact, I've found that just telling mothers about what happens in these cultures that support new mothers can be very liberating, and encourages them to seek out support for themselves postpartum.

You might also have to refer mothers for other types of help. That means finding resources available in your community, and even online. These types of resource can include support groups on various topics (breastfeeding, depression, difficult birth, premature babies, child-bearing loss, mothering multiples, or single mothering). In rural communities, websites can be very helpful as specialized groups may not exist locally. Mothers may also need referrals for therapy and/or medications. Organizations such as Postpartum Support International keep a list of professionals who specialize in the needs of postpartum women. Your state psychological or medical association can also provide you names of professionals in your community who can help depressed mothers. You may want to speak with these individuals before referring mothers, however. Also, be sure to find out what their payment policy is – especially for your low-income mothers.

## Conclusions

Intervention with new mothers can make a significant difference in their lives, and in the lives of their families. In closing, I'd like to share the words of Salle Webber, a postpartum doula who understands the pivotal role you can have in young families.

> Incredible as it seems, our culture, with its emphasis on education, has left young adults entirely unprepared to face the practical realities of parenting. And this may be the most important job they will ever hold. So, for those of us who are comfortable and happy in the work of parenting, we can serve the future of humanity through our humble sharing of our skills and our love for children and families.
>
> (Webber, 1992: 17)

I wish you great success in this important work.

# References

Abdel-Salam, O. M. (2005). Anti-inflammatory, antinociceptive, and gastric effects of Hypericum perforatum in rats. *Scientific World Journal, 5*: 586–95.

Abraham, S., Taylor, A. and Conti, J. (2001). Postnatal depression, eating, exercise, and vomiting before and during pregnancy. *International Journal of Eating Disorders, 29*: 482–7.

Abramowitz, J., Moore, K., Carmin, C., Wiegartz, P. S. and Purdon, C. (2001). Acute onset of obsessive-compulsive disorder in males following childbirth. *Psychosomatics, 42*: 429–31.

Abramowitz, J. S., Schwartz, S. A., Moore, K. M. and Luenzmann, K. R. (2002). Obsessive-compulsive symptoms in pregnancy and the puerperium: A review of the literature. *Anxiety Disorders, 426*: 1–18.

Abramson, L. Y., Seligman, M. E. P. and Teasdale, J. D. (1978). Learned helplessness in humans: Critique and reformulation. *Journal of Abnormal Psychology, 87*: 49–74.

Affleck, G., Tennen, H., Rowe, J., Roscher, B. and Walker, L. (1989). Effects of formal support on mothers' adaptation to the hospital-to-home transition of high-risk infants: The benefits and costs of helping. *Child Development, 60*: 488–501.

Affonso, D. D., De, A. K., Horowitz, J. A. and Mayberry, L. J. (2000). An international study exploring levels of postpartum depressive symptomatology. *Journal of Psychosomatic Research, 49*: 207–16.

Agency for Healthcare Research and Quality (2002). *S-Adenosyl-L-Methionine for treatment of depression, osteoarthritis, and liver disease* (Evidence Report/Technology Assessment No. 64). Rockville, MD: U.S. Department of Health and Human Services.

Ahlborg, T. and Strandmark, M. (2006). Factors influencing the quality of intimate relationships six months after delivery: First-time parents' own views and coping strategies. *Journal of Psychosomatic Obstetrics & Gynecology, 27*(3): 163–72.

Ahmed, A., Stewart, D. E., Teng, L., Wahoush, O. and Gagnon, A. J. (2008). Experience of immigrant new mothers with symptoms of depression. *Archives of Women's Mental Health, 11*(4): 295–303.

Ahokas, A., Aito, M. and Rimon, R. (2000). Positive treatment effect of estradiol in postpartum psychosis: A pilot study. *Journal of Clinical Psychiatry, 61*: 166–9.

Ahokas, A., Kaukoranta, J., Wahlbeck, K. and Aito, M. (2001). Estrogen deficiency in severe postpartum depression: Successful treatment with sublingual physiologic 17β Estradiol: A preliminary study. *Journal of Clinical Psychiatry, 62*: 332–6.

AHRQ, *see* Agency for Healthcare Research and Quality.

Akman, I., Kuscu, K., Ozdemir, N., Yurdakul, Z., Solakoglu, M., Orhan L., *et al.* (2006). Mothers' postpartum psychological adjustment and infantile colic. *Archives of Diseases of Childhood, 91*: 417–19.

Akman, I., Kuscu, K., Yurdakul, Z., Ozdemir, N., Solakoglu, M., Orhon L., *et al.* (2008). Breastfeeding duration and postpartum psychological adjustments: Role of maternal attachment styles. *Journal of Paediatrics and Child Health, 44*: 369–73.

Alder, J., Stadlmayr, W., Tschudin, S. and Bitzer, J. (2006). Post-traumatic symptoms after childbirth: What should we offer? *Journal of Psychosomatic Obstetrics & Gynecology, 27*(2): 107–12.

Alexander, J. L. (2007). Quest for timely detection and treatment of women with depression. *Journal of Managed Care Pharmacy, 13*(9): S3–S11.

Altemus, M., Deuster, P. A., Galliven, E., Carter, C. S. and Gold, P. W. (1995). Suppression of the hypothalmic-pituitary-adrenal axis responses to stress in lactating women. *Journal of Clinical Endocrinology & Metabolism, 80*(10): 2954–9.

American Psychiatric Association. (2000). *Diagnostic and statistical manual of mental disorders*, 4th ed., text revision. Washington, DC: American Psychiatric Association.

Amir, L. H., Dennerstein, L., Garland, S. M., Fisher, J. and Farish, S. J. (1996). Psychological aspects of nipple pain in lactating women. *Journal of Psychosomatic Obstetrics and Gynecology, 17*: 53–8.

Amorin, A. R., Linne, Y. M. and Lourenco, P. M. (2007). Diet or exercise, or both, for weight reduction in women after childbirth. *Cochrane Database Systematic Review, July 18*.

Anderson, G. C. (1991). Current knowledge about skin-to-skin (Kangaroo) care for preterm infants. *Journal of Perinatology, XI*: 216–26.

Anderson, L. N., Campbell, M. K., daSilva, O., Freeman, T. and Xie, B. (2008). Effect of maternal depression and anxiety on use of health services for infants. *Canadian Family Physician, 54*: 1718–19.

Andreozzi, L., Flanagan, P., Seifer, R., Brunner, S. and Lester, B. (2002). Attachment classifications among 18-month-old children of adolescent mothers. *Archives of Pediatric and Adolescent Medicine, 156*: 20–6.

Anghelescu, I. G., Kohnen, R., Szegedi, A., Klement, S. and Kieser, M. (2006). Comparison of Hypericum extract WS 5570 and paroxetine in ongoing treatment after recovery from an episode of moderate to severe depression: Results from a randomized multicenter study. *Pharmacopsychiatry, 39*: 213–19.

Ansara, D., Cohen, M. M., Gallop, R., Kung, R., Kung, R. and Schei, B. (2005). Predictors of women's physical health problems after childbirth. *Journal of Psychosomatic Obstetrics & Gynecology, 26*: 115–25.

Antonuccio, D., Danton, W. G. and DeNelsky, G. Y. (1995). Psychotherapy versus medication for depression: Challenging the conventional wisdom with data. *Professional Psychology: Research and Practice, 26*: 574–85.

Appleby, L., Warner, R., Whitton, A. and Faragher, B. (1997). A controlled study of fluoxetine and cognitive-behavioral counseling in the treatment of postnatal depression. *British Medical Journal, 314*: 932–6.

Appleby, L., Mortensen, P. B. and Faragher, E. B. (1998). Suicide and other causes of mortality after postpartum psychiatric admission. *British Journal of Psychiatry, 173*: 209–11.

Ashman, S. B., Dawson, G., Panagiotides, H., Yamada, E. and Wilkins, C. W. (2002). Stress hormone levels of children of depressed mothers. *Development and Psychopathology, 14*: 333–49.

Astbury, J., Brown, S., Lumley, J. and Small, R. (1994). Birth events, birth experiences, and social differences in postnatal depression. *Australian Journal of Public Health, 18*: 176–84.

Ayers, S. and Pickering, A. D. (2001). Do women get posttraumatic stress disorder as a result of childbirth? A prospective study of incidence. *Birth, 28*: 111–18.

Ayers, S., Wright, R. and Wells, N. (2007). Symptoms of post-traumatic stress disorder in couples after birth: Association with the couple's relationship and parent-baby bond. *Journal of Reproductive and Infant Psychology, 25*(1): 40–50.

Babyak, M., Blumenthal, J. A., Herman, S., Khatri, P., Doraiswamy, M., Moore, K., Craighead, W. E., Baldewicz, T. T. and Krishnan, R. R. (2000). Exercise treatment for major depression: Maintenance of therapeutic benefit at 10 months. *Psychosomatic Medicine, 62*: 633–8.

Badenhorst, W., Riches, S., Turton, P. and Hughes, P. (2006). The psychological effects of stillbirth and neonatal death on fathers: Systematic review. *Journal of Psychosomatic Obstetrics & Gynecology, 27*(4): 245–56.

Balch, P. (2002). *Prescription for herbal healing*. New York: Avery.

Barr, J. A. and Beck, C. T. (2008). Infanticide secrets: Qualitative study on postpartum depression. *Canadian Family Physician, 54*: 1716–17.

Baxter, L. R., Schwartz, J. M., Bergman, K. S. and Szuba, M. P. (1992). Caudate glucose metabolic rate changes with both drug and behavioral therapy for obsessive-compulsive disorders. *Archives of General Psychiatry*, *49*: 681–9.

Beach, S. R. H., Smith, D. A. and Fincham, F. D. (1994). Marital interventions for depression: Empirical foundation and future prospects. *Applied and Preventive Psychology*, *3*: 233–50.

Beck, C. T. (1995). The effects of postpartum depression on maternal-infant interaction: A meta-analysis. *Nursing Research*, *44*: 298–304.

Beck, C. T. (1996a). Postpartum depressed mothers' experiences interacting with their children. *Nursing Research*, *45*: 98–104.

Beck, C. T. (1996b). A meta-analysis of the relationship between postpartum depression and infant temperament. *Nursing Research*, *45*: 225–30.

Beck, C. T. (2001). Predictors of postpartum depression: An update. *Nursing Research*, *50*: 275–85.

Beck, C. T. (2002). Postpartum depression: A metasynthesis. *Qualitative Health Research*, *12*: 453–72.

Beck, C. T. (2006). Postpartum depression: It isn't just the blues. *American Journal of Nursing*, *106*(5): 40–50.

Beck, C. T. (2009). An adult survivor of child sexual abuse and her breastfeeding experience: A case study. *American Journal of Maternal Child Nursing*, *34*(2): 91–7.

Beck, C. T. and Gable, R. K. (2000). Postpartum Depression Screening Scale: Development and psychometric testing. *Nursing Research*, *49*: 272–82.

Beck, C. T. and Gable, R. K. (2001a). Further validation of the Postpartum Depression Screening Scale. *Nursing Research*, *50*: 155–64.

Beck, C. T. and Gable, R. K. (2001b). Comparative analysis of the performance of the Postpartum Depression Screening Scale with two other depression instruments. *Nursing Research*, *50*: 242–50.

Beck, C. T., Froman, R. D. and Bernal, H. (2005). Acculturation level and postpartum depression in Hispanic mothers. *American Journal of Maternal Child Nursing*, *30*(5): 299–304.

Beeghly, M., Weinberg, M. K., Olson, K. L., Kernan, H., Riley, J. and Tronick, E. Z. (2002). Stability and change in level of maternal depressive symptomatology during the first postpartum year. *Journal of Affective Disorders*, *71*: 169–80.

Beilin, B., Shavit, Y., Trabekin, E., Mordashev, B., Mayburd, E., Zeidel A., *et al.* (2003). The effects of postoperative pain management on immune response to surgery. *Anesthesia & Analgesia*, *97*: 822–7.

Belizan, J. M., Althabe, F., Barros, F. C. and Alexander, S. (1999). Rates and implications of caesarean sections in Latin America: Ecological study. *British Medical Journal*, *319*: 1397–1402.

Benedict, M., Paine, L. and Paine, L. (1994). *Long-term effects of child sexual abuse on functioning in pregnancy and pregnancy outcome*. Final report, National Center on Child Abuse and Neglect. Washington, DC: National Center on Child Abuse and Neglect.

Bick, D. E., MacArthur, C. and Lancashire, R. J. (1998). What influences the uptake and early cessation of breastfeeding? *Midwifery*, *14*: 242–7.

Black, M. M., Papas, M. A., Hussey, J. M., Dubowitz, H., Kotch, J. B. and Starr, R. H., Jr. (2002). Behavior problems among preschool children born to adolescent mothers: Effects of maternal depression and perceptions of partner relationships. *Journal of Clinical Child and Adolescent Psychology*, *31*: 16–26.

Bladt, S. and Wagner, H. (1994). Inhibition of MAO by fractions and constituents of hypericum extract. *Journal of Geriatric Psychiatry and Neurology*, *7 (Supplement)*: S57–9.

Bloch, M., Schmidt, P. J., Danaceau, M., Murphy, J., Niemann, L. and Rubinow, D. R. (2000). Effects of gonadal steroids in women with a history of postpartum depression. *American Journal of Psychiatry*, *157*: 924–30.

Blumenthal, J. A., Babyak, M. A., Doraiswamy, P. M., Watkins, L., Hoffman, B. M., Barbour K. A., *et al.* (2007). Exercise and pharmacotherapy in the treatment of major depressive disorder. *Psychosomatic Medicine*, *69*: 587–96.

Blyton, D. M., Sullivan, C. E. and Edwards, N. (2002). Lactation is associated with an increase in slow-wave sleep in women. *Journal of Sleep Research, 11*: 297–303.

Bond, M. J., Prager, M. A., Tiggemann, M. and Tao, B. (2001). Infant crying, maternal well-being and perceptions of caregiving. *Journal of Applied Health Behavior, 3*: 3–9.

Bonomi, A. E., Cannon, E. A., Anderson, M. L. and Rivara, F. P. (2008). Association between self-reported health and physical and/or sexual abuse experienced before age 18. *Child Abuse & Neglect, 32*: 693–701.

Bowen, E., Heron, J., Waylen, A., Wolke, D. and Team, A. S. (2005). Domestic violence risk during and after pregnancy: Findings from a British longitudinal study. *British Journal of Obstetrics and Gynecology, 112*(8): 1083–9.

Boyce, P. and Condon, J. (2001). Providing good clinical care means listening to women's concerns. *British Medical Journal, 322*: 928.

Bozoky, I. and Corwin, E. J. (2002). Fatigue as a predictor of postpartum depression. *Journal of Gynecologic, Obstetric, and Neonatal Nursing, 31*: 436–43.

Bratman, S. and Girman, A. M. (2003). *Handbook of herbs and supplements and their therapeutic uses.* St Louis, MO: Mosby.

Brennan, P. A., Hammen, C., Anderson, M. J., Bor, W., Najman, J. M. and Williams, G. M. (2000). Chronicity, severity, and timing of maternal depressive symptoms: Relationships with child outcomes at age 5. *Developmental Psychology, 36*: 759–66.

Britton, J. R. (2007). Postpartum anxiety and breast feeding. *Journal of Reproductive Medicine, 52*(8): 689–95.

Brown, M-A., Goldstein-Shirley, J., Robinson, J. and Casey, S. (2001). The effects of multi-modal intervention trial on light, exercise, and vitamins on women's mood. *Women & Health, 34*: 93–112.

Brown, S. and Lumley, J. (1994). Satisfaction with care in labor and birth: A survey of 790 Australian women. *Birth, 21*(1): 4–13.

Bugental, D. B., Beaulieu, D., and Schwartz, A. (2008). Hormonal sensitivity of preterm versus full-term infants to the effects of maternal depression. *Infant Behavior and Development, 31*: 51–61.

Buist, A. and Janson, H. (2001). Childhood sexual abuse, parenting, and postpartum depression: A 3-year follow-up study. *Child Abuse & Neglect, 25*: 909–21.

Bullock, L. F., Libbus, M. K. and Sable, M. R. (2001). Battering and breastfeeding in a WIC population. *Canadian Journal of Nursing Research, 32*: 43–56.

Callahan, S., Sejourne, N. and Denis, A. (2006). Fatigue and breastfeeding: An inevitable partnership? *Journal of Human Lactation, 22*(2): 182–7.

Canivet, C., Jakobsson, I. and Hagander, B. (2002). Colicky infants according to maternal reports in telephone interviews and diaries: A large Scandinavian study. *Journal of Developmental and Behavioral Pediatrics, 23*: 1–8.

Capuzzi, C. (1989). Maternal attachment to handicapped infants and the relationship to social support. *Research in Nursing & Health, 12*: 161–7.

Carmichael, C. L. and Reis, H. T. (2005). Attachment, sleep quality, and depressed affect. *Health Psychology, 24*: 526–31.

Carter, F. A., Frampton, C. M. and Mulder, R. T. (2006). Cesarean section and postpartum depression: A review of the evidence examining the link. *Psychosomatic Medicine, 68*(2): 321–30.

Centers for Disease Control (2008). Prevalence of self-reported postpartum depressive symptoms – 17 states, 2004–5. *Morbidity & Mortality Weekly Report, 57*(14): 361–6.

Cerutti, R., Sichel, M. P. and Perin, M. (1993). Psychological distress during puerperium: A novel therapeutic approach using S-adenosylmethionine. *Current Therapeutic Research, Clinical and Experimental, 53*: 707–16.

Chabrol, H. and Teissedre, J. (2004). Relation between Edinburgh Postnatal Depression Scale scores at 2–3 days and 4–6 weeks postpartum. *Journal of Reproductive and Infant Psychology, 22*(1): 33–9.

Chabrol, H., Teissedre, J., Armitage, M. D. and Walburg, V. (2004). Acceptability of psychotherapy and antidepressants for postnatal depression among newly delivered mothers. *Journal of Reproductive and Infant Psychology, 22*(1): 5–12.

Chandra, P. S., Vankatasubramanian, G. and Thomas, T. (2002). Infanticidal ideas and infanticial behavior in Indian women with severe postpartum psychiatric disorders. *Journal of Nervous and Mental Disease, 190*: 457–61.

Chaudron, L. H. (2007). Treating pregnant women with antidepressants: The gray zone. *Journal of Women's Health, 16*(4): 551–3.

Chaudron, L. H., Klein, M. H., Remington, P., Palta, M., Allen, C. and Essex, M. J. (2001). Predictors, prodromes and incidence of postpartum depression. *Journal of Psychosomatic Obstetrics and Gynaecology, 22*: 103–12.

Chaudron, L. H., Kitzman, H. J., Peifer, K. L., Morrow, S., Perez, L. M. and Newman, M. C. (2005). Prevalence of maternal depressive symptoms in low-income Hispanic women. *Journal of Clinical Psychiatry, 66*(4): 418–23.

Chen, E., Bloomberg, G. R., Fisher, E. B. and Strunk, R. C. (2003). Predictors of repeat hospitalizations in children with asthma: The role of psychosocial and socioenvironmental factors. *Health Psychology, 22*: 12–18.

Chess, S. and Thomas, A. (1977). Temperamental individuality from childhood to adolescence. *Journal of Child Psychiatry, 16*: 218–26.

Chi, T. C. and Hinshaw, S. P. (2002). Mother-child relationships of children with ADHD: The role of maternal depressive symptoms and depression-related distortions. *Journal of Abnormal Child Psychology, 30*: 387–400.

Cho, H. J., Kwon, J. H. and Lee, J. J. (2008). Antenatal cognitive-behavioral therapy for prevention of postpartum depression: A pilot study. *Yonsei Medical Journal, 49*(4): 553–62.

Chung, T. K., Lau, T. K., Yip, A. S., Chiu, H. F. and Less, D. T. (2001). Antepartum depressive symptomatology is associated with adverse obstetric and neonatal outcomes. *Psychosomatic Medicine, 63*: 830–4.

Cigoli, V., Gilli, G. and Saita, E. (2006). Relational factors in psychopathological responses to childbirth. *Journal of Psychosomatic Obstetrics & Gynecology, 27*(2): 91–7.

Cipriani, A., Geddes, J. R., Furukawa, T. A. and Barbui, C. (2007). Metareview on short-term effectiveness and safety of antidepressants for depression: An evidence-based approach to inform clinical practice. *Canadian Journal of Psychiatry, 52*: 553–62.

Cohen, L. S., Sichel, D. A., Dimmock, J. A. and Rosenbaum, J. F. (1994). Impact of pregnancy on panic disorder: A case series. *Journal of Clinical Psychiatry, 55*: 284–8.

Cooper, P. J., Tomlinson, M., Swartz, L., Woolgar, M., Murray, L. and Molteno, C. (1999). Postpartum depression and the mother-infant relationship in a South African peri-urban settlement. *British Journal of Psychiatry, 175*: 554–8.

Cooper, P. J., Landman, M., Tomlinson, M., Molteno, C., Swartz, L. and Murray, L. (2002). Impact of a mother-infant intervention in an indigent peri-urban South African context: Pilot study. *British Journal of Psychiatry, 180*: 76–81.

Cornish, A. M., McMahon, C. A., Ungerer, J. A., Barnett, B., Kowalenko, N. and Tennant, C. (2005). Postnatal depression and infant cognitive and motor development in the second postnatal year: The impact of depression chronicity and infant gender. *Infant Behavior and Development, 28*: 407–17.

Corral, M., Kuan, A. and Kostaras, D. (2000). Bright light therapy's effect on postpartum depression. *American Journal of Psychiatry, 157*: 303–4.

Corral, M., Wardrop, A. A., Zhang, H., Grewal, A. K. and Patton, S. (2007). Morning light therapy for postpartum depression. *Archives of Women's Mental Health, 10*: 221–4.

Corwin, E. J. and Arbour, M. (2007). Postpartum fatigue and evidence-based interventions. *American Journal of Maternal Child Nursing, 32*(4): 215–20.

Corwin, E. J. and Pajer, K. (2008). The psychoneuroimmunology of postpartum depression. *Journal of Women's Health, 17*(9): 1529–34.

Corwin, E. J., Bozoky, I., Pugh, L. C. and Johnston, N. (2003). Interleukin-1beta elevation during the postpartum period. *Annals of Behavioral Medicine, 25*: 41–7.

Coussons-Read, M. E., Okun, M. L., Schmitt, M. P. and Giese, S. (2005). Prenatal stress alters cytokine levels in a manner that may endanger human pregnancy. *Psychosomatic Medicine, 67*: 625–31.

Cox, J. L., Holden, J. M. and Sagovsky, R. (1987). Detection of postnatal depression: Development of the 10-item Edinburgh Postnatal Depression Scale. *British Journal of Psychiatry, 150*: 782–6.

Crouch, J. L., Skowronski, J. J., Milner, J. S. and Harris, B. (2008). Parental responses to infant crying: The influence of child physical abuse risk and hostile priming. *Child Abuse & Neglect, 32*: 702–10.

Cryan, E., Keogh, F., Connolly, E., Cody, S., Quinlan, A. and Daly, I. (2001). Depression among postnatal women in an urban Irish community. *Irish Journal of Psychological Medicine, 18*: 5–10. (Abstract.)

Currie, M. L. and Rademacher, R. (2004). The pediatrician's role in recognizing and intervening in postpartum depression. *Pediatric Clinics of North America, 51*: 785–801.

Cutler, C. B., Legano, L. A., Dreyer, B. P., Fierman, A. H., Berkule, S. B., Lusskin, S. I., *et al.* (2007). Screening for maternal depression in a low education population using a two-item questionnaire. *Archives of Women's Mental Health, 10*: 277–83.

Cutrona, C. E. and Troutman, B. R. (1986). Social support, infant temperament, and parenting self-efficacy: A mediational model of postpartum depression. *Child Development, 57*: 1507–18.

Czarnocka, J. and Slade, P. (2000). Prevalence and predictors of posttraumatic stress symptoms following childbirth. *British Journal of Clinical Psychology, 39*: 35–51.

Da Costa, D., Larouche, J., Dritsa, M. and Brender, W. (2000). Psychosocial correlates of prepartum and postpartum depressed mood. *Journal of Affective Disorders, 59*: 31–40.

Dagher, R. K., McGovern, P. M., Alexander, B. H., Dowd, B. E., Ukestad, L. K. and McCaffrey, D. J. (2009). The psychosocial work environment and maternal postpartum depression. *International Journal of Behavioral Medicine*, e-pub.

Daley, A. J., Macarthur, C. and Winter, H. (2007). The role of exercise in treating postpartum depression: A review of the literature. *Journal of Midwifery and Women's Health, 52*: 56–62.

Dalton, K. (1985). Progesterone prophylaxis used successfully in postnatal depression. *The Practitioner, 229*: 507–8.

Danaci, A. E., Dinc, G., Deveci, A., Sen, F. S. and Icelli, I. (2002). Postnatal depression in Turkey: Epidemiological and cultural aspects. *Social Psychiatry & Psychiatric Epidemiology, 37*: 125–9.

Danese, A., Pariante, C. M., Caspi, A., Taylor, A. and Poulton, R. (2007). Childhood maltreatment predicts adult inflammation in a life-course study. *Proceedings of the National Academy of Sciences USA, 104*(4): 1319–24.

Davidson, J. and Robertson, E. (1985). A follow-up study of post-partum illness, 1946–1978. *Acta Psychiatrica Scandanavica, 71*: 451–7.

Davis, E. P., Glynn, L. M., Schetter, C. D., Hobel, C., Chicz-Demet, A. and Sandman, C. A. (2007). Prenatal exposure to maternal depression and cortisol influences infant temperament. *Journal of the American Academy of Child & Adolescent Psychiatry, 46*(6): 737–46.

Dayan, J., Creveuil, C., Marks, M. N., Conroy, S., Herlicoviez, M., Dreyfus, M. and Tordjman, S. (2006). Prenatal depression, prenatal anxiety, and spontaneous preterm birth: A prospective cohort study among women with early and regular care. *Psychosomatic Medicine, 68*: 938–46.

de Jonge, P., van den Brink, R. H., Spijkerman, T. A. and Ormel, J. (2006). Only incident depressive episodes after myocardial infarction are associated with new cardiovascular events. *Journal of the American College of Cardiology, 48*(11): 2204–8.

Delatte, R., Cao, H., Meltzer-Brody, S. and Menard MK. (2009). Universal screening for postpartum depression: an inquiry into provider attitudes and practice. *American Journal of Obstetrics & Gynecology. 200*(5): 63–4.

Dell'Aica, I., Caniato, R., Biggin, S. and Garbisa, S. (2007). Matrix proteases, green tea, and St. John's wort: Biomedical research catches up with folk medicine. *Clinical Chimica Acta, 381*: 69–77.

Dennis, C-L. (2004a). Influence of depressive symptomatology on maternal health service utilization and general health. *Archives of Women's Mental Health, 7*: 183–91.

Dennis, C-L. (2004b). Can we identify mothers at risk for postpartum depression in the immediate postpartum period using the Edinburgh Postnatal Depression Scale? *Journal of Affective Disorders, 78*: 163–9.

Dennis, C-L. (2005). Psychosocial and psychological interventions for prevention of postnatal depression: Systematic review. *British Medical Journal, 331*: doi:10.1136/bmj.1331.7505. 1115.

Dennis, C-L. and Ross, L. E. (2005). Relationships among infant sleep patterns, maternal fatigue, and development of depressive symptomatology. *Birth, 32*(3): 187–93.

Dennis, C-L. and Chung-Lee, L. (2006). Postpartum depression help-seeking barriers and maternal treatment preferences: A qualitative systematic review. *Birth, 33*(4): 323–31.

Dennis, C-L. and Ross, L. E. (2006a). The clinical utility of maternal self-reported personal and familial psychiatric history in identifying women at risk for postpartum depression. *Acta Obstetricia et Gynecologica, 85*: 1179–85.

Dennis, C-L. and Ross, L. E. (2006b). Women's perceptions of partner support and conflict in the development of postpartum depressive symptoms. *Journal of Advanced Nursing, 56*(6): 588–99.

Dennis, C-L. and McQueen, K. (2007). Does maternal postpartum depressive symptomatology influence infant feeding outcomes? *Acta Paediatrica 96*(4): 590–4.

Dennis, C-L. and Allen, K. (2008). Interventions (other than pharmacological, psychosocial or psychological) for treating antenatal depression. *Cochrane Database Systematic Review* (4), CD006795. DOI:006710.001002/14651858.CD14006795.pub14651852.

Dennis, C-L. and Kingston, D. (2008). A systematic review of telephone support for women during pregnancy and the early postpartum period. *Journal of Obstetric, Gynecologic and Neonatal Nursing, 37*: 301–14.

Dennis, C-L. and McQueen, K. (2009). The relationship between infant-feeding outcomes and postpartum depression: A qualitative systematic review. *Pediatrics, 123*: e736–e751.

Dennis, C-L., Janssen, P. A. and Singer, J. (2004). Identifying women at-risk for postpartum depression in the immediate postpartum period. *Acta Psychiatrica Scandanavica, 110*: 338–46.

Dennis, C-L., Hodnett, E., Kenton, L., Weston, J., Zupancic, J., Stewart, D. E., *et al.* (2009). Effect of peer support on prevention of postnatal depression among high-risk women: Multisite randomised controlled trial. *British Medical Journal, 338*: a3064 doi:3010.1136/bmj. a3064.

Des Rivières-Pigeon, C., Séguin, L., Brodeur, J-M., Perreault, M., Boyer, G., Colin, C. and Goulet, L. (2000). The Edinburgh Postnatal Depression Scale: Validity for Quebec women of low socioeconomic status. *Canadian Journal of Community Mental Health, 19*: 201–14.

Des Rivières-Pigeon, C., Séguin, L., Goulet, L. and Descarries, F. (2001). Unraveling the complexities of the relationship between employment status and postpartum depressive symptomatology. *Women & Health, 34*: 61–79.

Desan, P. H., Weinstein, A. J., Michalak, E. E., Tam, E. M., Meesters, Y., Ruiter M. J., *et al.* (2007). A controlled trial of the Litebook light-emitting diode (LED) light therapy device for treatment of Seasonal Affective Disorder (SAD). *BMC Psychiatry, 7*: doi:10.1186/1471–1244X/1187/1138.

Devilly, G. J. and Spence, S. H. (1999). The relative efficacy and treatment distress of EMDR and cognitive behavioral trauma treatment protocol in the amelioration of posttraumatic stress disorder. *Journal of Anxiety Disorders, 13*: 131–58.

Dhabhar, F. D. and McEwen, B. S. (2001). Bidirectional effects of stress and glucocorticoid hormones on immune function: Possible explanations for paradoxical observations. In R. Ader, Felten, D. L. and Cohen, N. (eds.), *Psychoneuroimmunology*, 3rd ed., Vol. 1, pp. 301–38. New York: Academic Press.

di Scalea, T. L., Hanusa, B. H. and Wisner, K. L. (2009). Sexual function in postpartum women treated for depression: Results from a randomized trial of nortriptyline versus sertraline. *Journal of Clincal Psychiatry, 70*(3): 423–8.

Diego, M. A., Field, T. and Hernandez-Reif, M. (2005). Prepartum, postpartum and chronic depression effects on neonatal behavior. *Infant Behavior and Development, 28*: 155–64.

Dietz, P. M., Williams, S. B., Callaghan, W. M., Bachman, D. J., Whitlock, E. P. and Hornbrook, M. C. (2007). Clinically identified maternal depression before, during, and after pregnancies ending in live births. *American Journal of Psychiatry, 164*: 1515–20.

Ditzen, B., Hoppmann, C. and Klumb, P. (2008). Positive couple interactions and daily cortisol: On the stress-protecting role of intimacy. *Psychosomatic Medicine, 70*: 883–9.

Doan, T., Gardiner, A., Gay, C. L. and Lee, K. A. (2007). Breastfeeding increases sleep duration of new parents. *Journal of Perinatal & Neonatal Nursing, 21*(3): 200–6.

Doering, L. V., Cross, R., Vredevoe, D., Martinez-Maza, O. I. and Cowan, M. J. (2007). Infection, depression and immunity in women after coronary artery bypass: A pilot study of cognitive behavioral therapy. *Alternative Therapy, Health & Medicine, 13*: 18–21.

Doering, L. V., Martinez-Maza, O. I., Vredevoe, D. L. and Cowan, M. J. (2008). Relation of depression, natural killer cell function, and infections after coronary artery bypass in women. *European Journal of Cardiovascular Nursing, 7*(1): 52–8.

Dombrowski, M. A., Anderson, G. C., Santori, C. and Burkhammer, M. (2001). Kangaroo (skin-to-skin) care with a postpartum woman who felt depressed. *American Journal of Maternal Child Nursing, 26*: 214–16.

Douglas, A. R. (2000). Reported anxieties concerning intimate parenting in women sexually abused as children. *Child Abuse & Neglect, 24*: 425–34.

Downs, D. S., DiNallo, J. M. and Kirner, T. L. (2008). Determinants of pregnancy and postpartum depression: Prospective influences of depressive symptoms, body image satisfaction, and exercise behavior. *Annals of Behavioral Medicine, 36*(1): 54–63.

Dowrick, C., Dunn, G., Ayuso-Mateos, J. L., Dalgard, O. S., Page, H., Lehtinen V., *et al.* (2000). Problem solving treatment and group psychoeducation for depression: Multicentre randomised controlled trial. *British Medical Journal, 321*: 1450.

Dubois, B. (2003). Overcoming the past. *New Beginnings, March–April*: 50–1.

Dubowitz, H., Black, M. M., Kerr, M. A., Hussey, J. M., Morrel, T. M., Everson, M. D. and Starr, R. H. (2001). Type and timing of mothers' victimization: Effects on mothers and children. *Pediatrics, 107*: 728–35.

Dudley, M., Roy, K., Kelk, N. and Bernard, D. (2001). Psychological correlates of depression in fathers and mothers in the first postnatal year. *Journal of Reproductive & Infant Psychology, 19*: 187–202.

Dugoua, J.-J., Mills, E., Perri, D. and Koren, G. (2006). Safety and efficacy of St. John's wort (Hypericum) during pregnancy and lactation. *Canadian Journal of Clinical Pharmacology, 13*: e268–e276.

Dunham, C. (1992). *Mamatoto: A celebration of birth.* New York: Viking Penguin.

Dunstan, J. A., Mori, T. A., Barden, A., Beilin, L. J., Holt, P. G., Calder, P. C., Taylor, A. L. and Prescott, S. L. (2004a). Effects of n-3 polyunsaturated fatty acid supplementation in pregnancy on maternal and fetal erythrocyte fatty acid composition. *European Journal of Clinical Nutrition, 58*: 429–37.

Dunstan, J. A., Roper, J., Mitoulas, L., Hartmann, P. E., Simmer, K. and Prescott, S. L. (2004b). The effect of supplementation with fish oil during pregnancy on breast milk immunoglobulin A, soluble CD14: cytokine levels and fatty acid composition. *Clinical & Experimental Allergy, 34*: 1237–42.

Durik, A. M., Hyde, J. S. and Clark, R. (2000). Sequelae of cesarean and vaginal deliveries: Psychosocial outcomes for mothers and infants. *Developmental Psychology, 36*: 251–60.

Eaker, E. D., Sullivan, L. M., Kelly-Hayes, M., D'Agostino, R. B. and Benjamin, E. J. (2007). Marital status, marital strain, and risk of coronary heart disease or total mortality: The Framingham Offspring Study. *Psychosomatic Medicine, 69*: 509–13.

Eberhard-Gran, M., Eskild, A., Tambs, K., Schei, B. and Opjordsmoen, S. (2001). The Edinburgh Postnatal Depression Scale: Validation in a Norwegian community sample. *Nordic Journal of Psychiatry, 55*: 113–17. (Abstract.)

Eberhard-Gran, M., Tambs, K., Opjordsmoen, S., Skrondal, A. and Eskild, A. (2004). Depression during pregnancy and after delivery: A repeated measurement study. *Journal of Psychosomatic Obstetrics & Gynecology, 25*: 15–21.

Einarson, A., Choi, J., Einarson, T. R. and Koren, G. (2009). Rates of spontaneous and therapeutic abortions following use of antidepressants in pregnancy: Results from a large prospective database. *Journal of Obstetrics & Gynaecology Canada, 31*(5): 452–6.

Eisenach, J. C., Pan, P. H., Smiley, R., Lavand'homme, P., Landau, R. and Houle, T. T. (2008). Severity of acute pain after childbirth, but not type of delivery, predicts persistent pain and postpartum depression. *Pain, 140*: 87–94.

Elliot, S. A. and Leverton, T. J. (2000). Is the EPDS a magic wand?: 2. "Myths" and the evidence base. *Journal of Reproductive and Infant Psychology, 18*: 297–307.

Elliot, S. A., Leverton, T. J., Sanjack, M., Turner, H., Cowmeadow, P., Hopkins, J. and Bushnell, D. (2000). Promoting mental health after childbirth: A controlled trial of primary prevention of postnatal depression. *British Journal of Clinical Psychology, 39*: 223–41.

Ellis, K. K., Chang, C., Bhandari, S., Ball, K., Geden, E., Everett, K. D., *et al.* (2008). Rural mothers experiencing the stress of intimate partner violence or not: Their newborn health concerns. *Journal of Midwifery and Women's Health, 53*(6): 556–62.

Emery, C. F., Kiecolt-Glaser, J. K., Glaser, R., Malarky, W. B. and Frid, D. J. (2005). Exercise accelerates wound healing among healthy older adults: A preliminary investigation. *The Journals of Gerontology: Medical Sciences, 60A*: 1432–6.

Epperson, C. N., Czarkowski, K. A., Ward-O'Brien, D., Weiss, E., Gueorguieva, R., Jatlow, P. I., *et al.* (2001). Maternal sertraline treatment and serotonin transport in breast-feeding mother–infant pairs. *American Journal of Psychiatry, 158*: 1631–37.

Ernst, E. (2002). The risk-benefit profile of commonly used herbal therapies: Ginkgo, St. John's wort, ginseng, echinacea, saw palmetto, and kava. *Annals of Internal Medicine, 136*: 42–53.

Evans, J., Heron, J., Francomb, H., Oke, S. and Golding, J. (2001). Cohort study of depressed mood during pregnancy and after childbirth. *British Medical Journal, 323*: 257–60.

Evans, J., Heron, J., Patel, R. R. and Wiles, N. (2007). Depressive symptoms during pregnancy and low birth weight at term. *British Journal of Psychiatry, 191*: 84–5.

Ernst, E. (2006). Herbal remedies for anxiety: A systematic review of controlled clinical trials. *Phytomedicine, 13*: 205–8.

Feldman, R., Eidelman, A. I., Sirota, L. and Weller, A. (2002). Comparison of skin-to-skin (Kangaroo) and traditional care: parenting outcomes and preterm infant development. *Pediatrics, 110*: 16–26.

Ferber, S. G., Granot, M. and Zimmer, E. Z. (2005). Catastrophizing labor pain compromises later maternity adjustments. *American Journal of Obstetrics & Gynecology, 192*: 826–31.

Fergerson, S. S., Jamieson, D. J. and Lindsay, M. (2002). Diagnosing postpartum depression: Can we do better? *American Journal of Obstetrics and Gynecology, 186*: 899–902.

Fergusson, D. M., Boden, J. M. and Horwood, L. J. (2008). Exposure to childhood sexual and physical abuse and adjustment in early adulthood. *Child Abuse & Neglect, 32*: 607–19.

Ferrucci, L., Cherubini, A., Bandinelli, S., Bartali, B., Corsi A., Lauretani, F., Martin, A., Andres-Lacueva, C., Senin, U. and Guralnik, J. M. (2006). Relationship of plasma polyunsaturated fatty acids to circulating inflammatory markers. *Journal of Clinical Endocrinology & Metabolism, 91*: 439–46.

Field, T. (1992). Infants of depressed mothers. *Development and Psychopathology, 4*: 49–66.

Field, T. (1995). Infants of depressed mothers. *Infant Behavior and Development, 18*: 1–13.

Field, T. (2008). Breastfeeding and antidepressants. *Infant Behavior and Development, 31*: 481–87.

Field, T., Fox, N. A., Pickens, J. and Nawrocki, T. (1995). Relative right frontal EEG activation in 3- to 6-month-old infants of "depressed" mothers. *Developmental Psychology, 31*: 358–63.

Field, T., Diego, M., Hernandez-Reif, M., Schanberg, S. and Kuhn, C. (2002a). Relative right versus left frontal EEG in neonates. *Developmental Psychobiology, 41*: 147–55.

Field, T., Hernandez-Reif, M. and Feijo, L. (2002b). Breastfeeding in depressed mother-infant dyads. *Early Child Development and Care, 172*: 539–45.

Field, T., Diego, M., Dieter, J., Hernandez-Reif, M., Schanberg, S., Kuhn C., *et al.* (2004). Prenatal depression effects on the fetus and the newborn. *Infant Behavior & Development, 27*: 216–29.

Field, T., Diego, M. and Hernandez-Reif, M. (2006a). Prenatal depression effects on the fetus and newborn: A review. *Infant Behavior and Development, 29*(3): 445–55.

Field, T., Hernandez-Reif, M., Diego, M., Figueiredo, B., Schanberg, S. and Kuhn, C. (2006b). Prenatal cortisol, prematurity and low birthweight. *Infant Behavior and Development, 29*: 268–75.

Field, T., Diego, M., Hernandez-Reif, M., Figueiredo, B., Schanberg, S. and Kuhn, C. (2007). Sleep disturbance in depressed pregnant women and their newborns. *Infant Behavior and Development, 30*: 127–33.

Field, T., Diego, M., Hernandez-Reif, M., Figueiredo, B., Deeds, O., Ascencio A., *et al.* (2008).

Prenatal serotonin and neonatal outcome: Brief report. *Infant Behavior and Development, 31*(2): 316–20.

Figley, C. R. (1986). Traumatic stress: The role of the family and social support system. In C. R. Figley (ed.) *Trauma and its wake, Vol. II: Traumatic stress theory, research and intervention*, pp. 39–54. New York: Bruner/Mazel.

Finucane, A. and Mercer, S. W. (2006). An exploratory mixed methods study of the acceptability and effectiveness of mindfulness-based cognitive therapy for patients with active depression and anxiety in primary care. *BMC Psychiatry, 6*: doi:10.11186/1471–244X-6-14).

Fisher, J., Astbury, J. and Smith, A. (1997). Adverse psychological impact of operative obstetric interventions: A prospective longitudinal study. *Australian and New Zealand Journal of Psychiatry, 31*: 728–38.

Fisher, J. R., Feekery, C. J., Amir, L. H. and Sneddon, M. (2002a). Health and social circumstances of women admitted to a private mother-baby unit. A descriptive cohort study. *Australian Family Physician, 31*: 966–70, 973.

Fisher, J. R. W., Feekery, C. J. and Rowe-Murray, H. J. (2002b). Nature, severity and correlates of psychological distress in women admitted to a private mother-baby unit. *Journal of Paediatrics and Child Health, 38*: 140–5.

Foa, E. B. and Cahill, S. P. (2002). Specialized treatment for PTSD: Matching survivors with the appropriate modality. In R. Yehuda (ed.) *Treating trauma survivors with PTSD*. Washington, DC: American Psychiatric Publishing, pp. 43–62.

Folstein, M., Liu, T., Peter, I., Buell, J., Arsenault, L., Scott, T. and Qiu, W. W. (2007). The homocysteine hypothesis of depression. *American Journal of Psychiatry, 164*(6): 861–7.

Foss, G. F. (2001). Maternal sensitivity, posttraumatic stress, and acculturation in Vietnamese and Hmong mothers. *American Journal of Maternal Child Nursing, 26*: 257–63.

Frangou, S., Lewis, M. and McCrone, P. (2006). Efficacy of ethyl-eicosapentaenoic acid in bipolar depression: Randomized double-blind placebo-controlled study. *British Journal of Psychiatry, 188*: 46–50.

Franko, D. L., Blais, M. A., Becker, A. E., Delinsky, S. S., Greenwood, D. N., Flores, A. T., Ekelblad, E. R., Eddy, K. T. and Herzog, D. B. (2001). Pregnancy complications and neonatal outcomes in women with eating disorders. *American Journal of Psychiatry, 158*: 1461–6.

Frasure-Smith, N. and Lesperance, F. (2005). Reflections on depression as a cardiac risk factor. *Psychosomatic Medicine, 67*: S19–S25.

Freeman, M. P. (2007). Antenatal depression: Navigating the treatment dilemmas. *American Journal of Psychiatry, 164*: 1162–5.

Freeman, M. P. (2009). Complementary and alternative medicine for perinatal depression. *Journal of Affective Disorders, 112*: 1–10.

Freeman, M. P. and Sinha, P. (2007). Tolerability of omega-3 fatty acid supplements in perinatal women. *Prostaglandins, Leukotrienes, and Essential Fatty Acids, 77*: 203–8.

Freeman, M. P., Smith, K. W., Freeman, S. A., McElroy, S. L., Kmetz, G. F., Wright, R. and Keck, P. E. Jr. (2002). The impact of reproductive events on the course of bipolar disorder in women. *Journal of Clinical Psychiatry, 63*: 284–7.

Freeman, M. P., Wright, R., Watchman, M., Wahl, R. A., Sisk, D. J., Fraleigh L., *et al.* (2005). Postpartum depression assessments at well-baby visits: Screening feasibility, prevalence, and risk factors. *Journal of Women's Health, 14*(10): 929–35.

Freeman, M. P., Hibbeln, J. R., Wisner, K. L., Davis, J. M., Mischoulon, D., Peet, M., Keck, P. E. Jr., Marangell, L. B., Richardson, A. J., Lake, J. and Stoll, A. L. (2006a). Omega-3 fatty acids: Evidence basis for treatment and future research in psychiatry. *Journal of Clinical Psychiatry, 67*: 1954–67.

Freeman, M. P., Hibbeln, J. R., Wisner, K. L., Brumbach, B. H., Watchman, M. and Gelenberg, A. J. (2006b). Randomized dose-ranging pilot trial of omega-3 fatty acids for postpartum depression. *Acta Psychiatrica Scandanavica, 113*: 31–5.

Freeman, M. P., Davis, M., Sinha, P., Wisner, K. L., Hibbeln, J. R. and Gelenberg, A. J. (2008). Omega-3 fatty acids and supportive psychotherapy for perinatal depression: A randomized placebo-controlled study. *Journal of Affective Disorders, 110*: 142–8.

Friedman, M. J. (2001). *Posttraumatic stress disorder: The latest assessment and treatment strategies.* Kansas City, MO: Compact Clinicals.

Froese, C. L., Butt, A., Mulgrew, A., Cheema, R., Speirs, M. A., Gosnell C., *et al.* (2008). Depression and sleep-related symptoms in an adult, indigenous, North American population. *Journal of Clinical Sleep Medicine, 4*(4): 356–61.

Fuggle, P., Glover, L., Khan, F. and Haydon, K. (2002). Screening for postnatal depression in Bengali women: Preliminary observations from using a translated version of the Edinburgh Postnatal Depression Scale (EPDS). *Journal of Reproductive and Infant Psychology, 20*: 71–82.

Furman, L., Minich, N. and Hack, M. (2002). Correlates of lactation in mothers of very low birth weight infants. *Pediatrics, 109*: e57.

Galea, S., Vlahov, D., Resnick, H., Ahern, J., Susser, E., Gold J., *et al.* (2003). Trends of probable post-traumatic stress disorder in New York City after the September 11 terrorist attacks. *American Journal of Epidemiology, 158*: 514–24.

Galler, J. R., Harrison, R. H. and Ramsey, F. (2006). Bed-sharing, breastfeeding and maternal moods in Barbados. *Infant Behavior and Development, 29*(4): 526–34.

Gallo, L. C., Troxel, W. M., Matthews, K. A. and Kuller, L. H. (2003). Marital status and quality in middle-aged women: Associations with levels and trajectories of cardiovascular risk factors. *Health Psychology, 22*: 453–63.

Gamble, J. A., Creedy, D. K., Webster, J. and Moyle, W. (2002). A review of the literature on debriefing or non-directive counseling to prevent postpartum emotional distress. *Midwifery, 8*(1): 72–9.

Gay, C. L., Lee, K. A. and Lee, S.-Y. (2004). Sleep patterns and fatigue in new mothers and fathers. *Biological Nursing Research, 5*(4): 311–18.

Gaynes, B. N., Gavin, N., Meltzer-Brody, S., Lohr, K. N., Swinson, T., Gartlehner G., *et al.* (2005). Perinatal depression: Prevalence, screening, accuracy, and screening outcomes. *Agency for Healthcare Research and Quality, AHRQ Pub. No. 05-E006–1*(119).

Geddes, J. R., Furukawa, T. A., Cipriani, A. and Barbui, C. (2007). Depressive disorder needs an evidence base commensurate with its public health importance. *Canadian Journal of Psychiatry, 52*: 543–4.

Geller, P. A. (2004). Pregnancy as a stressful life event. *CNS Spectrums, 9*(3): 188–97.

Genevie, L. and Margolies, E. (1987). *The motherhood report: How women feel about being mothers.* New York: Macmillan.

George, L. and Elliot, S. A. (2004). Searching for antenatal predictors of postnatal depressive symptomatology: Unexpected findings from a study of obsessive-compulsive personality traits. *Journal of Reproductive and Infant Psychology, 22*(1): 25–31.

Geracioti, T. D. Jr., Carpenter, L. L., Owens, M. J., Baker, D. G., Ekhator, N. N., Horn, P. S., Strawn, J. R., Sanacora, G., Kinkead, B., Price, L. H. and Nemeroff, C. B. (2006). Elevated cerebrospinal fluid substance P concentrations in posttraumatic stress disorder and major depression. *American Journal of Psychiatry, 163*: 637–43.

Gilson, K. J. and Lancaster, S. (2008). Childhood sexual abuse in pregnant and parenting adolescents. *Child Abuse & Neglect, 32*(9): 869–77.

Gjerdingen, D. K. and Chaloner, K. M. (1994). The relationship of women's postpartum mental health to employment, childbirth, and social support. *Journal of Family Practice, 38*: 465–72.

Glover, V., Onozawa, K. and Hodgkinson, A. (2002). Benefits of infant massage for mothers with postnatal depression. *Seminars in Neonatalogy, 7*: 495–500.

Glynn, L. M., Davis, E. P., Schetter, C. D., Chicz-DeMet, A., Hobel, C. J. and Sandman, C. A. (2007). Postnatal maternal cortisol levels predict temperament in healthy breastfed infants. *Early Human Development, 83*(10): 675–81.

Glynn, L. M., Schetter, C. D., Hobel, C. J. and Sandman, C. A. (2008). Pattern of perceived stress and anxiety in pregnancy predicts preterm birth. *Health Psychology, 27*(1): 43–51.

Golden, R. N., Gaynes, B. N., Ekstrom, R. D., Hamer, R. M., Jacobsen, F. M., Suppes, T., Wisner, K. L.

and Nemeroff, C. B. (2005). The efficacy of light therapy in the treatment of mood disorders: A review and meta-analysis of the evidence. *American Journal of Psychiatry*, *162*: 656–62.

Goyal, D., Gay, C. L. and Lee, K. A. (2007). Patterns of sleep disruption and depressive symptoms in new mothers. *Journal of Perinatal & Neonatal Nursing*, *21*(2): 123–9.

Gracia, E. and Musitu, G. (2003). Social isolation from communities and child maltreatment: A cross-cultural comparison. *Child Abuse & Neglect*, *27*: 153–68.

Grandjean, P., Bjerve, K. S., Weihe, P. and Steuerwald, U. (2001). Birthweight in a fishing community: Significance of essential fatty acids and marine food contaminants. *International Journal of Epidemiology*, *30*: 1272–8.

Grazioli, R. and Terry, D. J. (2000). The role of cognitive vulnerability and stress in the prediction of postpartum depressive symptomatology. *British Journal of Clinical Psychology*, *39*: 329–47.

Grigoriadis, S. and Ravitz, P. (2007). An approach to interpersonal psychotherapy for postpartum depression: Focusing on interpersonal changes. *Canadian Family Physician*, *53*: 1469–75.

Grimstad, H. and Schei, B. (1999). Pregnancy and delivery for women with a history of child sexual abuse. *Child Abuse and Neglect*, *23*: 81–90.

Groer, M. W. (2005). Differences between exclusive breastfeeders, formula-feeders, and controls: A study of stress, mood, and endocrine variables. *Biological Nursing Research*, *7*(2): 106–17.

Groer, M. W. and Davis, M. W. (2006). Cytokines, infections, stress, and dysphoric moods in breastfeeders and formula feeders. *Journal of Obstetric, Gynecologic and Neonatal Nursing*, *35*: 599–607.

Groer, M. W. and Morgan, K. (2007). Immune, health and endocrine characteristics of depressed postpartum mothers. *Psychoneuroendocrinology*, *32*(2): 133–9.

Groer, M. W., Davis, M. W. and Hemphill, J. (2002). Postpartum stress: Current concepts and the possible protective role of breastfeeding. *Journal of Obstetric, Gynecologic and Neonatal Nursing*, *31*(4): 411–17.

Groer, M., Davis, K. and Casey, B. (2005). Neuroendocrine and immune relationships in postpartum fatigue. *The American Journal of Maternal Child Nursing*, *30*: 133–138.

Groer, M. W., Thomas, S. P., Evans, G. W., Helton, S. and Weldon, A. (2006). Inflammatory effects and immune system correlates of rape. *Violence and Victims*, *21*(6): 796–808.

Guedeney, N., Fermanian, J., Guelfi, J. D. and Kumar, R. C. (2000). The Edinburgh Postnatal Depression Scale (EPDS) and the detection of major depressive disorders in early postpartum: Some concerns about false negatives. *Journal of Affective Disorders*, *61*: 107–12.

Guo, S. F., Wu, J. L., Qu, C. Y. and Yan, R. Y. (2004). Physical and sexual abuse of women before, during and after pregnancy. *International Journal of Gynaecology and Obstetrics*, *84*(3): 281–6.

Haapasalo, J. and Petaja, S. (1999). Mothers who killed or attempted to kill their child: Life circumstances, childhood abuse, and types of killing. *Violence and Victims*, *14*: 219–39.

Hagan, R., Evans, S. F. and Pope, S. (2004). Preventing postnatal depression in mothers of very preterm infants: A randomized controlled trial. *British Journal of Obstetrics & Gynecology*, *111*: 641–7.

Hale, T. W. (2008). *Medications and mothers' milk*, Vol. 13. Amarillo, TX: Hale.

Hallahan, B. and Garland, M. R. (2005). Essential fatty acids and mental health. *British Journal of Psychiatry*, *186*: 275–7.

Hallahan, B., Hibbeln, J. R., Davis, J. M. and Garland, M. R. (2007). Omega-3 fatty acid supplementation in patients with recurrent self-harm: Single-centre double-blind randomized controlled trial. *British Journal of Psychiatry*, *190*: 118–22.

Hamazaki, K., Itomura, M., Huan, M., Nishizawa, H., Sawazaki, S., Tanouchi M., *et al.* (2005). Effect of omega-3 fatty acid-containing phospholipids on blood catecholamine concentrations in healthy volunteers: A randomized, placebo-controlled, double-blind trial. *Nutrition*, *21*: 705–10.

Hamer, M. and Steptoe, A. (2007). Association between physical fitness, parasympathetic control, and proinflammatory responses to mental stress. *Psychosomatic Medicine*, *69*: 660–6.

Hammen, C. and Brennan, P. (2002). Interpersonal dysfunction in depressed women: Impairments independent of depressive symptoms. *Journal of Affective Disorders*, *72*: 145–56.

Hanlon, C., Medhin, G., Alem, A., Araya, M., Abdulahi, A., Hughes M., *et al.* (2008). Detecting perinatal common mental disorders in Ethiopia: Validation of the self-reporting questionnaire and Edinburgh Postnatal Depression Scale. *Journal of Affective Disorders, 108*: 251–62.

Hannah, M. E., Hannah, W. J., Hodnett, E. D., Chalmers, B., Kung, R., Willan A., *et al.* (2002). Outcomes at 3 months after planned cesarean vs. planned vaginal delivery for breech presentation at term: The international randomized term breech trial. *Journal of the American Medical Association, 287*: 1822–31.

Harkness, R. and Bratman, S. (2003). *Handbook of drug-herb and drug-supplement interactions*. St. Louis, MO: Mosby.

Harris, B., Lovett, L., Newcombe, R. G., Read, G. F., Walker, R. and Riad-Fahmy, D. (1994). Maternity blues and major endocrine changes: Cardiff puerperal mood and hormone study II. *British Medical Journal, 308*: 949–53.

Harrykissoon, S. D., Rickert, V. I. and Wiemann, C. M. (2002). Prevalence and patterns of intimate partner violence among adolescent mothers during the postpartum period. *Archives of Pediatric and Adolescent Medicine, 156*(4): 325–30.

Haslam, D. M., Pakenham, K. I. and Smith, A. (2006). Social support and postpartum depressive symptomatogy: The mediating role of maternal self-efficacy. *Infant Mental Health Journal, 27*: 276–91.

Hassmen, P., Koivula, N. and Uutela, A. (2000). Physical exercise and psychological well-being: A population study in Finland. *Preventative Medicine, 30*: 17–25.

Hatton, D. C., Harrison-Hohner, J., Coste, S., Dorato, V., Curet, L. B. and McCarron, D. A. (2005). Symptoms of postpartum depression and breastfeeding. *Journal of Human Lactation, 21*(4): 444–9.

Hay, D. F., Pawlby, S., Sharp, D., Asten, P., Mills, A. and Kumar, R. (2001). Intellectual problems shown by 11-year-old children whose mothers had postnatal depression. *Journal of Child Psychology & Psychiatry & Allied Disciplines, 42*: 871–89.

Hay, D. F., Pawlby, S., Water, C. S. and Sharp, D. (2008). Antepartum and postpartum exposure to maternal depression: Different effects on different adolescent outcomes. *The Journal of Child Psychology and Psychiatry, 49*(10): 1079–88.

Hayes, B. A., Muller, R. and Bradley, B. S. (2001). Perinatal depression: A randomized controlled trial of an antenatal education intervention for primiparas. *Birth, 28*: 28–35.

Head, J. G., Storfer-Isser, A., O'Connor, K. G., Hoagwood, K. E., Kelleher, K. J., Heneghan, A. M., *et al.* (2008). Does education influence pediatricians' perceptions of physician-specific barriers for maternal depression? *Clinical Pediatrics, 47*: 670–8.

Health Quest Radio News & Science (2000). *SAMe*. Available online at: http://www.healthquestradio.com/libSAMe

Hearn, G., Iliff, A., Jones, I., Kirby, A., Ormiston, P., Parr, P., Rout, J. and Wardman, L. (1998). Postnatal depression in the community. *British Journal of General Practice, 48*: 1064–6.

Heh, S. S., Huang, L. H., Ho, S. M., Fu, Y. Y. and Wano, L. L. (2008). Effectiveness of an exercise support program in reducing the severity of postnatal depression in Taiwanese women. *Birth, 35*(1): 60–5.

Heinrichs, M., Meinlschmidt, G., Neumann, I., Wagner, S., Kirschbaum, C., Ehlert U., *et al.* (2001). Effects of suckling on hypothalamic-pituitary-adrenal axis responses to psychosocial stress in post-partum lactating women. *Journal of Clinical Endocrinology & Metabolism, 86*: 4798–4804.

Helland, I. B., Smith, L., Saarem, K., Saugstad, O. D. and Drevon, C. A. (2003). Maternal supplementation with very-long-chain n-3 fatty acids during pregnancy and lactation augments children's IQ at 4 years of age. *Pediatrics, 111*: e39–e44.

Heneghan, A. M., Chaudron, L. H., Storfer-Isser, A., Park, E. R., Kelleher, K. J., Stein, R. E. K., *et al.* (2007). Factors associated with identification and management or maternal depression by pediatricians. *Pediatrics, 119*: 444–54.

Hibbeln, J. R. (2002). Seafood consumption, the DHA content of mothers' milk and prevalence rates of postpartum depression: A cross-national, ecological analysis. *Journal of Affective Disorders, 69*: 15–29.

Hobbins, D. (2004). Survivors of childhood sexual abuse: Implications for perinatal nursing care. *Journal of Obstetric, Gynecologic and Neonatal Nursing, 33*: 485–97.

Hobfoll, S. E., Ritter, C., Lavin, J., Hulsizer, M. R. and Cameron, R. P. (1995). Depression prevalence and incidence among inner-city pregnant and postpartum women. *Journal of Consulting and Clinical Psychology, 63*: 445–53.

Hong, S., Nelesen, R. A., Krohn, P. L., Mills, P. J. and Dimsdale, J. E. (2006). The association of social status and blood pressure with markers of vascular inflammation. *Psychosomatic Medicine, 68*: 517–23.

Horowitz, J. A., Bell, M., Trybulski, J. A., Munro, B. H., Moser, D., Hartz, S. A., McCordic, L. and Sokol, E. S. (2001). Promoting responsiveness between mothers with depressive symptoms and their infants. *Journal of Nursing Scholarship, 33*: 323–9.

Hu, Z. P., Yang, X. X., Chan, S. Y., Xu A. L., Duan, W., Zhu Y. Z., *et al.* (2006). St. John's wort attenuates irinotecan-induced diarrhea via down-regulation of intestinal pro-inflammatory cytokines and inhibition of intestinal epithelial apoptosis. *Toxicology & Applied Pharmacology, 216*: 225–37.

Huang, C.-M., Carter, P. A. and Guo, J.-L. (2004). A comparison of sleep and daytime sleepiness in depressed and non-depressed mothers during the early postpartum period. *Journal of Nursing Research, 12*(4): 287–95.

Hughes, P., Turton, P. and Evans, C. D. H. (1999). Stillbirth as risk factor for depression and anxiety in the subsequent pregnancy: Cohort study. *British Medical Journal, 318*: 1721–4.

Hulme, P. A. (2000). Symptomatology and health care utilization of women primary care patients who experienced childhood sexual abuse. *Child Abuse and Neglect, 24*: 1471–84.

Humphrey, S. (2003). *The nursing mother's herbal*. Minneapolis, MN: Fairview Press.

Humphrey, S. (2007). Herbal therapeutics during lactation. In T. W. Hale and P. E. Hartmann (eds.), *Textbook of Human Lactation*. Amarillo, TX: Hale, pp. 629–54.

Hunker, D. F., Patrick, T. E., Albrecht, S. A. and Wisner, K. L. (2009). Is difficult childbirth related to postpartum maternal outcomes in the early postpartum period? *Archives of Women's Mental Health, DOI 10: 1007/s00737-009-0068-3.*

Hyde, J. S., Klein, M. H., Essex, M. J. and Clark, R. (1995). Maternity leave and women's mental health. *Psychology of Women Quarterly, 19*: 257–85.

Hypericum Depression Trial Study Group. (2002). Effect of Hypericum perforatum (St. John's Wort) in major depressive disorder. *Journal of the American Medical Association, 287*: 1807–14.

Ifabumuyi, O. I. and Akindele, M. O. (1985). Post-partum mental illness in Northern Nigeria. *Acta Psychiatrica Scandinavica, 72*: 63–8.

Institute for Clinical Systems Improvement (2000). *Health care guidelines: Major depression in specialty care in adults*. Available online at: http://www.icsi.org

Janssen, H. J., Cuisinier, M. C., Hoogduin, K. A. and de Graauw, K. P. (1996). Controlled prospective study on the mental health of women following pregnancy loss. *American Journal of Psychiatry, 153*: 226–30.

Johnson, M. P., and Baker, S. R. (2004). Implications of coping repertoire as predictors of men's stress, anxiety and depression following pregnancy, childbirth and miscarriage: A longitudinal study. *Journal of Psychosomatic Obstetrics & Gynecology, 25*: 87–98.

Johnstone, S. J., Boyce, P. M., Hickey, A. R., Morris-Yates, A. D. and Harris, M. G. (2001). Obstetric risk factors for postnatal depression in urban and rural community samples. *Australian and New Zealand Journal of Psychiatry, 35*: 69–74.

Jones, I. and Craddock, N. (2001). Familiality of the puerperal trigger in bipolar disorder: Results of a family study. *American Journal of Psychiatry, 158*: 913–17.

Jones, N. A., McFall, B. A. and Diego, M. A. (2004). Patterns of brain electrical activity in infants of depressed mothers who breastfeed and bottle feed: The mediating role of infant temperament. *Biological Psychology, 67*: 103–24.

Jotzo, M. and Poets, C. F. (2005). Helping parents cope with the trauma of premature birth: An evaluation of a trauma-preventive psychological intervention. *Pediatrics, 115*: 915–19.

Kabir, K., Sheeder, J. and Kelly, L. S. (2008). Identifying postpartum depression: Are 3 questions as good as 10? *Pediatrics, 122*: e696–e702.

Kallen, B. (2004). Neonate characteristics after maternal use of antidepressants in late pregnancy. *Archives of Pediatric & Adolescent Medicine, 158*(4): 312–16.

Kaneita, Y., Ohida, T., Uchiyama, M., Takemura, S., Kawahara, K., Yokoyama E., *et al.* (2006). The relationship between depression and sleep disturbances: A Japanese nationwide general population survey. *Journal of Clincal Psychiatry, 67*(2): 196–203.

Karlstrom, A., Engstrom-Olofsson, R., Norbergh, K. G., Sjoling, M. and Hidlingsson, I. (2007). Postoperative pain after cesarean birth affects breastfeeding and infant care. *Journal of Obstetric, Gynecologic and Neonatal Nursing, 36*(5): 430–40.

Kashaninia, Z., Sajedi, F., Rahgozar, M. and Noghabi, F. A. (2008). The effect of Kangaroo Care on behavioral responses to pain of an intramuscular injection in neonates. *Journal for Specialists in Pediatric Nursing, 13*(4): 275–80.

Kendall-Tackett, K. A. (2007). A new paradigm for depression in new mothers: The central role of inflammation and how breastfeeding and anti-inflammatory treatments protect maternal mental health. *International Breastfeeding Journal, 2*: 6. Available online at: http://www.internationalbreastfeeding journal.com/content/2/1/6

Kendall-Tackett, K. A. (2009). Psychological trauma and physical health: A psychoneuroimmunology approach to etiology of negative health effects and possible interventions. *Psychological Trauma, 1*: 35–48.

Keogh, E., Hughes, S., Ellery, D., Daniel, C. and Holdcroft, A. (2006). Psychosocial influences on women's experience of planned elective cesarean section. *Psychosomatic Medicine, 68*(1): 167–74.

Kersting, A., Dorsch, M., Kreulich, C., Reutemann, M., Ohrmann, P., Baez E., *et al.* (2005). Trauma and grief 2–7 years after termination of pregnancy because of fetal anomalies: A pilot study. *Journal of Psychosomatic Obstetrics & Gynecology, 26*(1): 9–14.

Kiecolt-Glaser, J. K. and Newton, T. L. (2001). Marriage and health: His and hers. *Psychological Bulletin, 127*: 472–503.

Kiecolt-Glaser, J. K., Preacher, K. J., MacCallum, R. C., Atkinson, C., Malarkey, W. B. and Glaser, R. (2003). Chronic stress and age-related increases in the proinflammatory cytokine IL-6. *Proceedings of the National Academy of Sciences USA, 100*(15): 9090–5.

Kiecolt-Glaser, J. K., Loving, T. J., Stowell, J. R., Malarky, W. B., Lemeshow, S., Dickinson, S. L. and Glaser, R. (2005). Hostile marital interactions, proinflammatory cytokine production, and wound healing. *Archives of General Psychiatry, 62*: 1377–84.

Kiecolt-Glaser, J. K., Belury, M. A., Porter, K., Beversdoft, D., Lemeshow, S. and Glaser, R. (2007). Depressive symptoms, omega-6: omega-3 fatty acids, and inflammation in older adults. *Psychosomatic Medicine, 69*: 217–24.

Kiernan, K. and Pickett, K. E. (2006). Marital status disparities in maternal smoking during pregnancy, breastfeeding and maternal depression. *Social Science & Medicine, 63*(2): 335–46.

Kim, J. J., Choi, S. S. and Ha, K. (2008). A closer look at depression in mothers who kill their children: Is it unipolar or bipolar depression? *Journal of Clinical Psychiatry, 69*(10): 1625–31.

Kitzinger, S. (1990). *The crying baby.* New York: Penguin.

Klier, C. M., Muzik, M., Rosenblum, K. L. and Lenz, G. (2001). Interpersonal psychotherapy adapted for the group setting in the treatment of postpartum depression. *Journal of Psychotherapy Practice and Research, 10*: 124–31.

Klier, C. M., Schafer, M. R., Schmid-Siegel, B., Lenz, G. and Mannel, M. (2002). St. John's wort (Hypericum Perforatum): Is it safe during breastfeeding? *Pharmacopsychiatry, 35*: 29–30.

Klier, C. M., Schmid-Siegel, B., Schafer, M. R., Lenz, G., Saria, A., Lee, A. and Zernig, G. (2006). St. John's wort (Hypericum perforatum) and breastfeeding: Plasma and breast milk concentrations of hyperforin for 5 mothers and 2 infants. *Journal of Clinical Psychiatry, 67*: 305–9.

Knipscheer, J. W., and Kleber, R. J. (2006). The relative contribution of posttraumatic and acculturative stress to subjective mental health among Bosnian refugees. *Journal of Clinical Psychology, 62*(3): 339–53.

Konsman, J. P., Parnet, P. and Dantzer, R. (2002). Cytokine-induced sickness behaviour: Mechanisms and implications. *Trends in Neuroscience, 25*: 154–8.

Kop, W. J. and Gottdiener, J. S. (2005). The role of immune system parameters in the relationship between depression and coronary artery disease. *Psychosomatic Medicine, 67*: S37–S41.

Kubera, M., Lin, A., Kenis, G., Bosmans, E., van Bockstaele, D. and Maes, M. (2001). Anti-inflammatory effects of antidepressants through suppression of the interferon-gamma/interleukin-10 production ratio. *Journal of Clinical Psychopharmacology, 21*(2): 199–206.

Kubera, M., Kenis, G., Bosmans, E., Kajta, M., Basta-Kalm, A., Scharpe S., *et al.* (2004). Stimulatory effect of antidepressants on the productioni of IL-6. *International Immunopharmacology, 4*(2): 185–92.

Kuhn, M. A. and Winston, D. (2000). *Herbal therapy and supplements: A scientific and traditional approach.* Philadelphia, PA: Lippincott.

Lam, R. W., Song, C. and Yatham, L. N. (2004). Does neuroimmune dysfunction mediate seasonal mood changes in winter depression? *Medical Hypotheses, 63*: 567–73.

Lam, R. W., Levitt, A. J., Levitan, R. D., Enns, M. W., Morehouse, R., Michalak, E. E. and Tam, E. M. (2006). The CAN-SAD Study: A randomized controlled trial of the effectiveness of light therapy and fluoxetine in patients with winter seasonal affective disorder. *American Journal of Psychiatry, 163*: 805–12.

Lane, A. M., Crone-Grant, D. and Lane, H. (2002). Mood changes following exercise. *Perceptual & Motor Skills, 94*: 732–4.

Lang, A. J., Rodgers, C. S. and Lebeck, M. M. (2006). Associations between maternal childhood maltreatment and psychopathology and aggression during pregnancy and postpartum. *Child Abuse & Neglect, 30*: 17–25.

Lappin, J. (2001). Time points for assessing perinatal mood must be optimized. *British Medical Journal, 323*: 1367a.

Lau, Y. and Chan, K. S. (2007). Influence of intimate partner violence during pregnancy and early postpartum depressive symptoms on breastfeeding among Chinese women in Hong Kong. *Journal of Midwifery and Women's Health, 52*(2): e15–e20.

Lavender, T. and Walkinshaw, S. A. (1998). Can midwives reduce postpartum psychological morbidity? A randomized trial. *Birth, 25*: 215–19.

Lawvere, S. and Mahoney, M. C. (2005). St. John's wort. *American Family Physician, 72*: 2249–54.

Lecrubier, Y., Clerc, G., Didi, R. and Kieser, M. (2002). Efficacy of St. John's wort extract WS 5570 in major depression: A double-blind, placebo-controlled trial. *American Journal of Psychiatry, 159*: 1361–6.

Lee, D. T., Yip, A. S., Chiu, H. F. and Chung, T. K. (2000). Screening for postnatal depression using a double-test strategy. *Psychosomatic Medicine, 62*(2): 258–63.

Lee, S.-Y., Lee, K. A., Rankin, S. H., Weiss, S. J. and Alkon, A. (2007). Sleep disturbance, fatigue, and stress among Chinese-American parents with ICU hospitalized infants. *Issues in Mental Health Nursing, 28*: 593–605.

Leibenluft, E. (2000). Women and bipolar disorder: An update. *Bulletin of the Menninger Clinic, 64*: 5–17.

Leppaemaeki, S. J., Partonen, T. T., Hurme, J., Haukka, J. K. and Loennqvist, J. K. (2002). Randomized trial of the efficacy of bright-light exposure and aerobic exercise on depressive symptoms and serum lipids. *Journal of Clinical Psychiatry, 63*: 316–21.

Lesperance, F. and Frasure-Smith, N. (2000). Depression in patients with cardiac disease: A practical review. *Journal of Psychosomatic Research, 48*: 379–91.

Letourneau, N., Duffett-Leger, L., Stewart, M., Hegadoren, K., Dennis, C.-L., Rinaldi, C. M., *et al.* (2007). Canadian mothers' perceived support needs during postpartum depression. *Journal of Obstetric, Gynecologic, and Neonatal Nursing, 36*: 441–9.

Leu, S. J., Shiah, I. S., Yatham, L. N., Cheu, Y. M. and Lam, R. W. (2001). Immune-inflammatory markers in patients with seasonal affective disorder: Effects of light therapy. *Journal of Affective Disorders, 63*: 27–34.

Leverton, T. J. and Elliot, S. A. (2000). Is the EPDS a magic wand?: 1. A comparison of the Edinburgh

Postnatal Depression Scale and health visitor report as predictors of diagnosis on the Present State Examination. *Journal of Reproductive and Infant Psychology, 18*: 279–96.

Lev-Wiesel, R. and Daphna-Tekoa, S. (2007). Prenatal posttraumatic stress symptoms in pregnant survivors of childhood sexual abuse: A brief report. *Journal of Loss and Trauma, 12*: 145–53.

Levy, V. (1987). The maternity blues in post-partum and post-operative women. *British Journal of Psychiatry, 151*: 368–72.

Lewis, T., Amini, F., and Lannon, R. (2000). *A general theory of love*. New York: Vintage.

Lieb, R., Isensee, B., Hofler, M., Pfister, H. and Wittchen, H-U. (2002). Parental major depression and the risk of depression and other mental disorders in offspring. *Archives of General Psychiatry, 59*: 365–74.

Lin, P. and Su, K.-P. (2007). A meta-analysis review of double-blinded, placebo-controlled trials of antidepressant efficacy of omega-3 fatty acids. *Journal of Clinical Psychiatry, 68*(7): 1056–61.

Linde, K., Ramirez, G., Mulrow, C. D., Pauls, A., Weidenhammer, W. and Melchart, D. (1996). St. John's wort for depression: An overview and meta-analysis of randomized clinical trials. *British Medical Journal, 313*: 253–8.

Lobel, M., DeVincent, C. J., Kaminer, A. and Meyer, B. A. (2000). The impact of prenatal maternal stress and optimistic disposition on birth outcomes in medically high-risk women. *Health Psychology, 19*: 544–53.

Lobel, M., Cannella, D. L., Graham, J. E., DeVincent, C., Schneider, J. and Meyer, B. A. (2008). Pregnancy-specific stress, prenatal health behaviors, and birth outcomes. *Health Psychology, 27*(5): 604–15.

Logsdon, M. C. and Usui, W. (2001). Psychosocial predictors of postpartum depression in diverse groups of women. *Western Journal of Nursing Research, 23*: 563–74.

Logsdon, M. C., Wisner, K. L. and Hanusa, B. H. (2009). Does maternal role functioning improve with antidepressant treatment in women with postpartum depression? *Journal of Women's Health, 18*(1): 85–90.

Looper, K. J. (2007). Potential medical and surgical complications of sertonergic antidepressant medications. *Psychosomatics, 48*: 1–9.

Louik, C., Lin, A. E., Werler, M. M., Hernandez-Diaz, S. and Mitchell, A. A. (2007). First-trimester use of selective serotonin-reuptake inhibitors and the risk of birth defects. *New England Journal of Medicine, 356*: 2675–83.

Lu, W., Mueser, K. T., Rosenberg, S. D. and Jankowski, M. K. (2008). Correlates of adverse childhood experiences among adults with severe mood disorders. *Psychiatric Services, 59*(9): 1018–26.

Lucas, A., Pizarro, E., Granada, M. L., Salinas, I. and Santmarti, A. (2001). Postpartum thyroid dysfunction and postpartum depression: Are they two linked disorders? *Clinical Endocrinology, 55*: 809–14.

Luce, G. G. (1966). *Current research on sleep and dreams* (Public Health Service Publication No. 1389). Washington, DC: Public Health Service.

Luoma, I., Tamminen, T., Kaukonen, P., Laippala, P., Puura, K., Salelin, R. and Almqvist, F. (2001). Longitudinal study of maternal depressive symptoms and child well-being. *Journal of the American Academy of Child and Adolescent Psychiatry, 40*: 1367–74.

Lutenbacher, M. (2002). Relationships between psychosocial factors and abusive parenting attitudes in low-income single mothers. *Nursing Research, 51*: 158–67.

Lutz, K. F. (2005). Abuse experiences, perceptions, and associated decisions during the childbearing cycle. *Western Journal of Nursing, 27*: 802–24.

Lutz, W. J. and Hock, E. (2002). Parental emotions following the birth of the first child: Gender differences in depressive symptoms. *American Journal of Orthopsychiatry, 72*: 415–21.

MacArthur, C., Winter, H. R., Bick, D. E., Knowles, H., Lilford, R., Henderson, C., Lancashire, R. J., Braunholtz, D. A. and Gee, H. (2002). Effects of redesigned community postnatal care on women's health 4 months after birth: A cluster randomized controlled trial. *Lancet, 359*: 378–85.

McCarter-Spaulding, D. and Horowitz, J. A. (2007). How does postpartum depression affect breastfeeding? *American Journal of Maternal Child Nursing, 32*(1): 10–17.

McCoy, S. J., Beal, M., Shipman, S. B. M., Payton, M. E. and Watson, G. H. (2006). Risk factors for postpartum depression: A retrospective investigation at 4-weeks postnatal and a review of the literature. *Journal of the American Osteopathic Association*, *106*: 193–8.

McDade, T. W., Hawkley, L. C. and Cacioppo, J. T. (2006). Psychosocial and behavioral predictors of inflammation in middle-aged and older adults: The Chicago Health, Aging, and Social Relations Study. *Psychosomatic Medicine*, *68*: 376–81.

McEwen, B. S. (2003). Mood disorders and allostatic load. *Biological Psychiatry*, *54*: 200–7.

McGarry, J., Kim, H., Sheng, X., Egger, M. and Baksh, L. (2009). Postpartum depression and help-seeking behavior. *Journal of Midwifery and Women's Health*, *54*(1): 50–9.

McGovern, P., Dowd, B., Gjerdingen, D., Gross, C. R., Kenney, S., Ukestad, L., McCaffrey, D. and Lundberg, U. (2006). Postpartum health of employed mothers 5 weeks after childbirth. *Annals of Family Medicine*, *4*: 159–67.

McGrath, J. M., Records, K. and Rice, M. (2008). Maternal depression and infant temperament characteristics. *Infant Behavior and Development*, *31*: 71–80.

McKee, M. D., Cunningham, M., Jankowski, K. R. and Zayas, L. (2001). Health-related functional status in pregnancy: Relationship to depression and social support in a multi-ethnic population. *Obstetrics and Gynecology*, *97*: 988–93.

McKim, M. K., Cramer, K. M., Stuart, B. and O'Connor, D. L. (1999). Infant care decisions and attachment security: The Canadian Transition to Child Care study. *Canadian Journal of Behavioural Science*, *31*: 92–106.

Maclean, L. I., McDermott, M. R. and May, C. P. (2000). Method of delivery and subjective distress: Women's emotional responses to childbirth practices. *Journal of Reproductive and Infant Psychology*, *18*(2): 153–62.

McLearn, K. T., Minkovitz, C. S., Strobion, D. M., Marks, E. and Hou, W. (2006a). Maternal depressive symptoms at 2 to 4 months postpartum and early parenting practices. *Archives of Pediatrics and Adolescent Medicine*, *160*(3): 279–84.

McLearn, K. T., Minkovitz, C. S., Strobino, D. M., Marks, E. and Hou, W. (2006b). The timing of maternal depressive symptoms and mothers' parenting practices with young children: Implications for pediatric practice. *Pediatrics*, *118*(1): e174–e182.

MacLennan, A., Wilson, D. and Taylor, A. (1996). The self-reported prevalence of postnatal depression. *Australian and New Zealand Journal of Obstetric and Gynecology*, *36*: 313.

McLennan, J. D. and Kotelchuck, M. (2000). Parental prevention practices for young children in the context of maternal depression. *Pediatrics*, *105*: 1090–5.

McLennan, J. D. and Offord, D. R. (2002). Should postpartum depression be targeted to improve child mental health? *Journal of the American Academy of Child and Adolescent Psychiatry*, *41*: 28–35.

McLennan, J. D., Kotelchuck, M. and Cho, H. (2001). Prevalence, persistence, and correlates of depressive symptoms in a national sample of mothers of toddlers. *Journal of the American Academy of Child and Adolescent Psychiatry*, *40*: 1316–23.

Maes, M. (2001). Psychological stress and the inflammatory response system. *Clinical Science*, *101*: 193–4.

Maes, M. and Smith, R. S. (1998). Fatty acids, cytokines, and major depression. *Biological Psychiatry*, *43*: 313–14.

Maes, M., Lin, A-H, Ombelet, W., Stevens, K., Kenis, G., de Jongh, R., Cox, J. and Bosmans, E. (2000). Immune activation in the early puerperium is related to postpartum anxiety and depression symptoms. *Psychoneuroendocrinology*, *25*: 121–37.

Maes, M., Verkerk, R., Bonaccorso, S., Ombelet, W., Bosmans, E. and Scharpe, S. (2002). Depressive and anxiety symptoms in the early puerperium are related to increased degradation of tryptophan into kynurenine, a phenomenon which is related to immune activation. *Life Science*, *71*(16): 1837–48.

Maes, M., Bosmans, E. and Ombelet, W. (2004). In the puerperium, primiparae exhibit higher levels of anxiety and serum peptidase activity and greater immune responses than multiparae. *Journal of Clincal Psychiatry*, *65*(1): 71–6.

Maina, G., Albert, U., Bogetto, F., Vaschetto, P. and Ravizza, L. (1999). Recent life events and obsessive-compulsive disorder (OCD): The role of pregnancy/delivery. *Psychiatry Research, 13*: 49–58.

Maloni, J. A., Kane, J. H., Suen, L. J. and Wang, K. K. (2002). Dysphoria among high-risk pregnant hospitalized women on bed rest: A longitudinal study. *Nursing Research, 51*: 92–9.

Manber, R., Schnyer, R. N., Allen, J. J. B., Rush, A. J. and Blasey, C. M. (2004). Acupuncture: A promising treatment for depression. *Journal of Affective Disorders, 83*: 89–95.

Mandl, K. D., Tronick, E. Z., Brennan, T. A., Alpert, H. R. and Home, C. J. (1999). Infant health care use and maternal depression. *Archives of Pediatric and Adolescent Medicine, 153*: 808–13.

Mann, J. R., McKeown, R. E., Bacon, J., Vesselinov, R. and Bush, F. (2008a). Do antenatal religious and spiritual factors impact the risk of postpartum depressive symptoms? *Journal of Women's Health, 17*(5): 745–55.

Mann, J. R., McKeown, R. E., Bacon, J., Vesselinov, R. and Bush, F. (2008b). Religiosity, spirituality and antenatal anxiety in Southern U.S. women. *Archives of Women's Mental Health, 11*: 19–26.

Manning, J. S. (2002). The brain-body connection and the relationship between depression and pain. Available online at: http://www.medscape.com/viewprogram/2166_pnt

Mantle, F. (2002). The role of alternative medicine in treating postnatal depression. *Complementary Therapies in Nursing and Midwifery, 8*: 197–203.

Marangell, L. B., Martinez, J. M., Zboyan, H. A., Chong, H. and Puryear, L. J. (2004). Omega-3 fatty acids for the prevention of postpartum depression: Negative data from a preliminary, open-label pilot study. *Depression & Anxiety, 19*: 20–3.

Martin, S. L., Mackie, L., Kupper, L. L., Buescher, P. A. and Moracco, K. E. (2001). Physical abuse of women before, during, and after pregnancy. *Journal of the American Medical Association, 285*(12): 1581–4.

Martinez, R., Johnston-Robledo, I., Ulsh, H. M. and Chrisler, J. C. (2000). Singing "the baby blues": A content analysis of popular press articles about postpartum affective disturbances. *Women and Health, 31*: 37–56.

Maschi, S., Clavenna, A., Campi, R., Schiavetti, B., Bernat, M. and Bonati, M. (2008). Neonatal outcome following pregnancy exposure to antidepressants: a prospective controlled cohort study. *British Journal of Obstetrics & Gynecology, 115*(2): 283–9.

Matthey, S., Barnett, B., Kavanagh, D. J. and Howie, P. (2001). Validation of the Edinburgh Postnatal Depression Scale for men, and comparison of item endorsement with their partners. *Journal of Affective Disorders, 64*(2–3): 175–84.

Meltzer-Brody, S., Payne, J. and Rubinow, D. (2008). Postpartum depression: What to tell patients who breast-feed. *Current Psychiatry, 7*(5): 87–95.

Meyer, C. L. and Oberman, M. (2001). *Mothers who kill their children: Understanding the acts of moms from Susan Smith to the "Prom Mom"*. New York: NYU Press.

Mezzacappa, E. S. and Katkin, E. S. (2002). Breastfeeding is associated with reduced perceived stress and negative mood in mothers. *Health Psychology, 21*: 187–93.

Mezzacappa, E. S. and Endicott, J. (2007). Parity mediates the association between infant feeding method and maternal depressive symptoms in the postpartum. *Archives of Women's Mental Health, 10*: 259–66.

Miceli, P. J., Goeke-Morey, M. C., Whitman, T. L., Kolberg, K. S., Miller-Loncar, C. and White, R. D. (2000). Birth status, medical complication, and social environment: Individual differences in development of preterm, very low birth weight infants. *Journal of Pediatric Psychology, 25*(5): 353–8.

Mick, E., Biederman, J., Prince, J., Fischer, B. A. and Faraone, S. V. (2002). Impact of low birth weight on attention-deficit hyperactivity disorder. *Journal of Developmental and Behavioral Pediatrics, 23*: 16–22.

Milgrom, J., Negri, L. M., Gemmill, A. W., McNeil, M. and Martin, P. R. (2005). A randomized controlled trial of psychological interventions for postnatal depression. *British Journal of Clinical Psychology, 44*: 529–42.

Miller, G. E., Cohen, S. and Ritchey, A. K. (2002). Chronic psychological stress and the regulation of pro-inflammatory cytokines: A glucocorticoid-resistance model. *Health Psychology, 21*: 531–41.

Miller, G. E., Rohleder, N., Stetler, C. and Kirschbaum, C. (2005). Clinical depression and regulation of the inflammatory response during acute stress. *Psychosomatic Medicine, 67*: 679–87.

Miller, L. J. (2002). Postpartum depression. *Journal of the American Medical Association, 287*: 762–5.

Mirowsky, J. and Ross, C. E. (2002). Depression, parenthood, and age at first birth. *Social Science and Medicine, 54*: 1281–98.

Misri, S., Kim, J., Riggs, K.W., and Kostaras, X. (2000a). Paroxetine levels in postpartum depressed women, breast milk, and infant serum. *Journal of Clinical Psychiatry, 6*: 828–32.

Misri, S., Kostaras, X., Fox, D. and Kostaras, D. (2000b). The impact of partner support in the treatment of postpartum depression. *Canadian Journal of Psychiatry, 45*: 554–8.

Misri, S., Reebye, P., Corral, M. and Mills, L. (2004). The use of paroxetine and cognitive-behavioral therapy in postpartum depression and anxiety: A randomized controlled trial. *Journal of Clinical Psychiatry, 65*: 1236–41.

Misri, S., Reebye, P., Milis, L. and Shah, S. (2006). The impact of treatment intervention on parenting stress in postpartum depressed women: A prospective study. *American Journal of Orthopsychiatry, 76*(1): 115–19.

Miyake, Y., Sasaki, S., Yokoyama, T., Tanaka, K., Ohya, Y., Fukushima W., *et al.* (2006). Risk of postpartum depression in relation to dietary fish and fat intake in Japan: The Osaka Maternal and Child Health Study. *Psychological Medicine, 36*: 1727–35.

Montgomery, S. M., Ehlin, A. and Sacker, A. (2006). Breast feeding and resilience against psychosocial stress. *Archives of Diseases of Childhood, 91*: 990–4.

Monti, F., Agostini, F., Fagandini, P., La Sala, G. B. and Blickstein, I. (2009). Depressive symptoms during late pregnancy and early parenthood following assisted reproductive technology. *Fertility & Sterility, 91*(3): 851–7.

Moore, G. A., Cohn, J. F. and Campbell, S. B. (2001). Infant affective responses to mother's still face at 6 months differentially predict externalizing and internalizing behaviors at 18 months. *Developmental Psychology, 37*: 706–14.

Mora, P. A., Bennett, I. M., Elo, I. T., Mathew, L., Coyne, J. C. and Culhane, J. F. (2009). Distinct trajectories of perinatal depressive symptomatology: Evidence from growth mixing modeling. *American Journal of Epidemiology, 169*(1): 24–32.

Morgan, J. F., Lacey, J. H. and Chung, E. (2006). Risk of postnatal depression, miscarriage, and preterm birth in bulimia nervosa: Retrospective controlled study. *Psychosomatic Medicine, 68*: 487–92.

Morrell, C. J., Spiby, H., Stewart, P., Walters, S. and Morgan, A. (2000). Costs and effectiveness of community postnatal support workers: Randomised controlled trial. *British Medical Journal, 321*: 593–8.

Morris-Rush, J. K. and Bernstein, P. S. (2002). Postpartum depression. *Medscape Ob/Gyn & Women's Health*. Available online at: http://www.medscape.com/viewarticle/433013

Moses-Kolko, E. L., & Roth, E. K. (2004). Antepartum and postpartum depression: Healthy mom, healthy baby. *Journal of the American Medical Women's Association, 59*: 181–91.

Moses-Kolko, E. L., Bogen, D., Perel, J. M., Bregar, A., Uhl, K., Levin B., *et al.* (2005). Neonatal signs after late in utero exposure to serotonin reuptake inhibitors. *Journal of the American Medical Association, 293*(19): 2372–83.

Mu, P-F, Wong, T-T, Chang, K-P and Kwan, S-Y. (2001). Predictors of maternal depression for families having a child with epilepsy. *Journal of Nursing Research, 9*: 116–26.

Mufson, L., Dorta, K. P., Wickramaratne, P., Nomura, Y., Olfson, M. and Weissman, M. M. (2004). A randomized effectiveness trial of interpersonal psychotherapy for depressed adolescents. *Archives of General Psychiatry, 61*: 577–84.

Muller, W. E. (2003). Current St. John's wort research from mode of action to clinical efficacy. *Pharmacology Research, 47*: 101–9.

Murray, L., Woolgar, M., Cooper, P. and Hipwell, A. (2001). Cognitive abilities to depression in 5-year-old children of depressed mothers. *Journal of Child Psychology and Psychiatry, 42*: 891–9.

Najman, J. M., Williams, G. M., Nikles, J., Spence, S., Bor, W., O'Callaghan, M., Le Brocque, R. and

Andersen, M. J. (2000). Mothers' mental illness and child behavior problems: Cause-effect association or observation bias? *Journal of the American Academy of Child & Adolescent Psychiatry, 39*: 592–602.

NAMI, *see* National Alliance on Mental Illness.

National Alliance on Mental Illness. (2007). Seasonal affective disorder. Available online at: http://www.nami.org

Noaghiul, S. and Hibbeln, J. R. (2003). Cross-national comparisons of seafood consumption and rates of bipolar disorders *American Journal of Psychiatry, 160*: 2222–7.

Oberlander, T. F., Misri, S., Fitzgerald, C. E., Kostaras, X., Rurak, D. and Riggs, W. (2004). Pharmacologic factors associated with transient neonatal symptoms following prenatal psychotropic medication exposure. *Journal of Clinical Psychiatry, 65*(2): 230–7.

Oberlander, T. F., Grunau, R. E., Fitzgerald, C., Papsdorf, M., Rurak, D. and Riggs, W. (2005). Pain reactivity in 2-month-old infants after prenatal and postnatal serotonin reuptake inhibitor medication exposure. *Pediatrics, 115*(2): 411–25.

Oberlander, T. F., Warburton, W., Misri, S., Aghajanian, J. and Hertzman, C. (2006). Neonatal outcomes after prenatal exposure to selective serotonin reuptake inhibitor antidepressants and maternal depression using population-based linked health data. *Archives of General Psychiatry, 63*(8): 898–906.

Oberlander, T. F., Reebye, P., Misri, S., Papsdorf, M., Kim, J. and Grunau, R. E. (2007). Externalizing and attentional behaviors in children of depressed mothers treated with a selective serotonin reuptake inhibitor antidepressant during pregnancy. *Archives of Pediatric & Adolescent Medicine, 161*: 22–9.

O'Brien, S. M., Scott, L. V., and Dinan, T. G. (2004). Cytokines: Abnormalities in major depression and implications for pharmacological treatment. *Human Psychopharmacology, 19*(6): 397–403.

O'Brien, S. M., Scott, L. V. and Dinan, T. G. (2006). Antidepressant therapy and C-reactive protein levels. *British Journal of Psychiatry, 188*: 449–52.

O'Connor, T. G., Thorpe, K., Dunn, J. and Golding, J. (1999). Parental divorce and adjustment in adulthood: Findings from a community sample. *Journal of Child Psychology and Psychiatry and Allied Disciplines, 40*: 777–89.

O'Hara, M. W. (1995). *Postpartum depression: Causes and consequences*. New York: Springer-Verlag.

O'Hara, M. W., Schlechte, J. A., Lewis, D. A. and Varner, M. W. (1991). Controlled prospective study of postpartum mood disorders: Psychological, environmental, and hormonal variables. *Journal of Abnormal Psychology, 100*: 63–73.

O'Hara, M. W., Stuart, S., Gorman, L. L., and Wenzel, A. (2000). Efficacy of interpersonal psychotherapy for postpartum depression. *Archives of General Psychiatry, 57*: 1039–45.

Olafsdottir, A. S., Skuladottir, G. V., Thorsdottir, I., Hauksson, A., Thorgeirsdottir, H. and Steingrimsdottir, L. (2006). Relationship between high consumption of marine fatty acids in early pregnancy and hypertensive disorders in pregnancy. *British Journal of Obstetrics & Gynecology, 113*: 301–9.

O'Leary, J. (2005). The trauma of ultrasound during a pregnancy following perinatal loss. *Journal of Loss and Trauma, 10*: 183–204.

Olfson, M., Marcus, S. C., Tedeschi, M. and Wan, G. J. (2006). Continuity of antidepressant treatment for adults with depression in the United States. *American Journal of Psychiatry, 163*: 101–8.

Onozawa, K., Glover, V., Adams, D., Modi, N. and Kumar, R. C. (2001). Infant massage improves mother-infant interaction for mothers with postnatal depression. *Journal of Affective Disorders, 63*: 201–7.

Oren, D. A., Wisner, K. L., Spinelli, M., Epperson, C. N., Peindl, K. S., Terman, J. S. and Terman, M. (2002). An open trial of morning light therapy for treatment of antepartum depression. *American Journal of Psychiatry, 159*: 666–9.

Orhon, F. S., Ulukol, B. and Soykan, A. (2007). Postpartum mood disorders and maternal perceptions of infant patterns in well-child follow-up visits. *Acta Paediatrica, 96*: 1777–83.

Orr, S. T., Reiter, J. P., Blazer, D. G. and James, S. A. (2007). Maternal prenatal pregnancy-related anxiety and spontaneous preterm birth in Baltimore, Maryland. *Psychosomatic Medicine, 69*: 566–70.

Pace, T. W., Hu, F. and Miller, A. H. (2007). Cytokine-effects on glucocorticoid receptor function: relevance to glucocorticoid resistance and the pathophysiology and treatment of major depression. *Brain, Behavior and Immunity*, *21*(1): 9–19.

Pajulo, M., Savonlahti, E., Sourander, A., Helenius, H. and Piha, J. (2001a). Antenatal depression, substance dependency, and social support. *Journal of Affective Disorders*, *6*: 9–17.

Pajulo, M., Savonlahti, E., Sourander, A., Ahlqvist, S., Helenius, H. and Piha, J. (2001b). An early report on the mother-baby interactive capacity of substance-abusing mothers. *Journal of Substance Abuse Treatment*, *20*: 143–51.

Park, E. R., Storfer-Isser, A., Kelleher, K. J., Stein, M. B., Heneghan, A. M., Chaudron, L. H., *et al.* (2007). In the moment: Attitudinal measure of pediatrician management of maternal depression. *Ambulatory Pediatrics*, *7*(3): 239–46.

Parker, G., Gibson, N. A., Brotchie, H., Heruc, G., Rees, A-M. and Hadzi-Pavlovic, D. (2006). Omega-3 fatty acids and mood disorders. *American Journal of Psychiatry*, *163*: 969–78.

Parmar, V. R., Kumar, A., Kaur, R., Parmar, S., Kaur, D., Basu S., *et al.* (2009). Experience with Kangaroo Mother Care in a neonatal intensive care unit (NICU) in Chandigarh, India. *Indian Journal of Pediatrics*, *76*(1): 25–8.

Patel, V. and Prince, M. (2006). Maternal psychological morbidity and low birth weight in India. *British Journal of Psychiatry*, *188*: 284–5.

Patel, V., Abas, M., Broadhead, J., Todd, C. and Reeler, A. (2001). Depression in developing countries: Lesson from Zimbabwe. *British Medical Journal*, *322*: 482–4.

Patel, V., Rodrigues, M. and DeSouza, N. (2002). Gender, poverty, and postnatal depression: A study of mothers in Goa, India. *American Journal of Psychiatry*, *159*: 43–7.

Pauli-Pott, U., Becker, K., Mertesacker, T. and Beckmann, D. (2000). Infants with "colic" – Mothers' perspectives on the crying problem. *Journal of Psychosomatic Research*, *48*: 125–32.

Payne, J. L. (2007). Antidepressant use in the postpartum period: Practical considerations. *American Journal of Psychiatry*, *164*: 1329–32.

Pedersen, C. A., Johnson, J. L., Silva, S., Bunevicius, R., Meltzer-Brody, S., Hamer M., *et al.* (2007). Antenatal thyroid correlates of postpartum depression. *Psychoneuroendocrinology*, *32*(3): 235–45.

Peet, M., and Stokes, C. (2005). Omega-3 fatty acids in the treatment of psychiatric disorders. *Drugs*, *65*: 1051–9.

Pelaez, M., Field, T., Pickens, J. N. and Hart, S. (2008). Disengaged and authoritarian parenting behavior of depressed mothers with their toddlers. *Infant Behavior and Development*, *31*: 145–8.

Perren, S., von Wyl, A., Burgin, D., Simoni, H. and von Klitzing, K. (2005). Depressive symptoms and psychosocial stress across the transition to parenthood: Associations with parental psychopathology and child difficulty. *Journal of Psychosomatic Obstetrics & Gynecology*, *26*(3): 173–83.

Peter, E. A., Janssen, P. A., Grange, C. S. and Douglas, M. J. (2001). Ibuprofen versus acetaminophen with codeine for the relief of perineal pain after childbirth: A randomized controlled trial. *Canadian Medical Association Journal*, *165*: 1203–9.

Philipp, M., Kohnen, R. and Hiller, K-O. (1999). Hypericum extract versus imipramine or placebo in patients with moderate depression: Randomized multicenter study of treatment for eight weeks. *British Medical Journal*, *319*: 1534–9.

Picardi, A., Battisti, F., Tarsitani, L., Baldassari, M., Copertaro, A., Mocchegiani E., *et al.* (2007). Attachment security and immunity in healthy women. *Psychosomatic Medicine*, *69*: 40–6.

Poleshuck, E. L., Talbot, N. L., Su, H., Tu, X., Chaudron, L. H., Gamble S., *et al.* (2009). Pain as a predictor of depression treatment outcomes in women with childhood sexual abuse. *Comprehesive Psychiatry*, *50*: 215–20.

Posmontier, B. (2008). Sleep quality in women with and without postpartum depression. *Journal of Obstetric, Gynecologic and Neonatal Nursing*, *37*(6): 722–37.

Prasko, J., Horocek, J., Zalesky, R., Kopecek, M., Novak, T., Paskova B., *et al.* (2004). The change of regional brain metabolism (18FDG PET) in panic disorder during the treatment with cognitive behavioral therapy or antidepressants. *Neuro Endocrinology Letters*, *25*: 340–8.

Prentice, J. C., Lu, M. C., Lange, L. and Halfon, N. (2002). The association between reported childhood sexual abuse and breastfeeding initiation. *Journal of Human Lactation, 18*: 219–26.

Preston, J. and Johnson, J. (2009). *Clinical psychopharmacology made ridiculously simple*, 6th ed. Miami, FL: MedMaster.

Punamaki, R-L., Repokari, L., Vilska, S., Poikkeus, P., Tiitinen, A., Sinkkonen J., *et al.* (2006). Maternal mental health and medical predictors of infant development and health problems from pregnancy to one year: Does former infertility matter? *Infant Behavior and Development, 29*: 230–42.

Quillin, S. I. M. and Glenn, L. L. (2004). Interaction between feeding method and co-sleeping on maternal-newborn sleep. *Journal of Obstetric, Gynecologic and Neonatal Nursing, 33*(5): 580–8.

Quinn, T. J. and Carey, G. B. (1999). Does exercise intensity or diet influence lactic acid accumulation in breast milk? *Medicine and Science in Sports and Exercise, 31*: 105–10.

Radestad, I., Nordin, C., Steineck, G. and Sjogren, B. (1996). Still birth is no longer managed as a nonevent: A nationwide study in Sweden. *Birth, 23*(4): 209–15.

Rampono, J., Hackett, L. P., Kristensen, J. H., Kohan, R., Page-Sharp, M. and Ilett, K. F. (2006). Transfer of escitalopram and its metabolite demethylescitalopram into breastmilk. *British Journal of Clinical Pharmacology, 62*(3): 316–22.

Ranjit, N., Diez-Roux, A. V., Shea, S., Cushman, M., Seeman, T., Jackson, S. A. and Ni, H. (2007). Psychosocial factors and inflammation in the Multi-Ethnic Study of Atherosclerosis. *Archives of Internal Medicine, 167*: 174–81.

Rapkin, A. J., Mikacich, J. A., Moatakef-Imani, B. and Rasgon, N. (2002). The clinical nature and formal diagnosis of premenstrual, postpartum, and perimenopausal affective disorders. *Current Psychiatry Reports, 4*: 419–28.

Reading, R. and Reynolds, S. (2001). Debt, social disadvantage and maternal depression. *Social Science and Medicine, 53*: 441–53.

Reay, R., Fisher, Y., Robertson, M., Adams, E., Owen, C. and Kumar, R. (2006). Group interpersonal psychotherapy for postnatal depression: A pilot study. *Archives of Women's Mental Health, 9*: 31–9.

Records, K. and Rice, M. (2007). Psychosocial correlates of depression symptoms during the third trimester of pregnancy. *Journal of Obstetric, Gynecologic and Neonatal Nursing, 36*: 231–42.

Rees, A-M., Austin, M-P. and Parker, G. (2005). Role of omega-3 fatty acids as a treatment for depression in the perinatal period. *Australia & New Zealand Journal of Psychiatry, 39*: 274–80.

Regmi, S., Sligl, W., Carter, D., Grut, W. and Seear, M. (2002). A controlled study of postpartum depression among Nepalese women: Validation of the Edinburgh Postpartum Depression Scale in Kathmandu. *Tropical Medicine and International Health, 7*: 378–82.

Remick, R. A. (2002). Diagnosis and management of depression in primary care: A clinical update and review. *Canadian Medical Association Journal, 167*: 253–60.

Rini, C., Manne, S., DuHamel, K., Austin, J., Ostroff, J., Boulad F., *et al.* (2008). Social support from family and friends as a buffer of low spousal support among mothers of critically ill children: A multilevel modeling approach. *Health Psychology, 27*(5): 593–603.

Ritter, C., Hobfoll, S. E., Lavin, J., Cameron, R. P. and Hulsizer, M. R. (2000). Stress, psychosocial resources, and depressive symptomatology during pregnancy in low-income, inner-city women. *Health Psychology, 19*: 576–85.

Roberts, J., Sword, W. S., Gafni, A., Krueger, P., Sheehan, D. and Soon-Lee, K. (2001). Costs of postpartum care: Examining associations from the Ontario mother and infant survey. *Canadian Journal of Nursing Research, 33*: 19–34.

Romieu, I., Torrent, M., Garcia-Esteban, R., Ferrer, C., Ribas-Fito, N., Anto, J. M., *et al.* (2007). Maternal fish intake during pregnancy and atopy and asthma in infancy. *Clinical & Experimental Allergy, 37*: 518–25.

Rondo, P. H. C. and Souza, M. R. (2007). Maternal distress and intended breastfeeding duration. *Journal of Psychosomatic Obstetrics & Gynecology, 28*(1): 55–60.

Rosenblum, K. L., McDonough, S., Muzik, M., Miller, A. and Sameroff, A. (2002). Maternal representations of the infant: Associations with infant response to the still face. *Child Development, 73*: 999–1015.

Ross, L. E. and Dennis, C-L. (2009). The prevalence of postpartum depression among women with substance use, an abuse history, or chronic illness: A systematic review. *Journal of Women's Health*, *18*(4): 475–86.

Ross, L. E., Murray, B. J. and Steiner, M. (2005). Sleep and perinatal mood disorders: A critical review. *Journal of Psychiatry & Neuroscience*, *30*: 247–56.

Rothman, B. K. (1982). *Giving birth: Alternatives in childbirth*. New York: Penguin.

Roubenoff, R. (2003). Exercise and inflammatory disease. *Arthritis Care & Research*, *49*(2): 263–6.

Roumestan, C., Michel, A., Bichon, F., Portet, K., Detoc, M., Henriquet C., *et al.* (2007). Anti-inflammatory properties of desipramine and fluoxetine. *Respiratory Research*, *8*: 35.

Roux, G., Anderson, C. and Roan, C. (2002). Postpartum depression, marital dysfunction, and infant outcome: A longitudinal study. *Journal of Perinatal Education*, *11*: 25–36.

Rowe-Murray, H. J. and Fisher, J. R. W. (2001). Operative intervention in delivery is associated with compromised early mother-infant interaction. *British Journal of Obstetrics and Gynaecology*, *108*: 1068–75.

Rupke, S. J., Blecke, D. and Renfrow, M. (2006). Cognitive therapy for depression. *American Family Physician*, *73*: 83–6.

Saisto, T., Salmela-Aro, K., Nurmi, J. E. and Halmesmaki, E. (2001). Psychosocial predictors of disappointment with delivery and puerperal depression: A longitudinal study. *Acta Obstetrica et Gynecologica Scandinavica*, *80*: 39–45.

Salmela-Aro, K., Nurmi, J-E., Saisto, T. and Halmesmaki, E. (2001). Goal reconstruction and depressive symptoms during the transition to motherhood: Evidence from two cross-lagged longitudinal studies. *Journal of Personality and Social Psychology*, *81*: 1144–59.

Salovey, P., Rothman, A. J., Detweiler, J. B. and Steward, W. T. (2000). Emotional states and physical health. *American Psychologist*, *55*: 110–21.

Sanderson, C. A., Cowden, B., Hall, D. M. B., Taylor, E. M., Carpenter, R. G. and Cox, J. L. (2002). Is postnatal depression a risk factor for sudden infant death? *British Journal of General Practice*, *52*: 636–40.

Sarris, J. (2007). Herbal medicines in the treatment of psychiatric disorders: A systematic review. *Phytotherapy Research*, *21*: 703–16.

Saunders, T. A., Lobel, M., Veloso, C. and Meyer, B. A. (2006). Prenatal maternal stress is associated with delivery analgesia and unplanned cesareans. *Journal of Psychosomatic Obstetrics & Gynecology*, *27*(3): 141–6.

Sayar, K., Arikan, M. and Yontem, T. (2002). Sleep quality in chronic pain patients. *Canadian Journal of Psychiatry*, *47*: 844–8.

Schiepers, O. J., Wichers, M. C. and Maes, M. (2005). Cytokines and major depression. *Progress in Neuropsychopharmacology and Biological Psychiatry*, *29*(2): 201–17.

Schuetze, P. and Das Eiden, R. (2005). The relationship between sexual abuse during childhood and parenting outcomes: Modeling direct and indirect pathways. *Child Abuse & Neglect*, *29*: 645–59.

Schultz, V. (2006). Safety of St. John's wort extract compared to synthetic antidepressants. *Phytomedicine*, *13*: 199–204.

Schwartz, E. B., Ray, R. M., Stuebe, A. M., Allison, M. A., Ness, R. B., Freiberg, M. S., *et al.* (2009). Duration of lactation and risk factors for maternal cardiovascular disease. *Obstetrics & Gynecology*, *113*(5): 974–82.

Seng, J. S., Oakley, D. J., Sampselle, C. M., Killion, C., Graham-Bermann, S. and Liberzon, I. (2001). Posttraumatic stress disorder and pregnancy complications. *Obstetrics and Gynecology*, *97*: 17–22.

Shaw, E., Levitt, C., Wong, S., Kaczorowski, J. and Group, T.M.U.P.R. (2006). Systematic review of the literature on postpartum care: Effectiveness of postpartum support to improve maternal parenting, mental health, quality of life, and physical health. *Birth*, *33*(3): 210–20.

Shaw, R. J., Deblois, T., Ikuta, L., Ginzburg, K., Fleisher, B. and Koopman, C. (2006). Acute stress disorder among parents of infants in the neonatal intensive care nursery. *Psychosomatics*, *47*(3): 206–12.

Shoji, H., Franke, C., Campoy, C., Rivero, M., Demmelmair, H. and Koletzko, B. (2006). Effect of docosahexaenoic acid and eicosapentaenoic acid supplementation on oxidative stress levels during pregnancy. *Free Radical Research*, *40*: 379–84.

Sichel, D. A., Cohen, L. S., Dimmock, J. A. and Rosenbaum, J. F. (1993). Postpartum obsessive compulsive disorder: A case series. *Journal of Clinical Psychiatry, 54*: 156–9.

Simkin, P. (1991). Just another day in a woman's life? Women's long-term perceptions of their first birth experience. Part I. *Birth, 18*: 203–10.

Simkin, P. (1992). Just another day in a woman's life? Part II: Nature and consistency of women's long-term memories of their first birth experiences. *Birth, 19*: 64–81.

Simon, G. E., VonKorff, M., Rutter, C. and Wagner, E. (2000). Randomised trial of monitoring, feedback, and management of care by telephone to improve treatment of depression in primary care. *British Medical Journal, 320*: 550–4.

Skouteris, H., Wertheim, E. H., Rallis, S., Milgrom, J. and Paxton, S. J. (2009). Depression and anxiety through pregnancy and the early postpartum: An examination of prospective relationships. *Journal of Affective Disorders, 113*: 303–8.

Small, R., Johnston, V. and Orr, A. (1997). Depression after childbirth: The views of medical students and women compared. *Birth, 24*: 109–15.

Small, R., Lumley, J., Donohue, L., Potter, A. and Waldenstrom, U. (2000). Randomised controlled trial of midwife led debriefing to reduce maternal depression after operative childbirth. *British Medical Journal, 321*: 1043–7.

Smyke, A. T., Boris, N. W. and Alexander, G. M. (2002). Fear of spoiling in at-risk African American mothers. *Child Psychiatry and Human Development, 32*: 295–307.

Smyth, J. M., Hockemeyer, J. R., Heron, K. E., Wonderlich, S. A. and Pennebaker, J. W. (2008). Prevalence, type, disclosure, and severity of adverse life events in college students. *Journal of American College Health, 57*(1): 69–76.

Spinelli, M. G. and Endicott, J. (2003). Controlled clinical trial of interpersonal psychotherapy versus parenting education program for depressed pregnant women. *American Journal of Psychiatry, 160*: 555–62.

Springate, B. A. and Chaudron, L. H. (2006). Mental health providers' self-reported expertise and treatment of perinatal depression. *Archives of Women's Mental Health, 9*: 60–1.

Starkweather, A. R. (2007). The effects of exercise on perceived stress and IL-6 levels among older adults. *Biological Nursing Research, 8*: 1–9.

Stefos, G., Staner, L., Kerkhofs, M., Hubain, P., Mendlewicz, J. and Linkowsik, P. (1998). Shortened REM latency as a psychobiological marker for psychotic depression? An age-, gender-, and polarity-controlled study. *Biological Psychiatry, 15*: 1314–20.

Stern, G. and Kruckman, L. (1983). Multi-disciplinary perspectives on post-partum depression: An anthropological critique. *Social Science and Medicine, 17*: 1027–41.

Stuart, S. and O'Hara, M. W. (1995). Interpersonal psychotherapy for postpartum depression. *Journal of Psychotherapy Practice and Research, 4*: 18–29.

Su, D., Zhao, Y., Binna, C., Scott, J. and Oddy, W. (2007). Breast-feeding mothers can exercise: Results of a cohort study. *Public Health Nutrition, 10*: 1089–93.

Su, K-P., Huang, S-Y., Chiu, T-H., Huang, K-C., Huang, C-L., Chang, H-C., *et al.* (2008). Omega-3 fatty acids for major depressive disorder during pregnancy: Results from a randomized, double-blind, placebo trial. *Journal of Clinical Psychiatry, 69*: 644–51.

Suarez, E. C. (2006). Sex differences in the relation of depressive symptoms, hostility, and anger expression to indices of glucose metabolism in nondiabetic adults. *Health Psychology, 25*: 484–92.

Suarez, E. C., Lewis, J. G., Krishnan, R. R. and Young, K. H. (2004). Enhanced expression of cytokines and chemokines by blood monocytes to in vitro lipopolysaccharide stimulation are associated with hostility and severity of depressive symptoms in healthy women. *Psychoneuroendocrinology, 29*: 1119–28.

Sullivan, B. and Payne, T. W. (2007). Affective disorders and cognitive failures: A comparison of seasonal and nonseasonal depression. *American Journal of Psychiatry, 164*: 1663–7.

Summers, A. L., & Logsdon, M. C. (2005). Web sites for postpartum depression. *Maternal Child Nursing, 30*(2): 88–94.

Suri, R., Altshuler, L., Hellemann, G., Burt, V. K., Aquino, A. and Mintz, J. (2007). Effects of antenatal depression and antidepressant treatment on gestational age at birth and risk of preterm birth. *American Journal of Psychiatry, 164*: 1206–13.

Swain, A. M., Tasgin, E., Mayes, L. C., Feldman, R., Constable, R. T. and Leckman, J. F. (2008). Maternal brain response to own baby-cry is affected by cesarean section delivery. *Journal of Child Psychology and Psychiatry, 49*(10): 1042–52.

Sword, W., Busser, D., Ganann, R., McMillan, T. and Swinton, M. (2008). Women's care-seeking experiences after referral for postpartum depression. *Qualitative Health Research, 18*(9): 1161–73.

Szajewska, H., Horvath, A. and Koletzko, B. (2006). Effect of n-3 long-chain polyunsaturated fatty acid supplementation of women with low-risk pregnancy outcomes and growth measures at birth: A meta-analysis of randomized controlled trials. *American Journal of Clinical Nutrition, 83*: 1337–44.

Szegedi, A., Kohnen, R., Dienel, A. and Kieser, M. (2005). Acute treatment of moderate to severe depression with hypericum extract WS 5570 (St. John's wort): Randomised controlled double blind non-inferiority trial versus paroxetine. *British Medical Journal, 330*: 503.

Szelenyi, J. and Vizi, E. S. (2007). The catecholamine cytokine balance: interaction between the brain and the immune system. *Annals of the New York Academy of Science, 1113*: 311–24.

Taj, R. and Sikander, K. S. (2003). Effects of maternal depression on breastfeeding. *Journal of the Pakistani Medical Association, 53*: 8–11.

Tam, L. W., Newton, R. P., Dern, M. and Parry, B. L. (2002). Screening women for postpartum depression at well baby visits: Resistance encountered and recommendations. *Archives of Women's Mental Health, 5*: 79–82.

Tammentie, T., Paavilainen, E., Astedt-Kurki, P. and Tarkka, M-T. (2004). Family dynamics of postnatally depressed mothers: Discrepancy between expectations and reality. *Journal of Clinical Nursing, 13*: 65–74.

Terman, M. and Terman, J. S. (2005). Light therapy for seasonal and nonseasonal depression: Efficacy, protocol, safety, and side effects. *CNS Spectrums, 10*: 647–63.

Terman, M. and Terman, J. S. (2006). Controlled trial of naturalistic dawn simulation and negative air ionization for Seasonal Affective Disorder. *American Journal of Psychiatry, 163*: 2126.

Thomas, A. and Chess, S. (1987). Commentary. In H. H. Goldsmith, A. H. Buss, R. Plomin, M. K. Rothbart, A. Thomas, S. Chess, R. R. Hinde and R. B. McCall (eds.). Roundtable: What is temperament? Four approaches. *Child Development, 58*: 505–29.

Thompson, J. F., Roberts, C. L., Currie, M. and Ellwood, D. A. (2002). Prevalence and persistence of health problems after childbirth: Associations with parity and method of birth. *Birth, 29*: 83–94.

Tolman, A. O. (2001). *Depression in adults: The latest assessment and treatment strategies*. Kansas City, MO: Compact Clinicals.

Tronick, E. Z. and Weinberg, M. K. (1997). Depressed mothers and infants: Failure to form dyadic states of consciousness. In L. Murray and P. Cooper (eds.) *Postpartum depression and child development*. New York: Guilford, pp. 54–81.

Troxel, W. M., Cyranowski, J. M., Hall, M., Frank, E. and Buysee, D. J. (2007). Attachment anxiety, relationship context, and sleep in women with recurrent major depression. *Psychosomatic Medicine, 69*: 692–9.

van de Pol, G., De Leeuw, J. R. J., van Brummen, H. J., Bruinse, H. W., Heintz, A. P. M. and van der Vaart, C. H. (2006). Psychosocial factors and mode of delivery. *Journal of Psychosomatic Obstetrics & Gynecology, 27*(4): 231–8.

van der Hulst, L. A. M., Bonsel, G. J., Eskes, M., Birnie, E., van Teijlingen, E. and Bleker, O. P. (2006). Bad experience, good birthing: Dutch low-risk pregnant women with a history of sexual abuse. *Journal of Psychosomatic Obstetrics & Gynecology, 27*(1): 59–66.

van der Kolk, B. A. (2002). Assessment and treatment of complex PTSD. In R. Yehuda (ed.) *Treating trauma survivors with PTSD*. Washington, DC: American Psychiatric Publishing, pp. 127–56.

van der Meer, Y. G., Loendersloot, E. W. and van Loenen, A. C. (1984). Effect of high-dose progesterone in post-partum depression. *Journal of Psychosomatic Obstetrics and Gynaecology, 3*: 67–8.

van der Watt, G., Laugharne, J. and Janca, A. (2008). Complementary and alternative medicine in the treatment of anxiety and depression. *Current Opinion in Psychiatry*, *21*(1): 37–42.

van Gurp, G., Meterissian, G. B., Haiek, L. N., McCusker, J. and Bellavance, F. (2002). St. John's wort or sertraline?: Randomized controlled trial in primary care. *Canadian Family Physician*, *48*: 905–12.

van Pampus, M. G., Wolf, H., Weijmar Schultz, W. C. M., Neeleman, J. and Aarnoudse, J. G. (2004). Posttraumatic stress disorder following preeclampsia and HELLP syndrome. *Journal of Psychosomatic Obstetrics & Gynecology*, *25*: 183–7.

Veddovi, M., Kenny, D. T., Gibson, F., Bowen, J. and Starte, D. (2001). The relationship between depressive symptoms following premature birth, mothers' coping style, and knowledge of infant development. *Journal of Reproductive & Infant Psychology*, *19*: 313–23.

Verdoux, H., Sutter, A. L., Glatigny-Dallay, E. and Minisini, A. (2002). Obstetrical complications and the development of postpartum depressive symptoms: A prospective survey of the MATQUID cohort. *Acta Psychiatrica Scandanavica*, *106*: 212–19.

Verkerk, G. J. M., Denollet, J., van Heck, G. L., van Son, M. J. M. and Pop, V. J. M. (2005). Personality factors as determinants of depression in postpartum women: A prospective 1-year follow-up study. *Psychosomatic Medicine*, *67*: 632–7.

Vesga-Lopez, O., Blanco, C., Keyes, K., Olfson, M., Grant, B. F. and Hasin, D. S. (2008). Psychiatric disorders in pregnant and postpartum women in the United States. *Archives of General Psychiatry*, *65*(7): 805–15.

Vollmar, P., Haghikia, A., Dermietzel, R. and Faustmann, P. M. (2007). Venlafaxine exhibits an anti-inflammatory effect in an inflammatory co-culture model. *International Journal of Neuropsychopharmacology*, 1–7.

Wang, C., Chung, M., Lichtenstein, A., Balk, E., Kupelnick, B., DeVine, D., *et al.* (2004). *Effects of omega-3 fatty acids on cardiovascular disease* (Vol. AHRQ Publication No. 04-E009–1). Rockville, MD: Agency for Healthcare Research and Quality.

Webber, S. (1992). Supporting the postpartum family. *The Doula*, *23*: 16–17.

Weber, K., Rockstroh, B., Borgelt, J., Awiszus, B., Popov, T., Hoffmann K., *et al.* (2008). Stress load during childhood affects psychopathology in psychiatric patients. *BMC Psychiatry*, *8*(63): doi: 10.1186/1471–1244X-1188-1163.

Webster, J., Linnane, J. W. J., Dibley, L. M. and Pritchard, M. (2000a). Improving antenatal recognition of women at risk for postnatal depression. *Australia and New Zealand Journal of Obstetrics and Gynaecology*, *40*: 409–12.

Webster, J., Linnane, J. W. J., Dibley, L. M., Hinson, J. K., Starrenburg, S. E. and Roberts, J. A. (2000b). Measuring social support in pregnancy: Can it be simple and meaningful? *Birth*, *27*: 97–101.

Webster, J., Pritchard, M. A., Linnane, J. W., Roberts, J. A., Hinson, J. K., and Starrenburg, S. E. (2001). Postnatal depression: Use of health services and satisfaction with healthcare providers. *Journal of Quality Clinical Practice*, *21*: 144–48.

Wei, G., Greaver, L. B., Marson, S. M., Herndon, C. H., Rogers, J. and Robeson Healthcare Corporation (2007). Postpartum depression: Racial differences and ethnic disparities in a tri-racial and bi-ethnic population. *Maternal Child Health Journal*, DOI 10.1007/s10995-10007-10287-z.

Weinberg, M. K. and Tronick, E. Z. (1998). Emotional characteristics of infants associated with maternal depression and anxiety. *Pediatrics*, *102 (Supplement)*: 1298–1304.

Weinberg, M. K., Tronick, E. Z., Beeghly, M., Olson, K. L., Kernan, H. and Riley, J. M. (2001). Subsyndromal depressive symptoms and major depression in postpartum women. *American Journal of Orthopsychiatry*, *71*: 87–97.

Weissman, A. M., Levy, B. T., Hartz, A. J., Bentler, S., Donohue, M., Ellingrod, V. L., *et al.* (2004). Pooled analysis of antidepressant levels in lactating mothers, breast milk, and nursing infants. *American Journal of Psychiatry*, *161*(6): 1066–78.

Weissman, M. M. (2007). Recent non-medication trials of interpersonal psychotherapy for depression. *International Journal of Neuropsychopharmacology*, *10*: 117–22.

Weissman, M. M., Pilowsky, D. J., Wickramaratne, P. J., Talati, A., Wisniewski, S. R., Fava M., *et al.*

(2006a). Remissions in maternal depression and child psychopathology. *Journal of the American Medical Association*, *295*(12): 1389–98.

Weissman, M. M., Wickramaratne, P., Nomura, Y., Warner, V., Pilowsky, D. and Verdeli, H. (2006b). Offspring of depressed parents: 20 years later. *American Journal of Psychiatry*, *163*: 1001–8.

Werneke, U., Turner, T. and Priebe, S. (2006). Complementary medicines in psychiatry: Review of effectiveness and safety. *British Journal of Psychiatry*, *188*: 109–21.

Wertz, R. W. and Wertz, D. C. (1989). *Lying in: A history of childbirth in America*, expanded ed. New Haven, CT: Yale University Press.

Williams, M. J., Williams, S. M. and Poulton, R. (2006). Breast feeding is related to C reactive protein concentration in adult women. *Journal of Epidemiology and Community Health*, *60*: 146–8.

Wisner, K. L., Perel, J. M. and Findling, R. L. (1996). Antidepressant treatment during breastfeeding. *American Journal of Psychiatry*, *153*: 1132–7.

Wisner, K. L., Peindl, K. S., Gigliotti, T. and Hanusa, B. H. (1999). Obsessions and compulsions in women with postpartum depression. *Journal of Clinical Psychiatry*, *60*: 176–80.

Wisner, K. L., Logsdon, M. C. and Shanahan, B. R. (2008). Web-based education for postpartum depression: Conceptual development and impact. *Archives of Women's Mental Health*, *11*: e-pub.

Wisner, K. L., Sit, D. K. Y., Hanusa, B. H., Moses-Kolko, E. L., Bogen, D. L., Hunker, D. F., *et al.* (2009). Major depression and antidepressant treatment: Impact of pregnancy and neonatal outcomes. *American Journal of Psychiatry*, ahead of publication.

Woelk, H. (2000). Comparison of St. John's wort and imipramine for treating depression: Randomised controlled trial. *British Medical Journal*, *321*: 536–9.

Wolf, A. W., De Andraca, I. and Lozoff, B. (2002). Maternal depression in three Latin American samples. *Social Psychiatry & Psychiatric Epidemiology*, *37*: 169–76.

Wolke, D., Rizzo, P. and Woods, S. (2002). Persistent infant crying and hyperactivity problems in middle childhood. *Pediatrics*, *109*: 1054–60.

Woods, A. B., Page, G. G., O'Campo, P., Pugh, L. C., Ford, D. and Campbell, J. C. (2005). The mediation effect of posttraumatic stress disorder symptoms on the relationship of intimate partner violence and IFN-gamma levels. *American Journal of Community Psychology*, *36*(1–2): 159–75.

Wurglies, M. and Schubert-Zsilavecz, M. (2006). Hypericum perforatum: A "modern" herbal antidepressant: Pharmacokinetics of active ingredients. *Clinical Pharmacokinetics*, *45*: 449–68.

Xu, Z., and Lu, B. (2001). Relationship between postpartum depression, life events, and social support. *Chinese Journal of Clinical Psychology*, *9*: 130, 132.

Yamashita, H., Yoshida, K., Nakano, H. and Tashiro, N. (2000). Postnatal depression in Japanese women: Detecting the early onset of postnatal depression by closely monitoring the postpartum mood. *Journal of Affective Disorders*, *58*: 145–54.

Yatham, L. N., Kennedy, S. H., Schaffer, A., Parikh, S. V., Beaulieu, S., O'Donovan, C., *et al.* (2009). Canadian Network for Mood and Anxiety Treatments (CANMAT) and International Society for Bipolar Disorders (ISBD) collaborative update of CANMAT guidelines for the management of patients with bipolar disorder: Update 2009. *Bipolar Disorders*, *11*: 225–55.

Yim, I. S., Glynn, L. M., Schetter, C. D., Hobel, C. J., Chicz-DeMet, A. and Sandman, C. A. (2009). Risk of postpartum depressive symptoms with elevated corticotropin-releasing hormone in human pregnancy. *Archives of General Psychiatry*, *66*(2): 162–9.

Yonkers, K. A. (2007). The treatment of women suffering from depression who are either pregnant or breastfeeding. *American Journal of Psychiatry*, *164*: 1457–9.

Yonkers, K. A., Ramin, S. M., Rush, A. J., Navarrete, C. A., Carmody, T., March, D., Heartwell, S. F. and Leveno, K. J. (2001). Onset and persistence of postpartum depression in an inner-city maternal health clinic system. *American Journal of Psychiatry*, *158*: 1856–63.

Zanoli, P. (2004). Role of hyperforin in the pharmacological activities of St. John's wort. *CNS Drug Reviews*, *10*: 203–18.

Zelkowitz, P. and Milet, T. H. (2001). The course of postpartum psychiatric disorders in women and their partners. *Journal of Nervous and Mental Disease*, *189*: 575–82.

Zhou, C., Tabb, M. M., Sadatrafiei, A., Grun, F., Sun, A. and Blumberg, B. (2004). Hyperforin, the active component of St. John's wort, induces IL-8 expression in human intestinal epithelial cells via a MAPK-dependent, NF-kappaB-independent pathway. *Journal of Clinical Immunology, 24*: 623–36.

Zlotnick, C., Miller, I. W., Pearlstein, T., Howard, M. and Sweeney, P. (2006). A preventive intervention for pregnant women on public assistance at risk for postpartum depression. *American Journal of Psychiatry, 163*: 1443–5.

# Index

Page numbers in **bold** refer to figures and tables.

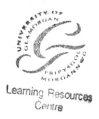